INTRODUCTION TO
PHYSICS IN
MODERN
MEDICINE

SECOND EDITION

INTRODUCTION TO
PHYSICS IN MODERN MEDICINE
SECOND EDITION

SUZANNE AMADOR KANE
Haverford College
Pennsylvania, USA

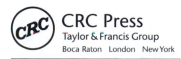

CRC Press
Taylor & Francis Group
Boca Raton   London   New York

CRC Press is an imprint of the
Taylor & Francis Group, an **informa** business

A TAYLOR & FRANCIS BOOK

CRC Press
Taylor & Francis Group
6000 Broken Sound Parkway NW, Suite 300
Boca Raton, FL 33487-2742

© 2009 by Taylor & Francis Group, LLC
CRC Press is an imprint of Taylor & Francis Group, an Informa business

---

Library of Congress Cataloging-in-Publication Data

Amador Kane, Suzanne.
    Introduction to physics in modern medicine / Suzanne Amador Kane. -- 2nd ed.
        p. cm.
    Includes bibliographical references and index.
    ISBN 978-1-58488-943-4 (pbk. : alk. paper)
    1. Medical physics. I. Title.

R895.A518 2009
610.1'53--dc22   2009011772

Visit the Taylor & Francis Web site at
http://www.taylorandfrancis.com

and the CRC Press Web site at
http://www.crcpress.com

To my husband, Charlie

Contents

Instructor's preface

While the physics community devotes a major portion of its teaching effort to educating premedical students and nonscience majors, most introductory textbooks devote relatively little time to the medical applications that hold great interest for these audiences. This book is intended to address this lack in part. Its intended audience is mainly premedical students, allied health students who need an elementary background in physics, and students not majoring in the natural sciences. However, many of our physics majors have appreciated it as a relatively nonmathematical introduction to this important area of applied physics. Although not designed as an introduction to medical physics for advanced students, its simple explanations of topics such as MRI can also serve as a useful introduction to more mathematical treatments.

This book grew out of a one-semester course on medical physics for students not majoring in the natural sciences. I ordinarily cover most of the book's contents in one semester, in the order indicated by the chapters. In teaching our two-semester premedical introductory physics sequence, I have used this material as a supplement that provides examples, problems, and images related to medical applications. For the most part, I have assumed little or no previous acquaintance with physics, biology, or chemistry, although some students may be somewhat familiar with these topics from earlier high school or college courses. In general the discussion adheres to simple qualitative explanations, using examples and illustrations to convey the science. The mathematics is confined to elementary applications of algebra and (sometimes) trigonometry, and the analysis of graphical information.

Each chapter in this book includes a short, self-contained explanation of the necessary scientific background, with occasional cross-references to previous chapters. I have tried to provide in one place much of what one needs to teach such a course without an extensive prior background in the subject, including problems, suggested readings, references to multimedia resources, and ideas for classroom demonstrations. Our course has also benefited (in its various incarnations) from hospital field trips and visits from physicians and medical physicists.

Student preface

Several years ago I developed sharp, severe pains in my lower abdomen. My physician felt a lump in the painful region and immediately ordered an ultrasound exam. In spite of the uncomfortable situation, I watched in fascination as a sonographer examined the inside of my body, my organs showing up as flickering, ghostly gray outlines on a television screen. As the exam proceeded, my scientific curiosity (and a healthy sense of self-preservation) began to raise many questions.

What exactly does one see on the television screen during ultrasound? How can it distinguish between a cancerous tumor (the feared outcome) and the actual diagnosis (a common and benign [noncancerous] cyst)? How safe are ultrasound exams? Before performing the exam, the sonographer smeared a gel onto the head of the ultrasound sensor—what was its function? In an ideal world, I would have had ample opportunities to have my questions answered on the spot. Under the circumstances, I was not likely to get answers unless I sought them out myself.

Since that experience, I have learned that many people are curious about these devices. Many have questions about the safety of these technologies as well as how they work, but assume that extensive training is required to understand such complicated medical devices as surgical lasers or computed tomography (CT) scanners. Obviously, physicians and other healthcare workers undergo years of specialized schooling in order to understand how to diagnose and treat disease using such tools. However, there is no reason the average person cannot comprehend and benefit from a *basic* understanding of these technologies. This book represents an attempt to provide this necessary background. In writing it, I have focused on those physical principles necessary to understand how these technologies work. This work grew out of an introductory course on this subject I have taught at Haverford College for many years to college students with no prior college-level training in the natural sciences. Its writing was influenced by extensive feedback from numerous students of widely varying backgrounds.

The reason you can tackle this material without an advanced degree is that, surprisingly, the answers to many questions do not lie in a sophisticated understanding of medicine and science. Rather, the basic concepts behind many techniques derive from very simple applications of physics, biology, and chemistry. Each chapter in this book includes a short, self-contained explanation of the necessary scientific background. I have assumed at most a familiarity with these topics at the high school level. The discussion adheres to simple explanations, using examples and illustrations to convey the science. Indeed, the topics covered are exactly those most people find most appealing about elementary science: sound, the science of light, genetics, and the mysterious structure of atoms and molecules.

Our study will focus on physics, rather than biology and chemistry. Medicine owes obvious debts to biology and chemistry; these fields have yielded essential insights into the development of drugs and vaccines, and into an understanding of organisms that cause infectious diseases, physiology at the molecular level, and—more recently—the immune system and genetics. Everyone knows that physicians diagnose and treat diseases using laboratory tests and drugs. However, it is not as widely appreciated how important medical physics is to medicine, especially through the imaging and therapeutic methods discussed above. Interestingly enough, the discoverers of these technologies did not aim at solving important problems in medicine. Roentgen's accidental discovery of x-rays touched off a medical revolution by making the body's interior visible for the first time, but his goal was to investigate the fundamental properties of matter. Lasers were invented by physicists fascinated by the properties of atoms and light. The basic science behind MRI was discovered first in the context of understanding the fundamental structure of the atomic nucleus. The mathematics used in computed tomography was first derived for applications in astronomy—and the list goes on. These examples powerfully illustrate how useful technologies can arise unexpectedly from basic scientific research into the fundamental properties of matter. No easy dividing line exists between "curiosity-driven" research and applied research aimed at a useful biomedical outcome.

In this book you will learn enough about the science behind medical technologies to demystify them and to allow you to better understand what they can offer. However, I hope that at the same time you may also discover how the unity and wonder of physics extend beyond its unexpected benefits.

Preface to the second edition

For the updated second edition, I have reviewed and included many new developments that have emerged since the first edition: camera pills that can film the inside of the digestive track, hybrid PET/CT scanners for improved cancer imaging, portable ultrasound scanners smaller than a laptop computer, an enhanced emphasis on digital imaging and computers in medicine, three-dimensional image reconstruction and display capabilities that have become an integral part of many different forms of medical imaging, robotic surgery devices, IMRT, proton therapy and other new forms of cancer radiation therapy are among the many new topics now covered in special sections, along with reflections on how the use of imaging technologies plays out in developing countries. The challenge of staying up to date in this field illustrates how key a role physics has come to play throughout modern medicine.

Acknowledgments

This project would never have come to fruition without many sources of support of various types. The National Science Foundation provided funding during the writing and development both of the original course and the book that resulted from it through a Course and Curriculum Development grant, DUE-9354422. The Howard Hughes Medical Institute (HHMI) provided invaluable assistance through a grant from its Undergraduate Biological Sciences Education Initiative. My perspectives were broadened immeasurably during the sabbatical leave made possible by a TriCollege New Directions Fellowship from the Andrew W. Mellon Foundation. I have appreciated, as well, the support of the administration of Haverford College and my colleagues in the biology, chemistry, and physics departments. Although many colleagues and acquaintances have helped me with the textbook, course, and various related activities along the way, I wish to thank in particular the late John R. Cameron, Peter Collings, John G. Truxal, John Brockway, Rufus Neal, Kaye Edwards, Steven Fischer, Becky Compton, Amy Slaton, Joseph Dumit, Patrician Allen, Rod Millbrandt, Dean Zollman, and Dr. Eric Rassmussen. Ted Ducas played an essential role in inspiring me to teach the original course. My students at Haverford have provided detailed and extremely helpful evaluations of the textbook as it evolved, as well as suggesting new topics for the second edition. Jody Forlizzi and Carrie Lebow ably crafted much of the original artwork. I learned a great deal from visitors to our course and professional contacts, including David Rose, Michael Cannon, Lewis Kinter, Jacqueline Tanaka, Gregory L. McIntire, Felice Frankel, Leon Mitchell, Geoffrey Aguirre, Arjun Yodh, and David K. Johnson. Hospitals in our area that have graciously hosted visits during the course's development include the HHMI Program at the Hospital of the University of Pennsylvania, Lankenau Hospital, and Bryn Mawr Hospital.

My agent, Edward Knappman of New England Publishing Associates, provided essential advice and support throughout. For this second edition, John Navas provided invaluable support and guidance throughout the entire process. I also appreciate the expert production editorial work by Amber Donley and others at Taylor & Francis.

My deepest debt of gratitude goes to my husband, Charlie. This book is dedicated to him.

Suzanne Amador
Haverford College

1 Introduction and overview

Physicians now possess the uncanny ability to see deep within the body without incisions, peering through skin and bone to gaze at the unborn child sucking its thumb, or to detect the potentially deadly action of a tumor. They "see" through the eyes of revolutionary new technologies: endoscopy, ultrasound imaging, computed tomography (CT or CAT), nuclear medicine imaging techniques, magnetic resonance imaging (MRI), and many others. At the same time, the science and technology that so dramatically reveal the body's anatomy and function have been harnessed for healing in techniques such as endoscopic surgery, laser surgery, and radiation therapy. These technologies are increasingly being combined with methods drawn from our growing knowledge of the human genome and molecular biology to produce a new age of individualized "molecular" medicine.

Writing at the dawn of the modern age of technology, the science fiction writer Isaac Asimov envisioned surgery under highly unusual circumstances in his novel *Fantastic Voyage*. As the novel's jacket explains the plot:

> Four men and one woman, reduced to a microscopic fraction of their original size, boarding a miniaturized atomic sub and being injected into a dying man's carotid artery. Passing through the heart, entering the inner ear, where even the slightest sound would destroy them, battling relentlessly into the cranium. Their objective...to reach a blood clot and destroy it with the piercing rays of a laser. At stake the fate of the entire world.

> Isaac Asimov, *Fantastic Voyage*, Bantam Books, New York, 1966

For the most part, Asimov's vision remains a fantasy. While modern surgeons can employ lasers to destroy blood clots, they do so without being shrunk to the size of a pinhead! However, physicians using medical endoscopes (Chapter 2) see essentially the same view as would Asimov's tiny heroes while cruising the body in their microscopic submarine (Figure 1.1). Endoscopes consist of slender tubes equipped with special optics and cameras for viewing far inside the body, even around curving passages; their size allows them to be inserted through natural body openings, or through

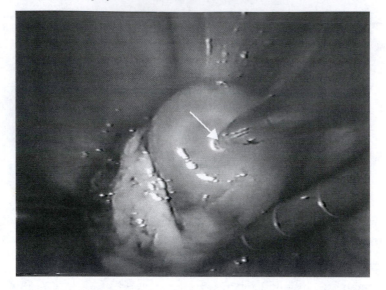

Figure 1.1 Image taken during laparoscopic laser surgery used to treat a woman for infertility. The goal of this operation was to remove growths caused by the disease endometriosis. The view shown of the inside of the body is that seen by the surgeon while performing the laparoscope procedure. The long rod at the center (white arrow) is a fiber optic guide for laser light used to cut through tissue, and the tool at bottom right is a forceps.

incisions the size of a buttonhole. The surgeon watches the endoscope's images on a television screen while manipulating tiny surgical tools, much as though playing a videogame. You may be more familiar with these devices by their specific names: laparoscopes for abdominal surgery; sigmoidoscopes and colonoscopes for colon cancer screening; arthroscopes for performing surgery on the knee, shoulder, and other joints; and many others.

Today, many types of surgery are often performed using lasers as a cutting tool, both reducing blood loss and dramatically increasing the precision of the incisions (Chapter 3) (Figure 1.1). This idea of employing light as a tool for surgery becomes especially exciting in ophthalmology, since the eye can often be treated without incisions due to the ability of laser light to pass directly through the lens and pupil and onto the diseased region. Lasers thus not only play a role in lifesaving surgery, they also provide treatments that enhance the quality of life, especially for senior citizens threatened with loss of vision from cataracts, diabetes, and glaucoma. In dermatologic laser surgery, light penetrates the skin to erase birthmarks, tattoos, age spots, and other blemishes. Physicians have long known of methods for fighting skin diseases using chemicals extracted from common plants, which concentrate in diseased tissue and are activated by sunlight. A modern version of this idea, called photodynamic therapy, offers the potential of someday destroying tumors with laser light.

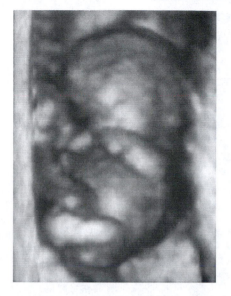

Figure 1.2 Ultrasound image of a human fetus at 16 weeks' gestation. The head (top left) and limbs (left) are visible in this three-dimensional reconstruction. (Reproduced with permission courtesy of Dr. Joseph Woo.)

Ultrasound imaging (Chapter 4) borrows a simple idea from nature—the ability of dolphins and bats to navigate using sound echoes—to create video images of the inside of the body. Because only low-intensity, very high-pitched sound is used, this technique is considered safe enough to use even in imaging the developing fetus during pregnancy (Figure 1.2), providing many parents with their first view of the child to come. Cardiac ultrasound exams (echocardiography, Doppler, or color flow ultrasound) provide a convenient bedside technique for visualizing the beating heart, major blood vessels, and faulty valves.

Chapter 5 surveys that great-grandparent of medical imaging, diagnostic radiography—the x-rays you get at the dentist's or when you break your leg. Innovations in x-ray imaging, such as digital radiography or CT scanning, are among the most exciting of new developments in diagnostic medicine (Figure 1.3). After a description of the basics of how x-ray images are formed, the discussion then moves on to what actually happens during such common exams as barium studies to visualize the digestive system and x-ray imaging of the heart during cardiac catheterization procedures. Advances in how x-rays are produced and detected are covered and used to explain how modern mammography makes possible effective screening for breast cancer. This chapter also gives a simple treatment of the complex topic of tomography, the formation of fully three-dimensional images of the body in CT scanning. The final section describes how x-rays are used to diagnose osteoporosis, a bone-embrittling condition of the elderly.

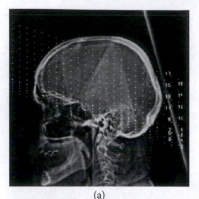

(a)

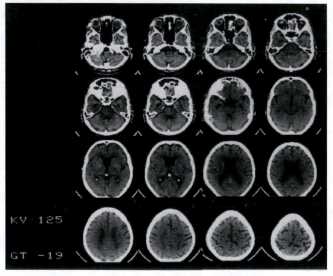

(b)

Figure 1.3 (a) X-ray image taken of the head prior to performing a CT scan. This image shows how standard x-rays are essentially shadows, which do not distinguish between overlapping tissues. Dotted lines indicate the planes at which cross-sectional CT images (b) were then taken. Each cross section gives an image of the tissues contained in that plane within the patient's head. (Reproduced with permission courtesy of Siemens Medical Systems.)

Minute amounts of injected radioactive substances are routinely used in medical diagnoses and treatments, yielding enormous medical benefits for a large number of patients. Chapter 6 describes the science behind radionuclide imaging, which uses radioactive tracer chemicals to study the heart, map the flow of body fluids, or highlight tumors (Figure 1.4). Using tomographic reconstruction—a computerized method for imaging "slices" within the body—doctors can use single photon emission computed tomography

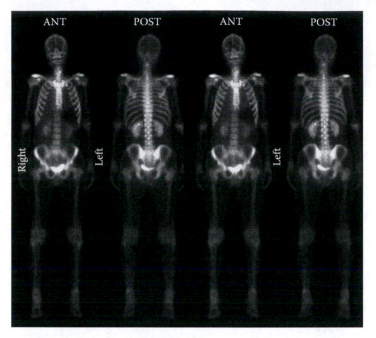

Figure 1.4 Gamma camera images, such as the bone scans shown here, are examples of radionuclide imaging. They are made by measuring maps of the distribution of radioactive sources located inside the body. (Reproduced with permission courtesy of Picker International.)

(SPECT) and positron emission tomography (PET) imaging to help diagnose Alzheimer's disease or to create colored maps of the brain in action.

Chapter 7 describes how radiation can be utilized to cure cancer in radiation therapy, not merely diagnose its presence (Figure 1.5). To explain how this technique works, the chapter opens with a summary of our present understanding of the biological effects of radiation, then proceeds to a more detailed explanation of how radiation doses are measured, radiation safety, and the radiation doses associated with common medical procedures. It closes with a discussion of innovations in improving cancer treatments using radiation.

Finally, we consider the abilities of magnetic resonance imaging (MRI), in some ways the most remarkable of all imaging technologies (Chapter 8) (Figure 1.6). This chapter uses simple and easily visualized experiments with compasses and magnets in order to help you understand the complex phenomenon of nuclear magnetism that underlies the operation of MRI. Sections review applications in which MRI can indeed offer important advantages in medical imaging. For example, functional MRI can detect brain activity, allowing researchers to image the actual physiological processes that occur during mental processes. This work may answer age-old questions about the mind, such as how the brain processes faces and language.

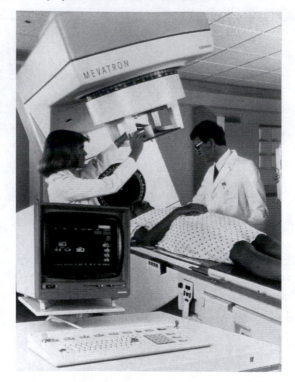

Figure 1.5 Sources of x-ray and gamma radiation can also be targeted to destroy tumor cells in cancer radiation therapy. (Reproduced with permission courtesy of Siemens Medical Systems.)

In addition to exploring the specifics of each technology, each chapter develops unifying themes that emerge naturally from the discussion. For example, the application of the law of conservation of energy is a constant in all areas of physics, including medical physics. The resulting consideration of how energy is transformed into various forms illuminates such diverse questions as why lasers are superior to ordinary lightbulbs for performing surgery, and how radioactivity can be used to image brain function. Other topics that recur throughout include the physics of waves (both electromagnetic and in media), optics (the science of light), the atomic theory of matter, and a basic understanding of subatomic physics.

Another persistent theme threading through each chapter is the question of each technology's safety. The media regularly report the results of studies that present evidence for or against the safety and effectiveness of various drugs and procedures. Rarely does this reporting include the background necessary to understanding the results and placing them in context. Since it is impractical to prove a technology totally safe, we consider how physicians determine the balance between the expected risks and benefits from each technology. We will see how necessary the relevant physics is to understanding fully, for example, the debate over the effectiveness of

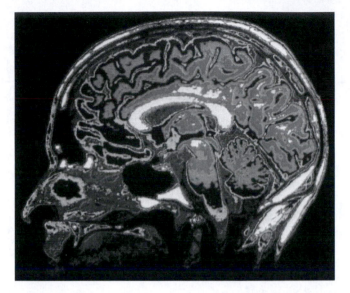

Figure 1.6 (*See color figure following page 78*.) Magnetic resonance imaging (MRI) permits detailed studies of the anatomy and physiological functioning of virtually the entire body, including the human brain. In this image, color is used to distinguish the different tissues of the brain and head, seen in cross section. (Reproduced with permission courtesy of Siemens Medical Systems.)

performing mammograms for breast cancer screening in women under age 50.

At the same time these medical physics techniques were exploding on the scene, our knowledge of the genome and biochemistry was undergoing a similar revolution. The result is molecular medicine—not a single field, but the synergy that results when all fields of medicine become informed by techniques resulting from our new understanding of genetics and molecular biology. Imaging technologies now can monitor the time course of body metabolism, explore the biology of specific receptors for brain chemicals or drugs, or map the response of different tumors to a program of chemotherapy for cancer to make sure each is responding and alternative therapies are not warranted.

Even so, for many who most desperately need medical care, the prospect is dim for taking advantage of developments at the forefront of modern medicine. We also will explore how medical technologies such as these play out in countries of the world where access to medicine is limited by economics, geography, and availability of trained personnel.

Although prophecy is a quite uncertain undertaking for science and medicine, each chapter concludes with a section on recent developments and likely future directions for each technology.

Our exploration of these medical technologies truly will be a fantastic voyage, one that will take us on a tour of the mysteries of the body and contemporary science. We will now begin our journey by exploring the simplest and most direct of techniques: medical fiber endoscopes—telescopes for inner space.

SUGGESTED READING

Other books that treat related topics in medical physics and the physics of the body at a similar (or somewhat more advanced) level

George B. Benedek and Felix M.H. Villars, *Physics with Illustrative Examples from Medicine and Biology, volumes 1, 2, and 3*. AIP Press, 2000.

Paul Davidovits, *Physics in Biology and Medicine*. Academic Press, 2008.

Irving P. Herman, *Physics of the Human Body*. Springer-Verlag, Berlin, 2007.

Russel K. Hobbie and Bradley J. Roth, *Intermediate Physics for Medicine and Biology* (excellent, but more advanced). Springer-Verlag, 2007.

J.A. Tuszynski and J.M. Dixon, *Biomedical Applications of Introductory Physics*. J. Wiley & Sons, 2002.

Introductory physics textbooks with some emphasis on coverage of medical physics & biophysics topics include

Alan Giambattista, Betty McCarthy Richardson, and Robert C. Richardson, *College Physics*. McGraw-Hill, Boston, 2004.

Morton M. Sternheim, Joseph W. Kane, *General Physics*, 2nd Edition. J. Wiley & Sons, 1991.

James S. Walker, *Physics*. Person/Prentice Hall, 2004.

Selected medical physics texts

Jerrold T. Bushberg, J. Anthony Seibert, Edwin M. Leidholdt Jr., and John M. Boone, *The Essential Physics of Medical Imaging*. Lippincott Williams & Wilkins, 2001.

Chris Guy and Dominic ffytche, *An Introduction to the Principles of Medical Imaging*. Imperial College Press, London, Hackensack, NJ: Distributed by World Scientific Publishing, 2005.

William R. Hendee and E. Russell, *Medical Imaging Physics*. Wiley-Liss, New York, 2002.

Harold Elford Johns and John R. Cunningham, *Solutions to Selected Problems: From the Physics of Radiology*. Charles C. Thomas Publishing, 1991.

Perry Sprawls, Jr., *Physical Principles of Medical Imaging*. Medical Physics Publishing, Madison, Wisconsin, 1995.

Medical physics videos

Jeff Hildebrand, *The Vision of Modern Medicine*, Morris Plains, NJ: Distributed by Lucerne Media, 1993.

Bill Hayes, Jim Colman, and Mona Kanin, *21st Century Medicine: Operating in the Future*, Advanced Medical Productions, Inc.; a production of Discovery Health Channel; New York: Ambrose Video Publishing, Inc., 2001.

The Learning Channel, The Operation: Knee Surgery, Discovery Communications, 1993.

Scientific American Frontiers: 21st Century Medicine, PBS Home Video, 2000.

A history of medical imaging that covers most of the techniques discussed here

Bettyann Kevles, *Naked to the Bone*. Rutgers University Press, New Brunswick, NJ, 1997.

Multimedia and Internet resources

Multimedia resources for studying this subject can be found on the World Wide Web, under the subject headings "Medical Physics" and "Radiology," among many others. By using the standard search engines, readers should be able to locate many up-to-date websites maintained by hospital and medical school imaging departments across the nation.

"Modern Medical Miracles," Kansas State Website on Medical Imaging, with various resources: http://web.phys.ksu.edu/mmmm/.

2 Telescopes for inner space
Fiber optics and endoscopes

2.1 INTRODUCTION

One of the earliest genes to be discovered was a hereditary defect popularly dubbed the colon cancer gene. A person possessing such a defective gene has a strong likelihood of developing a common form of cancer of the colon, or large intestine, as well as an enhanced risk of other forms of cancer (Figure 2.1). Even in the absence of a family history of this disease, this person is at risk. Since the first discovery, a variety of such hereditary factors have been identified. Some researchers estimate that up to 85% of those persons carrying some types of colon cancer gene will eventually contract the disease. However, many people who will contract colon cancer have no detectable genetic defects—and even those who do carry the gene have no way of knowing who will be in the unlucky 85%. Genetic testing can put you on alert, but not detect or cure colon cancer.

Colon (also called colorectal) cancer is the third most common cancer in the U.S. (apart from skin cancers) with 154,000 new cases in 2007. It is also the second most deadly form of cancer in the U.S., after lung cancer, causing around 52,000 deaths per year. However, even if genetic testing gives you advanced notice by establishing that you have a genetic predisposition, no drug currently exists to safeguard you from eventually developing the disease. Your only recourse is to maintain a healthy lifestyle and to have regular screenings for precancerous growths. These growths, called **polyps** or **adenomas**, can be removed safely before they have progressed into malignant tumors. By searching for and removing polyps at an early stage, physicians hope to virtually eliminate this painful and deadly disease. Indeed, the death rate from colon cancer has dropped significantly over the past 15 years, and early detection and treatment is thought to play a major role in this decline—this is one case where physicians can *prevent* cancer with advanced notice.

How can doctors know when a precancerous growth exists? To thoroughly search for polyps, a physician must completely examine the contorted length of the large intestine. As you can see from Figure 2.1(a), this presents an immediate problem: how can one see inside so small and twisting a passage? If you look down the length of a bent tube, you see that a simple

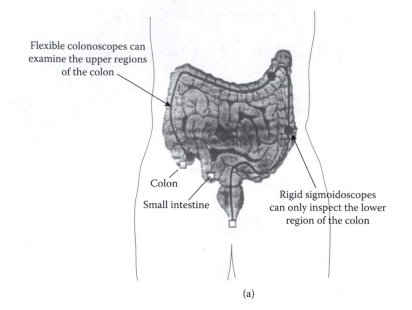

Flexible colonoscopes can examine the upper regions of the colon

Colon

Small intestine

Rigid sigmoidoscopes can only inspect the lower region of the colon

(a)

Figure 2.1 (*See color figure following page 78.*) (a) The large intestine (or colon) is the final stage of the digestive tract. (b) Colon cancer can be detected in its early, most readily treatable stages, by examinations that use endoscopes like the instrument shown in (b) to examine the lining of the colon for precancerous growths. (c) A view of the inside of the colon as it normally appears when viewed through an endoscope. (d) Time sequence showing the removal of a precancerous growth (or polyp). The first image shows, at lower left, a polyp growing within the colon, as seen through an endoscope. In the middle two images, a lasso-like tool called a snare is used to hook and remove the polyp. The final picture shows the site after the removal. Note that no bleeding occurs during the procedure. (Figure 2.1b reproduced with permission courtesy of Peter B. Cotton and Christopher B. Williams, *Practical Gastrointestinal Endoscopy*, Blackwell, Oxford, U.K., 1990. Figure 2.1c and d reproduced with permission from http://www.gastro.com/index.htm, courtesy of Drs. Peter W. Gardner and Stuart Waldstreicher. This website contains much useful information about, and interesting images of, common endoscopic procedures.)

tube does not allow one to see around corners. In addition, the inside of the colon must be illuminated during the inspection. How can this be accomplished? The light from a simple flashlight shone into the body would not reach around corners in the windings of the intestines. It is also not feasible to introduce a light source directly into the body because the lamp needed would generate appreciable heat as well as being much too bulky.

Devices called **sigmoidoscopes** and **colonoscopes** have been developed to overcome these problems. They belong to a large class of medical instruments called **endoscopes** (Figure 2.1b). Endoscopes utilize slender, flexible viewing tubes provided with a source of illumination; they can be

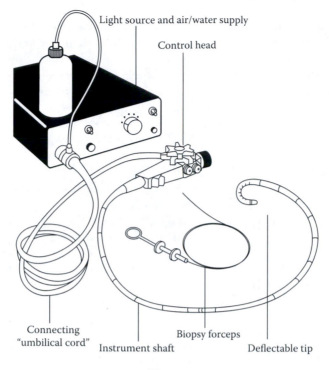

Light source and air/water supply

Control head

Connecting "umbilical cord"

Instrument shaft

Biopsy forceps

Deflectable tip

(b)

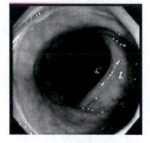

(c)

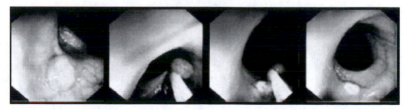

(d)

Figure 2.1 (continued).

equipped with tiny surgical tools with which physicians can remove pre-cancerous growths in procedures such as colon cancer screening (Figure 2.1c–d). Endoscopes can illuminate the inside of the body and see around corners, because they utilize tiny videocameras and **fiber optics**, slender strands of glass that act like pipes for lights. Fiber optics have many applications in addition to these medical uses. They can transmit information—such as telephone calls, video images, or computer data—over high-speed fiber optic communications lines. Electronic computer networks depend on extensive fiber optic links nationwide, and telephone companies have already converted many existing phone lines to this technology.

Many areas of medicine now make use of fiber optic scopes for both surgery and examination; the tiniest can go virtually anywhere a needle can. The **laparoscope** (named after the Greek word for flank) can be used for surgery in the abdomen, including gynecological procedures, as well as gallbladder removals, hernia repairs, and stomach surgery. Surgeons can often achieve equally good success rates and lower complication rates compared to conventional, or **open surgery**, which requires large incisions in the abdomen. Similarly, **arthroscopes** are widely used for operations on the knee, ankle, shoulder, and other joints (Figure 2.2). Patients who have undergone laparoscopic and arthroscopic surgery generally require much shorter hospital stays and fewer days of recovery time. In fact, after undergoing arthroscopic surgery a person can usually leave the hospital the same

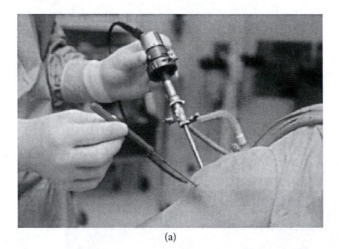

(a)

Figure 2.2 (a) Rather than cutting the knee wide open, doctors use tiny arthroscopic surgical tools to perform knee surgery. (b) The surgeons see inside the knee using an arthroscope; images from inside the knee are viewed on a television monitor. (c) Keyhole view inside the knee during arthroscopic surgery. A tiny surgical tool is seen in the center of the picture. (Reproduced with permission courtesy of John B. McGinty, Richard B. Caspari, Robert W. Jackson, and Gary G. Poehling, eds., *Operative Arthroscopy*, Raven Press, New York, 1996.)

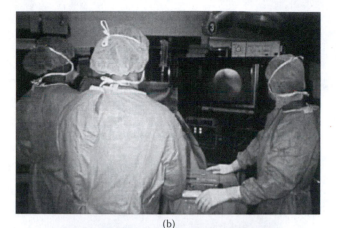

(b)

(c)

Figure 2.2 (continued).

day. This is in part because the surgery is performed through tiny keyhole-sized incisions that leave equally small scars.

Underlying the operation of all endoscopes is optics, the science of light. In this chapter we will explore the physics of fiber optics, then discuss several specific applications of medical endoscopes.

2.2 OPTICS: THE SCIENCE OF LIGHT

2.2.1 How to see around corners

Geometrical optics concerns itself with the physics of light: how light travels within various materials, how it interacts with matter, and how light can be manipulated to perform various useful functions. Our starting point

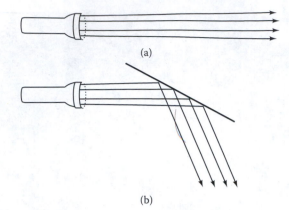

Figure 2.3 (a) The rays emitted from a source of light, such as the flashlight shown here, travel through a uniform medium, such as air, in straight lines without bending. (b) After being reflected from a mirror (or shiny mirrorlike surface) each ray of light continues to follow a straight line.

is the travel of light within a uniform medium. By **medium**, we mean any material, such as air, water, glass, blood, fat, or other human tissue. In the cases we study first, light can be thought of as traveling in straight lines, or rays, from its source to a distant point (Figure 2.3a), so long as it stays within the same medium. A narrow shaft of sunlight breaking through a cloud is a good approximation to a ray of light.

Light does not flow like a fluid, curving around as it travels. Instead, when light encounters an obstacle, it is **transmitted, reflected,** or **absorbed**. Transmitted light continues to travel into the medium, although often with a direction different from the original ray. Reflected rays rebound from the interface like a ball bouncing off a wall, as shown for rays of light reflecting from a mirror in Figure 2.3(b). If the light is absorbed, some of its energy is transferred to the medium, resulting in a gradual dimming of the light along its pathway.

How does this bear on the problem of illuminating the inside of the colon? If we shine a bright light down one end of a long, twisted tube, virtually no light comes out the other end (Figure 2.4). This is because the light's rays simply hit and reflect from the sides of the tube. At each reflection, part of the light is absorbed and part is reflected. After bouncing several times off of the tube's sides, the light is entirely absorbed, and none is left to shine through to the other end. Thus, a simple tube won't suffice for guiding light into the body.

It is just as impossible to view objects through an ordinary twisting tube as to get illumination from one end to another. For the tube discussed above, absorption also prevents the light from an object from reaching the viewer. However, what if the inside of the tube is shiny like a mirror, so that most of the light is reflected from end to end? Even if it were not very difficult to construct such a device, a simple mirrored tube could not be used for viewing objects inside the body. To see why, we first ask how we see

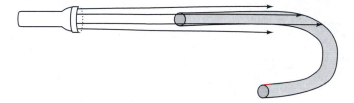

Figure 2.4 If a source of light, such as a flashlight, shines down a tube, the rays of light will reflect off of the sides of the tube. Some of the light will be absorbed at each reflection, resulting in only a very small amount of light (if any) reaching the other end.

any object. For objects that generate their own light, such as the flashlight above or the sun, our eyes intercept rays of light emitted by the object. For all other objects there must be a source of light nearby for illumination. We then see the object by means of the light reflected from its surface. Think of any visible object as emitting or reflecting many rays of light from each point on its surface. Our eyes collect only a tiny fraction of these rays and form them into an image of the object (Figure 2.5); we will soon see how such optical images are formed. However, the eye can only recombine these rays into an image of the original object if the ray's directions have been carefully preserved.

We can now understand why one cannot see objects through a mirrored twisted tube. Rays from an object present at one end can indeed bounce through to the other end. Unfortunately, the ray's directions are completely scrambled by their multiple reflections inside the tube, and cannot be reassembled into an image. You can see this by carefully rolling a tube of aluminum foil, and then gently curving the tube. Looking through the tube, you see images distorted like those in a funhouse mirror because of the confusing multiple reflections.

This is the predicament that faces physicians wishing to examine the windings of the large intestine. They need a means for guiding light rays around corners without losing information about their original directions.

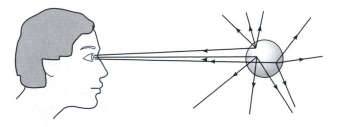

Figure 2.5 Your eyes intercept only a small fraction of the rays reflecting off a visible object, such as the ball shown here. These rays are focused by the lens of your eye to make the image you perceive. (The source of illumination is not shown.)

Optics gives us a method for solving this problem, and we will now study the solution.

2.2.2 Reflecting and bending light

Light travels in straight lines so long as it stays in a single medium, such as air or glass, but it can change direction when it meets a new material. The boundary between two media is called an **interface**. For the moment, we only consider **transparent** media, those which do not significantly absorb light. (The absorption of light is discussed later in Chapter 3, as it is extremely important for understanding laser surgery.) Light rays encounter two fates at an interface: (1) a fraction of the light is reflected from the interface, and (2) the remainder is transmitted, or **refracted**, into the next medium, potentially with a different direction. If we follow the pathway of a single ray of light across an interface between air and water, it splits into refracted and reflected rays as shown in Figure 2.6.

The rules of geometrical optics predict the new direction of the refracted light, so we can use refraction to change the pathway of light at will. Indeed, this idea underlies the construction of lenses used in eyeglasses and microscopes, as we will see shortly.

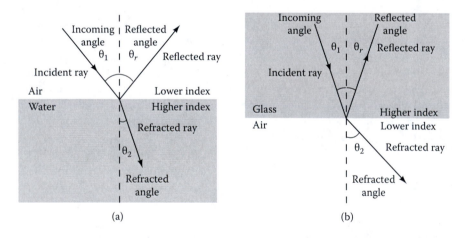

(a)   (b)

Figure 2.6 (a) The situation resulting when a ray of light travels from a medium of lower index of refraction, air in this case, to one of higher index of refraction, such as water. The original incident ray splits into two new rays of light, one reflected from the surface and the other, called the refracted ray, transmitted through the surface but with a new angle. The reflected ray makes the same angle with an imaginary line drawn perpendicular to (i.e., normal to) the surface, while the refracted ray makes an angle smaller than the incident ray. (b) The reverse situation, in which a ray of light travels from a higher to a lower index of refraction medium. Here, the refracted ray makes a larger angle with the normal than does the original, incident ray. Note that the same result holds as in part (a) for the reflected ray.

The direction of each ray of light is described by the angle it makes with the direction perpendicular to the interface. These angles are indicated in Figure 2.6 for the incoming or **incident**, θ_1, reflected, θ_r, and refracted rays, θ_2. The reflected ray *always* makes the same angle as the incident ray: $\theta_r = \theta_1$. This is true for mirror-like surfaces, where almost all of the light is reflected, as well as transparent materials with smooth surfaces. On the other hand, in general the refracted angle, θ_2, is different from the direction of the original ray, causing the ray's direction to change as it enters the second medium.

Most surfaces are not flat, but have curved or rough areas. How can we extend our statements above to cover these more realistic cases? The solution is to look at a very small region of an uneven area. Even a rough or curved surface looks flat over a sufficiently small patch. We can then consider the phenomena of reflection and refraction occurring as previously described at each small, flat region of the overall rough or curved surface.

2.2.3 Why does light bend? The index of refraction

The change in the speed of light as it crosses from one material to another determines how the angle of refraction differs from the incident angle. To understand this surprising statement, think first of a mechanical analogy. Consider a car traveling from a roadway onto mud (Figure 2.7a). At first, one front wheel becomes partly mired in the mud and moves more slowly than the front wheel still on the roadway, causing the vehicle to rotate. A similar situation occurs when the rear tires straddle the road and mud. Consequently, by the time all four wheels are on the mud, the car is

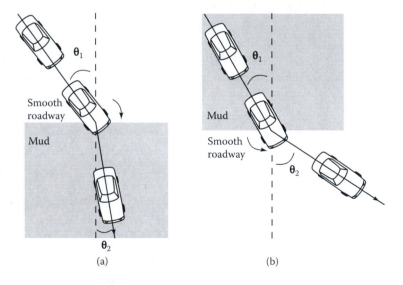

Figure 2.7 A simple mechanical analogy to refraction. (See explanation in the text.)

traveling in a new direction. In the language of light rays, we say that the car's refractive angle is *smaller* than its incident angle because it traveled into a medium with a *slower* speed. (Here, the car's front or rear wheel base corresponds to the width of a beam of light, and the speed of the car on different surfaces is analogous to the speed of light in different materials.)

If the car begins on the mud and then encounters a smooth surface where its speed *increases*, the reverse situation occurs. This results in the refractive angle of the car *increasing* (Figure 2.7b). Similarly for light, if the new speed of light is less than that of the original medium, the refractive angle is also less than the incident angle (Figure 2.6a). When a light ray travels across an interface into a medium with a *greater* speed of light, the refractive angle is *greater* than the incident angle (Figure 2.6b).

In fact, the speed of light does vary from medium to medium. In a vacuum, light moves at the extremely high speed of about 3.00×10^8 meter/second (3.00×10^8 m/s or 186,000 miles/s); this value is represented by the letter *c*. However, whenever light travels through a medium other than a vacuum, its interactions with the material result in a lower speed. This is because the light actually is continually being absorbed and re-emitted many times as it travels through the medium, reducing the effective speed of transmission of the light. The travel of light within a particular material is consequently described by the ratio between the speed of light in a vacuum, *c*, and the speed of light in that medium. This ratio is called the medium's **index of refraction, *n*.** The index of refraction of a medium in which the speed of light is equal to *v* is given by:

$$n = \frac{\text{speed of light in vacuum}}{\text{speed of light in medium}} = \frac{c}{v} \tag{2.1}$$

This ratio is always greater than or equal to 1 because light travels at a higher speed in a vacuum than in any other medium. Some typical values of the index of refraction are listed in Table 2.1 for common transparent materials. For example, in water light travels at a speed of only $c/n = (3.00 \times 10^8 \text{ m/s})/1.33$, or 2.26×10^8 m/s.

Table 2.1 Index of refraction of common materials

Medium	Index of refraction, n
Air	1.00
Oil	1.47
Water	1.33
Vitreous humor (the clear, jellylike filling of the eyeball)	1.336
Crystalline lens in the eye	1.437
Alcohol	1.36
Various types of glass	Roughly 1.5 to 1.7

The exact relation between the incident and refracted angle is given by a mathematical formula that depends upon the ratio between the indices of refraction in the two media. This equation, known as **Snell's law**, can be used to find the angle at which light travels after crossing any interface:

$$n_1 \sin\theta_1 = n_2 \sin\theta_2 \tag{2.2}$$

The refraction of light rays corresponds to the change of direction described for the car in Figure 2.7: rays passing from a medium with lower index to one with a higher index have an angle of refraction *lower* than the incident angle, while if the ray passes from higher to lower index, it is bent at a *greater* refractive angle (Figure 2.6a–b). The first case corresponds, for example, to light passing from air into water, while the second describes exiting from glass into air.

Sample calculation: To make clear the concepts embodied in Snell's law, we consider two specific calculations. In the first case, a ray of light with incident angle $\theta_1 = 15°$ passes from air into a glass with an index of refraction of 1.5, and we wish to know the refracted angle, θ_2. The values of the index of refraction in Equation 2.2 refer to the index of the medium the light ray travels *from* as n_1, and that of the medium it passes *into* as n_2. In our case, $n_1 = 1.00$ for air and $n_2 = 1.50$ for the glass:

$$n_1 \sin\theta_1 = n_2 \sin\theta_2$$

$$\sin\theta_2 = \frac{n_1 \sin\theta_1}{n_2}$$

$$\sin\theta_2 = \frac{1.00 \times \sin 15°}{1.50} = \frac{1.00 \times 0.26}{1.50}$$

$$\theta_2 = \sin^{-1}(\sin\theta_2) = \sin^{-1}(0.173) = 9.9°$$

The refracted angle is $\theta_2 = 9.9°$. Note that since the ray travels from a faster speed of light (higher index) medium into a slower (lower index) medium, the ray is bent to lower angles (away from the interface). (To check whether a refracted angle has been calculated correctly, try using it in Snell's law directly to make sure Equation 2.2 is satisfied. That is, confirm that $1.00 \times \sin 15° = 1.50 \times \sin 9.9°$.)

(continued on next page)

What would happen if a ray of light with the same incident angle had instead started out from the glass side of the interface? In this case, the light ray travels from glass, making $n_1 = 1.50$, into air, making $n_2 = 1.00$. The angle of incidence is the same, so we still have $\theta_1 = 15°$, but the angle of refraction is different. We must repeat our previous calculation, but with the new, correct value of the indices of refraction. (Make sure you understand how these new values were chosen!)

$$\sin\theta_2 = \frac{n_1 \sin\theta_1}{n_2}$$

$$\sin\theta_2 = \frac{1.50 \times \sin 15°}{1.00} = \frac{1.50 \times 0.26}{1.00}$$

$$= 0.39$$

$$\theta_2 = \sin^{-1}(0.39) = 23°$$

This time, the ray is bent toward the interface to a higher refracted angle as it travels from a slower (high index) to faster (low index) medium.

While Snell's law determines the direction of the refracted light rays, we have not discussed what *fraction* of the original light is reflected or transmitted. These quantities also can be computed from the rays' angles and values of the index of refraction.

These results for reflection and refraction allow the use of lenses and mirrors to shape the pathway of light and form magnified images. The operation of mirrors is solely determined by the reflection rule and the shape of the mirror. The mirror's optics are determined by drawing sample rays of light and tracing their pathways upon reflection, using the rule that the reflected ray's angle is equal to that of the original ray. Lenses are specially ground pieces of glass, plastic, or quartz (Figure 2.8a); their operation can be understood by considering the way they refract the light that falls on them. Lenses are constructed to utilize this refraction to *focus* rays. This is shown in Figure 2.8(b), where parallel light impinging on the lens to the left is concentrated down to a small **focal point** by this effect, before once again diverging. The distance from the lens to the point where the light rays are brought together is called the **focal length, f,** of the lens.

This focusing of light has two consequences for future discussions. First, it allows light to be concentrated down to a small spot—so small its intensity can be used to damage human tissue (Figure 2.8b). We will return to this

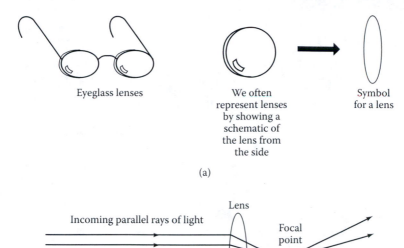

(a)

(b)

Figure 2.8 (a) Lenses are curved pieces of a transparent material such as glass or plastic. One of the more common examples are the lenses used in eyeglasses or contact lenses. Scientists typically represent lenses using the schematic side view shown. (b) A convex (converging) lens uses refraction to bend the pathways of rays of light hitting it so that they are bent toward a line drawn through the center of the lens (dashed line). Parallel rays of light incident on the lens will be focused to a focal point at a distance equal to the focal length, f.

fact in Chapter 3 in the discussion of laser surgery. Second, it allows light to be manipulated to form magnified images using one or more lenses.

2.2.4 Optional: How lenses form images

To see how lenses can be used to produce magnified images of objects, we will discuss in detail one particular case of image formation using converging lenses. (See Figure 2.9a–b.) First, note that a lens can only intercept a thin pencil of all of the many rays of light reflecting from the surface of an object, such as the house in Figure 2.9(a). We will only consider what happens to a few representative rays from this narrow range; for ease of understanding, we will only follow the paths of rays emanating from one point on the object.

The formation of images proceeds from a direct application of Snell's law, since this is the fundamental reason the rays of light have new directions

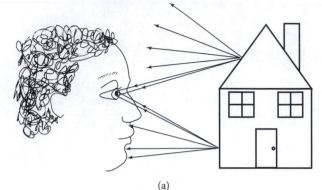

(a)

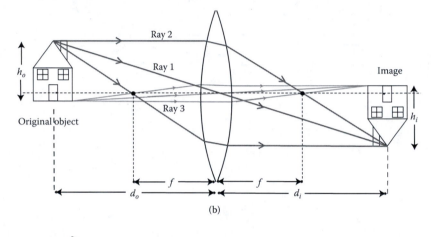

(b)

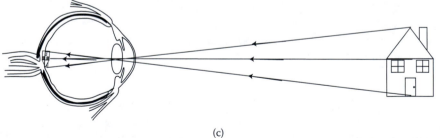

(c)

Figure 2.9 (a) Only a thin pencil of light rays from an object can enter the lens of an imaging system, such as that found in the eye. (b) Illustration of image formation with a converging lens. The lens axis is shown as a dashed line. The figure shows the paths followed by rays of light emanating from a point on the object (at right), which are refracted by the lens and focused to form an image (at left). (See explanation in text.) (c) The process of image formation shown in (b) is the same as that used in the eye to form images on the retina, using the eye's cornea and lens as the focusing element. (For clarity, only the rays that pass approximately straight through the lens and cornea are shown.)

after passing through the lens. You might expect that determining the new paths of the rays would be very difficult, since there are many different possible rays with many different incident and refracted angles to account for. However, very thin converging lenses can be very accurately described by a few simple rules that altogether avoid the complexity of a case-by-case application of Snell's law. Before describing these rules, it is useful to first define the **lens axis**, a line running through the center of the lens and perpendicular to its face, indicated by a dashed line in Figure 2.9(b). The rules for image formation are then as follows: (1) Rays of light which pass *through the center of the lens* can be treated as though they travel without refraction. Their new path after the lens is then simply an extension of their original path before the lens, as shown for ray 1 in Figure 2.9(b). (In fact, their paths are very slightly shifted, but for a thin lens this is not an important effect.) (2) Rays of light that *travel parallel to the axis* of the lens are focused by the lens so as to pass through the lens axis exactly one focal point away from the lens, as shown for ray 2 in Figure 2.9(b). (3) Rays of light that *pass through a point one focal length away* from the lens are refracted so as to travel parallel to the lens axis, as shown for ray 3 in Figure 2.9(b).

Figure 2.9(b) shows the net effect of these ray-tracing rules on rays of light emanating from the same point on the object a distance d_o from the lens. These rays are focused to the same point on the other side of the lens at a distance d_i. (Note that while we've only considered three rays here, *all rays* emitted from the same point on the original object that pass through the lens are also focused at the same new point as these three particular rays.) In other words, rays of light coming from each point on the original image are focused by the lens at a new location. Figure 2.9(b) shows that this new location is different for different points on the original object; in fact, by applying these rules to rays from each point on the original object, we could prove that the light is always focused at the new location so as to always preserve the shape of the original image. This new location is that of the image. We call this location an **image** because rays of light exit from it just as they would from an actual object present at that location. We call it a **real image** because you could actually project a picture of the object on a screen at that location.

While our discussion so far has focused on lenses in general, exactly the same process occurs in the human eye. There, the combination of the cornea of the eye and the lens provides the refraction needed to form images on the retina of the eye (Figure 2.9c). The muscles of the eye can be used to change the focal length of the eye's lens in order to maintain the image's position at the retina for objects at varying distances. The rod and cone light-sensing cells within the retina then detect a pattern of light color and intensity that accurately describe that of the original object.

Other examples of commonly encountered real images include the images projected by a computer projector, and those formed by cameras on film and by videocameras on electronic light sensors, respectively. (There is a second class of images, called **virtual images**, which we will not discuss here. They include examples such as the image seen through a magnifying glass or eyeglasses, or the eyepiece of an endoscope. Virtual images differ from real images in that they cannot be projected on a screen; the rules for their construction are a simple extension of those we have discussed here for real images.)

As you can see from Figure 2.9(b) and (c), the image is often not the same size as the original object. In fact, depending upon the position of the object and the lens' focal length, the image formed can be larger or smaller than the original object. The ratio of the image's size, h_i, to that of the original object, h_o, is called the **magnification, $M = h_i/h_o$**. In our example, it is possible to show, using trigonometry, that $M = d_i/d_o$. (This is true because the ray through the center of the lens travels without deflection, so it makes the same angle with the lens axis on either side of the lens. Because the angles are similar, we can conclude that $h_i/d_i = h_o/d_o$. Rearranging this last relation, we can find that $d_i/d_o = h_i/h_o$, and hence $M = d_i/d_o$.) The rules described above for ray tracing can be extended to cover multiple lenses. This framework allows the construction of optical imaging systems used to create the images formed in endoscopy.

2.2.5 Making pipes for light

The rules of geometrical optics enable the construction of light pipes: structures that allow us to guide light along a winding pathway. Such devices are commonly called **optical fibers**. They are encountered in nature as well as in medical technology: seedlings use their semitransparent stems as effective fiber optic guides to direct light underground to the developing plant. Using our knowledge of optics, we can now understand how optical fibers work.

Consider the following sequence of events (Figure 2.10) that happens when rays of light hit an interface at glancing angles. At the top of each diagram, light is incident on an interface between glass (the top medium) and air (the bottom medium). A typical value for the index of refraction of glass is 1.5, and that of air is very close to 1.00, so the light travels from a high index (low speed) to low index (high speed) medium. For each of the incident angles, the reflected ray always makes an angle equal to the original ray. However, as the rays of light pass through the interface, the refracted rays are bent into angles *greater* than those of the incident rays. Eventually, an incident angle is reached for which the refracted ray is bent almost 90°, skimming the surface (Figure 2.10d). If the incident angle becomes even greater, what happens to the refracted ray then? It has been bent as far as it can go without re-entering the original medium! In fact, for angles greater than the angle shown in Figure 2.10(d), there is no refracted light. *All* of the incoming light is reflected, a phenomenon called **total internal reflection**. In fact, even though we ordinarily think of the interface between air and glass as transparent, for a special range of angles, the light is reflected from the interface as if from a perfect mirror!

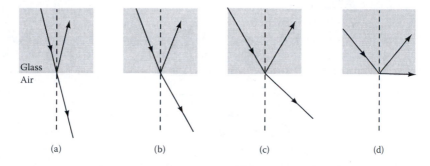

Glass
Air

(a)   (b)   (c)   (d)

Figure 2.10 Rays of light are both reflected and refracted when moving from a higher to a lower index medium (in this case, from glass to air). The angle of refraction is greater than the angle of incidence, and it increases as the angle of incidence increases. (a through c). At some angle of incidence, the refracted angle is equal to 90°, and the refracted ray is at the largest angle it can achieve before crossing the interface (d). For larger angles, no refraction occurs, and all of the original light is reflected.

We can use Snell's law to compute the incoming angle at which this happens. When the refracted angle has reached the highest value it can attain without crossing the interface, it is equal to 90°, so $\sin \theta_2 = \sin 90° = 1.00$. This corresponds to an incoming angle, θ_1, called the *critical angle*, θ_{crit}; for values of θ_1 greater than the critical angle, no refracted ray exists. Snell's law relates the critical angle to the indices of refraction of the two media using the equation:

$$\sin \theta_{crit} = \frac{n_2}{n_1} \tag{2.3a}$$

This is just Snell's law written for the special case where the incoming angle $\theta_1 = \theta_{crit}$ and the refracted ray would have $\sin \theta_2 = \sin 90° = 1.00$. The higher index is n_1 and the lower n_2 in this equation, since the ray enters from the higher index medium.

$$n_1 \sin \theta_{crit} = n_2 \sin \theta_2$$

$$= n_2 \sin 90°$$

$$= n_2 \times 1.00 \tag{2.3b}$$

$$\sin \theta_{crit} = \frac{n_2}{n_1}$$

$$\theta_{crit} = \sin^{-1}\left(\frac{n_2}{n_1}\right)$$

Total internal reflection cannot happen when light is moving *from* a lower index medium *into* a higher index medium. This is because the refracted light is bent in the opposite direction, making the outgoing ray's angle always less than that of the incoming ray (Figure 2.7a). The situation shown in Figure 2.10(d) consequently can never occur in that case.

Sample calculation: Let us compute the critical angle for an air–glass interface as an example. The situation we are interested in involves rays of light traveling from glass into the air. (As the earlier sample calculation showed, for a light ray passing from air into glass, the angle of incidence always decreases, so total internal reflection never takes place in that case.) This corresponds to having glass as the medium at the top of the diagram in Figure 2.11 and air as the medium at the bottom. (There is nothing special about this orientation of the two interfaces, and the same results hold for any other orientation so long as the rays pass from glass into air.) We can compute the critical angle, θ_{crit}, for total internal reflection using Equation 2.3, using a value of $n_1 = 1.50$ for the index of glass and $n_2 = 1.00$ for air.

$$\sin \theta_{crit} = \frac{n_2}{n_1} = \frac{1.0}{1.5} = 0.66$$

$$\theta_{crit} = \sin^{-1} 0.66 = 42°$$

This turns out to be 42° for air and glass. All light incident from the glass side at angles greater than 42° is totally internally reflected at this glass–air interface.

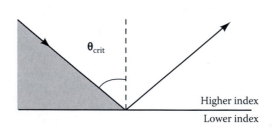

Figure 2.11 Geometry for total internal reflection. In order for total internal reflection to occur, the incident ray must be traveling from a medium of higher index to one of lower index of refraction. Incident rays with incident angles greater than the critical angle, θ_{crit} will be totally reflected, with no refraction occurring. All of the incident light is reflected in this case. Rays with angles of incidence smaller than θ_{crit} will undergo ordinary reflection and refraction, as discussed earlier in this chapter.

The geometry for total internal reflection is illustrated in Figure 2.11. Light rays with incoming angles greater than the critical angle are totally reflected. Ordinary refraction and reflection occur for incoming angles less than the critical angle.

For example, consider again the interface between glass and air. If light rays coming from glass hit an interface between glass and air at angles greater than the critical angle of 42°, then the rays undergo total internal reflection. This is illustrated for a glass rod surrounded by air in Figure 2.12. Unless the rod is bent sharply, the incident angle at each bounce of the light ray is within the total reflection condition, even if the rod is curved. As a result, *all* of the light bounces from end to the end of the rod *even when the rod is bent*, a situation illustrated in Figure 2.12.

What happens as you make the light pipe thinner and thinner? The total internal reflection condition still holds in this case. We call such very thin light pipes optical fibers. Many of the light rays entering the fiber do so at angles that exceed the critical angle, so that they are totally reflected. The light entering the fiber bounces many times against the sides, finally exiting from the other end. Since these rays are continually totally reflected, with no losses out the sides, virtually the same amount of light leaves the optical fiber as entered.

In addition, glass becomes much less rigid when it is stretched into thin fibers, just as steel is less rigid when formed into slender wires. Consequently, glass optical fibers are extremely flexible and easily bent around corners. This does not interfere with total internal reflection unless the bending angle is extremely sharp. To ensure that the optical fiber is surrounded by a lower index material—without which total internal reflection cannot occur—optical fibers are often manufactured with a **cladding**, a coating of lower index glass (Figure 2.13). In many cases, the entire fiber is then coated with a tough plastic layer to resist damage. The materials used to construct optical fibers must be extremely pure and free of colors or defects

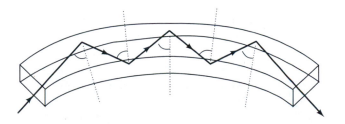

Figure 2.12 Illustration of total internal reflection within a glass rod surrounded by air, for which the critical angle is 42°. Each time the ray of light reflects from the sides of the rod it satisfies the total internal reflection criterion, so it is totally reflected. Thus, even though the rod is curved, the light can travel from one end of the rod to the other without loss.

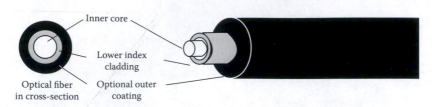

Inner core

Lower index
cladding

Optical fiber
in cross-section

Optional outer
coating

Figure 2.13 Typical construction of an optical fiber. The inner core, made of
glass, quartz, or some other transparent material, has a higher index
of refraction than the surrounding cladding, which is made of some
similar material. In some applications, a protective outer coating surrounds the fiber.

to ensure high transparency. This ensures that very little light is absorbed
by the optical fiber itself. Various types of glasses are used as well as quartz
and silica.

If a bundle of optical fibers is gathered together, each of the fibers can
separately transmit light efficiently from one end to the other (Figure 2.14a).
If the bundle is assembled so as to carefully preserve the orientation of each
fiber with respect to its neighbors, we say the bundle is **coherent**; such a
bundle is sometimes referred to as an **image conduit** (Figure 2.14b–c). If
we place the image conduit close to an object, each of its constituent fibers
collects light emitted by that point on the object nearest the fiber. Total
internal reflection carries that light to the other end of the bundles of fibers,
where it emerges at the corresponding fiber's exit end. At this end, the fibers
are arranged in the same pattern as the input. As the piped light exits each
fiber, the image of the object is reconstructed exactly, with the original size
and colors preserved (Figure 2.14b–c).

As shown in Figure 2.14(b), the image is transmitted one fiber at a time,
each fiber collecting light from that part of the image closest to it. Just
as was the case with the mirrored tube discussed at the beginning of this
chapter, each individual fiber scrambles the light rays traveling within it.
Overall, the bundle keeps the image straight by using different fibers for
each part of the image. (However, because of this scrambling within a
fiber, the smallest feature visible on the reconstructed image is no smaller
than the fibers themselves.) This method of assembling an image from
many separate dots, each dot corresponding to the end of a single optical
fiber, resembles the way your television screen or computer monitor builds
images. Their pictures are constructed from tiny, colored dots called pixels (for picture element). Similarly, newspaper photographs are assembled
from many dots. If you look carefully at a television screen using a magnifying glass or tiny drop of water on the screen, you can distinguish the
individual pixels.

If an optical fiber bundle is assembled so that the fibers have random
orientations at opposite ends, then an image is not formed, much as though
the pixels on your television set were scrambled to make a random pattern

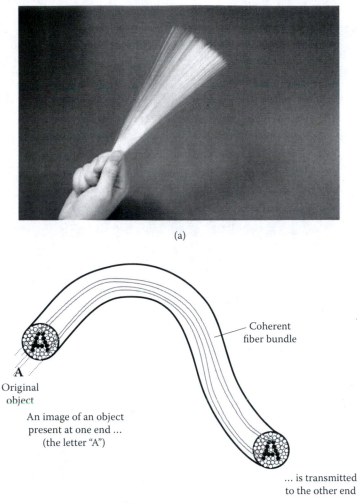

(a)

Coherent
fiber bundle

A
Original
object

An image of an object
present at one end ...
(the letter "A")

... is transmitted
to the other end

(b)

Figure 2.14 (a) Fiber bundles consist of many closely packed optical fibers bound
together. (b) Image conduit made of a coherent bundle of optical
fibers. Light from each point on the original object (in this case the
letter "A") is collected by individual optical fibers in the conduit. (c) A
fiber directly above a point on the white paper transmit rays of white
light from that region, while those above a point on the dark ink of the
letter collect and transmit rays from only that point. (d) By contrast, if
the orientation of the optical fibers is not preserved from end to end,
no image is apparent at the opposite end, as occurs for incoherent optical fiber bundles.

(Figure 2.14d). Such bundles are called **incoherent** fiber optics; although
they are useful for transmitting light for illumination, they cannot be used
for image formation.

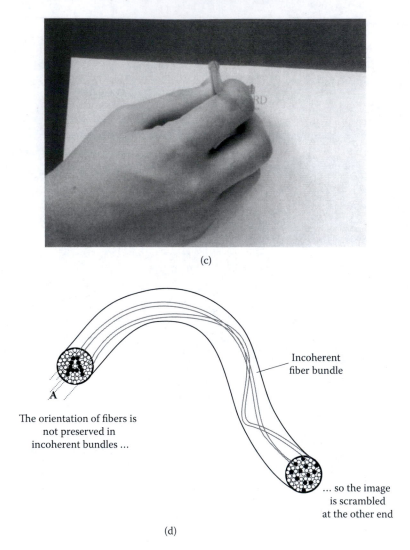

(c)

(d)

Incoherent
fiber bundle

The orientation of fibers is
not preserved in
incoherent bundles ...

... so the image
is scrambled
at the other end

Figure 2.14 (continued).

   One useful application that involves only illumination is the use of fiber optic blankets for treating **jaundice** in newborn babies. This common condition results when an excessive amount of bilirubin (a waste product produced during the breakdown of red blood cells) is present in the bloodstream. Light can be used to chemically break down the bilirubin so it can be more readily cleared from the blood, but this phototherapy entails exposing the newborn to long periods of high intensity light. One method of delivering this light entails having the infant lie unclothed under lamps in the hospital's nursery for a set period of time each day. In many cases, the infant can instead receive phototherapy at home by being wrapped in a

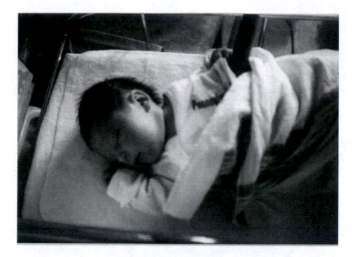

Figure 2.15 (See color figure following page 78.) Fiber optic blankets can enable parents to treat jaundice at home rather than in the hospital; here a newborn baby rests while receiving phototherapy from the biliblanket swaddling her.

special blankets into which optical fibers have been embedded. This allows the high intensity light to shine directly on the newborn's skin while the parents hold and care for their child (Figure 2.15).

Thus, fiber optics can transmit images over long distances and along curving pathways when assembled into coherent bundles. By joining the fibers only at the ends, and leaving them as separate strands in between, one can form bundles that retain the flexibility of individual fibers. This provides one way to build an endoscope: a device that can be threaded through even the twisting passages of the large intestine for a close, detailed look.

2.3 FIBER OPTICS APPLICATIONS IN MEDICINE: ENDOSCOPES AND LAPAROSCOPES

2.3.1 Different types of endoscopes and their typical construction

Medical endoscopes go by specific names that are determined by which parts of the body each scope is used to image. A partial listing is given in Table 2.2. Many different types exist, each designed for a specific application. Endoscopes are used for examining the inside of the body; examples include the colonoscopes and sigmoidoscopes mentioned earlier. Other surgical procedures performed on the gastrointestinal tract use endoscopes inserted through the mouth and esophagus, while bronchoscopes allow access to the larger passages of the respiratory tract.

Table 2.2 Some types of medical fiber optic scopes

Type of scope	Used for imaging of
Endoscope	Hollow organs: the gastrointestinal tract, the eye, etc.; this is also a generic term
Laparoscope	Abdominal cavity, used for gynecological surgery, gallbladder removals, appendectomies, hernia repair, etc.
Bronchoscope	Bronchial passages of the lung
Cystoscope	Urinary bladder
Colonoscope	Large intestine
Sigmoidoscope	Outer regions of the large intestine
Thoracoscope	Chest cavity
Laryngoscope	Larynx
Angioscope	Blood vessels
Arthroscope	Interior of joints: knee, ankle, shoulder, elbow

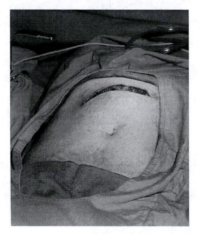

(a)

Figure 2.16 (a) Example of the wide incision required for open surgery on the abdomen. (b) By comparison, surgeons perform laparoscopic procedures through several tiny incisions, using laparoscopes and additional tools. The laparoscope and various specialized surgical instruments are inserted through these small incisions after the abdomen is inflated with an inert gas. (c) Laparoscopic surgery in progress. (Figures a and c reproduced with permission courtesy of John N. Graber, Leonard S. Schultz, Joseph J. Pietrafitta, and David F. Hickock, *Laparoscopic Abdominal Surgery*, McGraw-Hill, New York, 1993.)

Laparoscopes are used to examine, and perform surgery on, the abdomen (Figure 2.16a–c). The earliest use of laparoscopy was in gynecological procedures. Laparoscopes inserted through an abdominal incision can be used to inspect a woman's reproductive organs for any of a number of

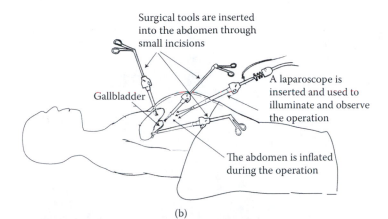

Surgical tools are inserted into the abdomen through small incisions

Gallbladder

A laparoscope is inserted and used to illuminate and observe the operation

The abdomen is inflated during the operation

(b)

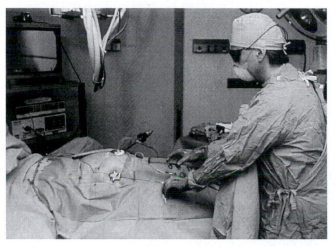

(c)

Figure 2.16 (continued.)

reasons, including ectopic pregnancy (a pregnancy that forms in a fallopian tube rather than the uterus) and endometriosis (a condition in which the endometrial tissue that lines the uterus grows elsewhere in the abdomen, often causing pain and infertility). Many types of gynecological surgery are also normally performed by laparoscopy, including treatments for these conditions. Special endoscopes, called **hysteroscopes**, which are inserted through the vagina, permit inspection of the inside of the uterus, and can also be used for surgical procedures such as hysterectomies (surgical removal of the uterus).

Many other types of abdominal surgery can be successfully accomplished by laparoscopy. Examples include examinations of tumors within the abdomen, gallbladder removals, appendectomies, and hernia repairs. Surgeons are experimenting with this evolving technology to evaluate which

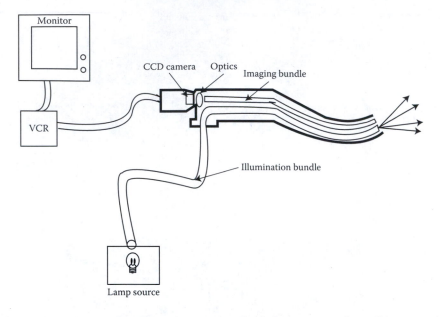

Figure 2.17 A typical endoscope consists of a light source, a long fiber optical conduit for the illuminating light, a headpiece that controls the actions of the scope head and any surgical tools used, a video (CCD) camera (either attached to the headpiece or incorporated into the tip of the instrument), and a long flexible shaft inserted into the body.

procedures can safely take advantage of this possibility and which are better performed by traditional, or "open," surgical techniques (Figure 2.16a). For some types of operations, open surgery may always be the best choice, but specific types of endoscopes have become the dominant method in many types of surgery.

The basic requirements for an endoscope's operation are shown in Figure 2.17. Since the body cavities to be examined are naturally quite dark, a source of light must be introduced. A bright lamp or LED (light emitting diode) source of light must be used, and its light guided into the body using an **illuminating** incoherent fiber optic bundle. Although only some endoscopes use imaging bundles, all make use of fiber optics for illumination.

For instruments such as arthroscopes and laparoscopes, a straight viewing pathway suffices and fiber optics are used only for illumination of the dark interior cavity. For these straight scopes, several lenses are used to make a telescope for looking within the body. When access must be made through a curving pathway, for example, for colonoscopes, there are two options for how images can be transmitted outside. For large-enough endoscopes, a tiny video camera only several millimeters square can be attached to the tip of the endoscope for what is called **direct** (or **local**) imaging. The same integrated circuit chips used as the imaging elements in commercial video cameras are employed in these endoscopes. One common type, **CCD** (**charge-coupled device**) integrated circuits, consists of a rectangular grid of thousands of tiny electronic light sensors that detect the light intensity at each point on an image. This information is then conveyed outside the body via slender electrical wires. The resulting image can be viewed directly on a monitor, and stored for future reference.

By contrast, **indirect** endoscopes use the **imaging** fiber optic bundles described above, which are typically 2 to 3 mm in diameter. For short examinations, physicians can view the resulting image directly through an eyepiece. For surgery and for longer procedures, it is usually more convenient to connect the outside face of the imaging bundle to a CCD camera, and project the image on a television monitor. The latter configuration is much more flexible, as it allows several persons to view the image and allows the physician to move more freely. For either type of endoscope, lenses are used to magnify the image viewed by approximately 4 to 40 times.

The total diameter of the scopes ranges from roughly 15 mm to only a few millimeters. (Extremely tiny versions can be as small as 0.3 mm in diameter!) Endoscopes for certain applications can be over one and a half meters in length. The apparatus can be made out of plastic, glass, and steel, and the entire scope must be designed so it can be thoroughly disinfected. The various inserts and related tools are often made disposable for sanitary reasons.

For endoscopes that use imaging bundles, the size of the individual optical fibers limits the smallest feature one can discern, a limit called the **spatial resolution** of the device. (A typical spatial resolution for colonoscopes using direct imaging would be a few tenths of a millimeter.) Presently, optical fibers can be made as small as a few microns, roughly one-hundredth the diameter of a human hair. Modern viewing bundles contain several thousand to tens of thousands of such tiny optical fibers. You might wonder whether this could be improved to allow the viewing of even individual cells, which are typically about one micron in size. However, limitations due to the wavelike aspects of light prevent the size of optical fibers from being further reduced, so the present size of an optical fiber very likely gives the best spatial resolution possible with this technique.

The preceding discussion covered only the optics necessary for *viewing* tissues. Of course, many applications involve actual surgery on internal organs and consequently most endoscopes are also equipped with various mechanical inserts and surgical tools. These can either be guided through channels in the scope's main tube or introduced through auxiliary tubes. Examples of the types of inserts used on an endoscope for examining the gastro-intestinal tract are shown in Figure 2.18(a–c). Because the body's organs naturally settle compactly together, leaving no clear air-filled spaces, a gas channel is usually included and used to inflate the region to be examined with inert carbon dioxide gas to lift and separate the tissues (Figures 2.16b and 2.18b). Similarly, another insert is used for injecting water and suctioning off fluid and debris.

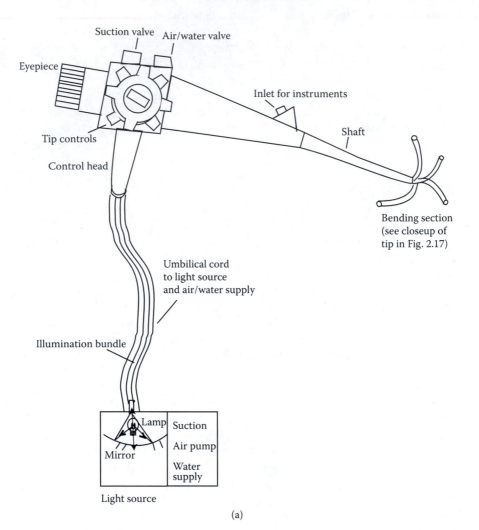

Suction valve   Air/water valve

Eyepiece

Inlet for instruments

Tip controls

Shaft

Control head

Bending section
(see closeup of
tip in Fig. 2.17)

Umbilical cord
to light source
and air/water supply

Illumination bundle

Lamp Suction

Air pump

Mirror

Water
supply

Light source

(a)

Figure 2.18 (a) The hand piece of an endoscope has controls used to steer the
head and to control the operations of the various tools used. (b) The
end of the endoscope inserted into the body contains several ports
through which the illuminating optical bundle transmits light and
through which the image is transmitted to the physician outside. In
the video endoscope shown, the CCD camera is located near the tip of
the endoscope. Other ports are used to introduce water or gases into
the patient, for suctioning out fluids and for inserting surgical tools of
various types. (c) Examples of the miniature surgical instruments used
in endoscopic and laparoscopic procedures. A biopsy forceps can be
used to take tissue samples for analysis. A thin loop of wire called a
snare can be used to remove precancerous growths from the colon.

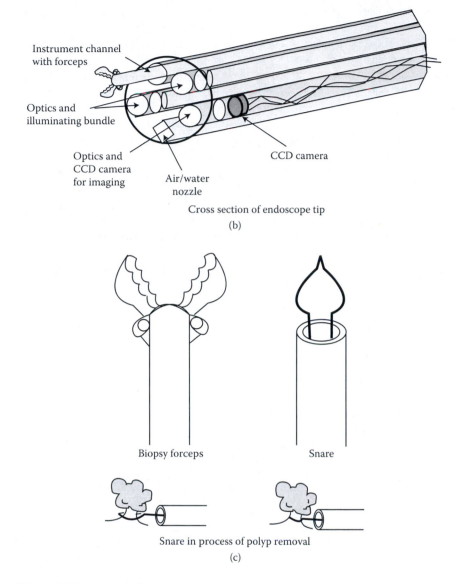

Instrument channel
with forceps

Optics and
illuminating bundle

Optics and
CCD camera
for imaging

Air/water
nozzle

CCD camera

Cross section of endoscope tip

(b)

Biopsy forceps

Snare

Snare in process of polyp removal

(c)

Figure 2.18 (continued).

The head of the endoscope (Figure 2.18a) can be moved using a control knob that manipulates a steerable head, allowing the operator to look around inside the body. Other common tools include forceps for manipulating and removing tissue for examination, tiny scalpels, miniaturized staple guns, tools for making sutures, and snares for both cutting and heating tissue (Figure 2.18c). The snare works by being looped around a region of tissue while an electric current is passed through the wire. This heats the wire, causing the tissue to heat up as well, and destroy tissue and seal off blood vessels at the same time, an effect called **cauterization**.

While the gastrointestinal tract can be examined by endoscopes introduced through the rectum or throat, for laparoscopic surgery, the instruments must be inserted through the wall of the abdomen. In this case, several incisions roughly one centimeter in length are made near the same site for inserting the laparoscope and its associated surgical instruments (Figure 2.16b and c). Most of these tools are similar in nature to those discussed above, with the difference that they are inserted through several separate incisions.

For example, presently colon cancer screening is mainly accomplished by regular endoscopic exams. For colon cancer prevention, persons over age 50 are recommended to undergo regular exams every few years, performed with either sigmoidoscopes, which can only access the outermost regions of the large intestine, or colonoscopes, which can see along its entire length. (Two other x-ray screening methods for colon cancer—double-contrast barium studies and CT or virtual colonoscopy—are discussed in Chapter 5.) While not a comfortable prospect, these exams are fast and can be done as an outpatient procedure using sedation only. The colonoscopy allows the physician to examine the walls of the colon for precancerous grows, and to biopsy and remove them in one step using, e.g., the snares and forceps described above. The documented success of this regimen means that many cases of potential or actual colon cancer can either be prevented or cured through early detection.

New developments in endoscopic imaging are aimed at improving the images available. For example, chromoendoscopy involves the uses of stains or pigments introduced to distinguish the appearance of polyps or other abnormal features from normal tissues. Narrow Band Imaging involves using optical filters (Chapter 3) to change the way colors are imaged, resulting in better detection of fine blood vessels, features useful in classifying polyps, for example.

An alternative to using endoscopes for imaging parts of the gastrointestinal tract is **video capsule endoscopy** employing a self-contained "camera pill" (Figure 2.19). Just as it sounds, this device is a tiny self-contained camera, light source, and video transmitter all in one compact, roughly 1-cm-long package. Patients swallow the camera pill in a doctor's office, then go about their daily activities while it makes its way through the digestive tract, moving by the natural method of peristalsis and taking a series of images two times a second as it goes. The patient wears about the waist a data recorder that receives and records transmitted images from the camera pill for later analysis. Video capsule endoscope is useful for imaging parts of the digestive tract, such as the deeper reaches of the small intestine, difficult to access using endoscopes, and has FDA approval for such examinations in the U.S. Despite its small size, the resolution of the camera pill is 0.1 mm,

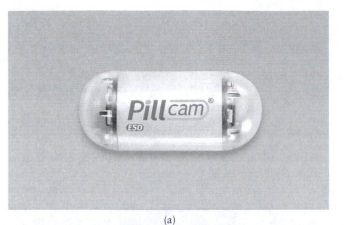

(a)

(b)

Figure 2.19 (*See color figure following page 78.*) (a) Video capsule endoscopy. The camera pill (PillCam™) is an alternative to using a flexible endoscope for some examinations of the gastrointestinal tract. (b) Camera pill image of an inflamed esophagus in esophagitis. (Images used with permission courtesy of Given Imaging.)

only somewhat coarser than regular endoscopy. Some drawbacks relative to colonoscopy or endoscopy of the upper gastrointestinal tract include the lack of ability to select the orientation of images, the inability to sample tissues for biopsy, and clinical approval only for small intestine imaging thus far. The next generation of **active capsule endoscopy** is slated to address some of these problems with devices that can propel and steer themselves.

2.3.2 Some advantages and disadvantages

The most striking advantages of laparoscopic surgery and other endoscopic procedures are apparent in many studies that have shown reduced hospital stays and faster recovery times for these procedures relative to open surgery. This is in part because the incisions required for the endoscope's insertion are much smaller than would be required for open surgery. In addition, patients can sometimes rely on only local or topical anesthesia for short examinations, thus reducing the risk associated with general anesthesia. The reduction in invasiveness, bleeding (and subsequent need for blood transfusions), risk of infection, and overall stress can turn some types of surgery that once required a hospital stay into outpatient procedures performed in a physician's office. Not all uses of endoscopes necessarily involve surgery. Examinations of the gastrointestinal tract (e.g., for colon cancer screening) or of the other abdominal organs can be made without the risks involved in open surgery.

However, problems unique to endoscopes have emerged as their use has spread. For example, in laparoscopy the need to inflate the abdomen with gas can lead to discomfort afterward, sometimes resulting in pain for days after the procedure. Devices called **abdominal retractors** allow an insert to be placed on the skin above the site to be examined, lifting up the abdominal wall to create a space in which the surgeon can work. Physicians hope this in some cases will replace the need for inflating the operating site with gas and hence will allow quicker recoveries with less pain.

A more serious problem involves the constricted access and unfamiliar motions required to operate with only a video monitor for feedback. Small, unnatural manipulations of inserted laparoscopic tools replace the more intuitive and direct applications of the hands and manually wielded tools used in open surgery. The surgeon loses the sense of touch that both provides feedback about how much force is being exerted, and facilitates the coordination of complex motions such as suturing wounds. The world of the video monitor is flat and fails to give a feeling for the depth of the surgical site; important features may simply be hidden from view. Physicians require considerable training to master these new methods, and must attend specialized training sessions in which surgery is practiced on models and animals (often pigs) before moving on to people. Worries that these complicating factors may result in fewer, but more serious, complications have been allayed, but not completely laid to rest, by studies documenting no increases in the rates of complications, now that laparoscopic techniques have been in use for several years. We will now consider laparoscopic gall-bladder removals, one of the more intensively studied new uses of laparo-scopic surgery, to see how these trade-offs have played out in practice in two success stories.

2.3.3 Laparoscopic gallbladder removals

The gallbladder stores bile produced by the liver and resecretes it when needed into the small intestine, thus aiding in the digestion of fatty foods. In some persons, cholesterol crystals, called gallstones, form within the gallbladder. Large ones can potentially block the bile ducts and cause sharp pains in the abdomen. Sometimes medication alone can dissolve these gall-stones. Failing this treatment, persons suffering from this can live with occasional abdominal pain while maintaining a restricted low fat diet, or they can undergo surgery to have their gallbladder removed, an operation called **cholecystectomy**. In spite of the often acute abdominal pain, many persons once opted to live with the condition indefinitely when faced with the prospect of open surgery, which typically entails a one-week hospital stay, an extended recovery period lasting an average of six weeks, and a six-inch-wide surgical scar.

Laparoscopic cholecystectomy was introduced to the U.S. in 1987 and soon became the dominant method for gallbladder removal for most cases. The reasons for its popularity are clear: the laparoscopic operation entails only a one- to two-day hospital stay, a return to normal activity after one week, little pain, and minimal scarring. The healthcare costs per proce-dure can be reduced, potentially saving money for the hospital and health insurer, and a greater saving to society can result because of the recipient's faster return to normal activity.

However, the actual way the introduction of this technology played out held some unexpected lessons. In the early 1990s, the success of lap-aroscopic gallbladder operations led to a dramatic increase in the overall number of removals. Much of this increase was tied convincingly to the introduction of laparoscopic procedures and the greater willingness of suf-ferers to elect optional surgery. In fact, in many regions, patient demand for the new technology was one of the major factors fueling its introduction. At the same time, mortality rates decreased for gall bladder operations as the risk of dying from laparoscopic procedures was less than that from open surgery on average. However, the overall picture represents a more mixed blessing. Even though the mortality *rate* was lower for the laparo-scope procedure, the *same total number* of deaths resulted as before (simply because a greater number of people were operated on). That is, the increase in the number of operations offset the benefits due to the decreased risk for each procedure. In addition, although the cost per procedure has fallen, the *total* healthcare bill due to gallbladder removals has risen steadily as the number of procedures has increased. An economic analysis of the effects of new medical technologies thus must take into account this increase when considering the benefits accrued by apparent gains, such as shorter hospital stays and faster recoveries.

2.4 NEW AND FUTURE DIRECTIONS

2.4.1 Robotic surgery and virtual reality in the operating room

The drawbacks of endoscopic and laparoscopic techniques mentioned above mostly concern the limitations imposed by the need for unnatural video–eye–hand coordination and the crudeness of surgical techniques available. In traditional laparoscopic surgery, physicians operate on parts of the body and manipulate tools that can only be seen via a computer monitor. This disconnect eliminates direct hand–eye coordination and forces the surgeon to operate at a remove, through narrow openings. Rather than performing intuitive motions, such as cutting directly with a scalpel, physicians must manipulate awkward special laparoscopic tools that sometimes must be moved in directions opposite their apparent motion on the video screen. Physicians and researchers are trying to overcome these problems by developing new technologies that both give the surgeon a better picture of the inside of the body and provide a better feel for the operation. **Virtual reality** is a computer-based technology that gives a person the vivid impression that he or she is seeing and handling a real object. Often the object is projected onto the field of vision using special goggles that allow the viewer to see images that look fully three dimensional. At the same time, robotic manipulators, or even gloves fitted with special sensors, reproduce for the user the sensations of handling objects.

This technology is being investigated as part of **robotic surgery** devices that combine virtual reality visualization with robotic surgical tools. In this technology, a robot does not perform operations, but instead assists a skilled human surgeon. For example, in the da Vinci™ robotic surgery system, motions of the surgeon's hand are translated into corresponding motions of miniaturized surgical tools within the patient's body (Figure 2.20). Meanwhile, the surgeon's hand experiences force feedback from the tools that mimics the sensation of touch in open surgery. The surgeon wears special goggles to view a three-dimensional, highly magnified image of the surgical site. Instead of the tiny motions required for laparoscopic surgery, the surgeon uses more comfortable and natural motions to perform the surgery, while the image viewed displayed the motions in their actual positions within the body. Thus, the surgeon gets the same "look and feel" of open surgery while being able to see directly a magnified view and operate with precise, delicate motions. The surgeon can operate from a console while in a relaxed, seated position, making for a more ergonomic stance for lengthy operations. The robotic system can remove any tremors from fine hand motions, and the surgeon can use both hands and feet to operate devices. Hundreds of such

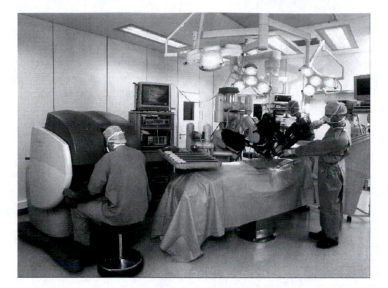

Figure 2.20 Photo of the da Vinci™ robot-assisted surgical system, showing a surgeon seated at the operating console at left, while the patient, surgical support team, and robotic surgical tools are at right. (Images used with permission courtesy Intuitive Surgical, Inc.)

devices are now in use across the U.S. and internationally, with their use growing in procedures including prostate surgery, heart surgery, and various gynecological, thoracic, and urological procedures. Other current-day systems include surgical robots for prosthetic implants and brain surgery.

These robotic techniques are also accomplished using all the tools of laparoscopic surgery described above, in addition to a team of surgical support staff. Because the surgeon is "connected" to the robotic surgery system only by electrical connections, it's possible for a surgeon to operate from another room, or even a remote location.

These technologies can be used in training surgeons in new operating techniques on **endoscopic surgery simulators**, allowing opportunities for extensive practice and reducing the reliance on animal models. **Virtual reality assisted surgery planning** allows physicians to make dry runs of a proposed surgery on a computer model. Surgeons use realistic models to try out an operation in advance while seeking to optimize goals such as the complete removal of a tumor without damaging sensitive, neighboring **organs.** The virtual reality display can create an image of the body with superimposed maps of the extent of the diseased regions gleaned from MRI, CT, or other imaging technologies discussed in later chapters. These maps are then projected onto the actual laparoscopic images to guide the surgeon during the real operation. One example is the need to operate on the prostate gland while avoiding damage to the male reproductive organs, bladder, and urethra.

The case of robotic surgery devices raises fascinating issues about the proper way to adopt new technologies. With a robotic surgery unit costing over one million dollars in 2008, hospitals must make a serious financial commitment to even experiment with these methods. However, this innovation can mean that procedures previously performed by, e.g., open heart surgery can be done in a minimally invasive fashion, with all the advantages previously outlined. However, these technologies have been adopted widely in advance of large-scale clinical trials to compare their effectiveness compared to open and standard laparoscopic surgery. This means that it is unknown whether these advantages are a reality in practice. So far, small-scale studies seem to bear out their effectiveness for procedures such as prostate removals, with lower blood loss, reduced complication rates, and shorter hospital stays being reported.

2.4.2 Telemedicine and military applications

In **telemedicine** (literally, medicine-at-a-distance), physicians monitor the health of patients and provide healthcare through a combination of remote video links and robotic tools. In one example that has been tried in practice, dermatology patients can consult with a physician in a remote location with images of any suspicious skin lesions being transmitted by video. In **telepresence surgery**, a surgeon can both monitor and affect the progress of endoscopic surgery taking place in a remote location. The surgeon watches the surgery on a television screen while manipulating robotic controls, just as if it were being performed in the same room. The motions of the robotic surgical tools are communicated by communications links to the remote operating room, where they would be received by a second apparatus that would translate them into motions of the actual surgical tools. Using telemedicine, surgeons can train distant physicians and advise them during surgery. This technology is already in use for allowing physicians to consult with patients in remote locations far from major medical centers, or to allow specialists from large medical centers to advise local physicians, as well as a handful of actual remote surgeries. For obvious reasons, the military has been very interested in developing these capabilities, with an eye to reducing the response time in battlefield medical care. This also has led to speculation that astronauts on space flights who encounter a medical emergency might be operated on by Earth-based surgeons.

The military is particularly interested in telemedicine and telepresence surgery because time is of the essence in treating traumatic battlefield injuries, with most combat fatalities resulting within a half hour of the injury. However, the battlefield is dangerous for healthcare workers and a difficult environment in which to provide healthcare. Treatments that can staunch uncontrolled bleeding, correct respiratory problems, prevent shock and stabilize the soldier for transport to a base are the goal. Lessons from these efforts can then feed back into civilian trauma care for accidents and disasters. At the moment, the most important tools in reducing battlefield fatalities are not advanced technology but basic trauma care combined with an efficient organization for rapidly conveying soldiers to bases and hospitals farther from the front.

Even so, the practice of medicine in the military is being revolutionized by the advent of these new technologies. On the scene of conflict, laptop personal computers can access special satellite communications links with remote military hospitals. This allows physicians to consult with one another, or with patients, including allowing specialists to consult on cases in forward surgical units located one step removed from combat. Images taken as the soldier/patients are in transit can be sent ahead to allow advanced planning. The communications system allows the coordination of a multi-stage military medical team involving small forward surgical teams.

In 2005, the U.S. Defense Advanced Research Projects Agency (DARPA) and SRI International began developing futuristic, fortified mobile unmanned operating rooms called **Trauma Pods**, a name drawn from a Robert Heinlein science fiction novel (Figure 2.21). Trauma Pods are meant to accompany squadrons at the front, providing rapid medical care and telecommunications links that allow distant physicians to interact with the unit. In one scenario envisioned by DARPA, a soldier with severe shrapnel wounds would be quickly transported to the Trauma Pod. Each unit is equipped with mobile CT scanners and other imaging and diagnostic devices to determine the extent of injury. The results are sent to remote physicians while the soldier receives anesthesia, antibiotics, and other treatments. The remote surgeon then operates using a Trauma Pod surgical robot to remove the shrapnel, stabilize the bleeding, and suture the wound.

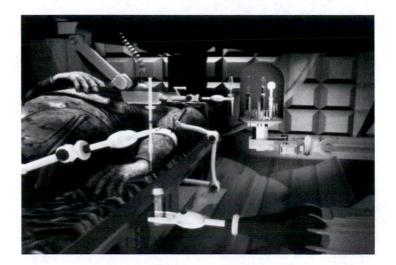

Figure 2.21 (*See color figure following page 78.*) Conceptual image of the Trauma Pod, showing an injured soldier lying prone on an operating table while robotic surgery is performed. (Image used with permission courtesy SRI International.)

If all goes well, the soldier is now stable enough to be transported safely to a distant base for further care. Of course, a unit developed for battlefield care is also useful for disaster relief in similarly demanding conditions. For example, recovery from a tsunami or devastating hurricane is difficult in part because the local healthcare infrastructure is damaged or absent, but Trauma Pods could be rapidly imported and linked to distant physicians.

One of many complications in developing the trauma pod is the disconnect between present surgical robots, which are meant to be used in a hospital operating room rather than a Humvee in a hostile battlefield located in hot, humid, or sandy environments, with only gasoline-powered generators to provide electricity. Also, hospital surgical robots are designed for minimally invasive surgery—not repairing traumatic injuries. Another is the time delay between sending signals between the physician and the trauma pod, a quantity called the **latency**. If this time is too long, surgeons cannot effectively control the robotic surgical tools. However, this time is fixed by the basic physics of the time required for light and radiowaves to travel between the trauma pod and the remote hospital. If satellites are used to bounce signals from the doctor to the Trauma Pod, these delays can be as long as a half-second or more—too long for effective remote control. Scientists are developing ways to use unmanned aerial vehicles (UAVs) to convey these signals from lower altitudes, reducing the signal's travel time to acceptable values.

2.4.3 Innovations on the horizon

More speculative uses of endoscope are being explored by the medical profession, including a new method for abdominal surgery that avoids external incisions altogether. Called **Natural Orifice Translumenal Endoscopic Surgery,** or **NOTES,** these procedures instead involve surgery performed by endoscopes inserted through the mouth or anus and incisions made through the stomach or colon wall. The surgical procedure then is performed with the endoscope being threaded internally to the site of surgery for, e.g., gallbladder removals. Why might this be advantageous? Cutting the skin and the walls of the abdomen in open or laparoscopic surgery excites a vigorous emergency response, including triggering nerves, the immune system, and chemical messengers that promote the body's defenses—but the same is less true for internal incisions. Thus, NOTES holds out the prospect of surgery with minimal pain, no need for general anesthesia, no external scarring, and reduced recovery time.

Some physicians are concerned that this method would not represent an advance over standard laparoscopic methods, worrying the potential gains are not significant enough to warrant the risk of serious infection, the cost of new technologies, and yet another learning curve as surgeons train in new methods. At the time of writing, this initiative is being investigated by the American Society for Gastrointestinal Endoscopy and the Society for American Gastrointestinal Endoscopic Surgeons, but only animal studies and a handful of successful human surgeries have been performed to evaluate its actual effectiveness.

Also under development are new endoscopes equipped with the ability to propel themselves, thus avoiding the risk of injury when physicians must blindly push the endoscope deep into body cavities. Instead, these devices are meant to crawl along the colon like an inchworm, gently negotiating their way deep inside.

Even more speculative are efforts to create tiny robots that would be introduced into the body laparoscopically, orally or via injections, with the goal of performing surgery at microscopic scales. These devices could be programmed to release drugs, destroy cells, or repair tissues under the instructions of physicians watching from outside the body. While these ideas may seem fanciful now, remember that the same could have been said of robotic surgery devices or video capsule endoscopy only a decade ago. However, the use of lasers in surgery is now a medical reality, one that is particularly well suited to endoscopic surgical techniques. In the next chapter, we further explore the science of light to see how a laser beam can be turned into a scalpel for surgery.

RESOURCES

Multimedia resources

Two Internet sites with useful information about endoscopic procedures and laparoscopy are http://www.laparoscopy.com and *The Atlas of Gastrointestinal Endoscopy* at http://www.endoatlas.com/atlas_1.html.

Carol E.H. Scott-Conner, "Laparoscopic general surgery," *Med. Clin. N. Am.* 86 (2002) 1401–1422.

Mitchell S. Cappell and David Friedel, "The role of sigmoidoscopy and colonoscopy in the diagnosis and management of lower gastrointestinal disorders: endoscopic findings, therapies and complications," *Med. Clin. N. Am.* 86 (2002) 1253–1288.

Article on the uses of endoscopes in surgery

Nathaniel J. Soper, L. Michael Brunt, and Kurt Kerbl, "Laparoscopic general surgery," *New Engl. J. Med.*, Vol. 330 (1994), pp. 409–419.

Medical texts containing more advanced discussions of endoscopes and surgery

Peter B. Cotton and Christopher B. Williams, *Practical Gastrointestinal Endoscopy*. Blackwell, Oxford, U.K., 1990.

John N. Graber, Leonard S. Schultz, Joseph J. Pietrafitta, and David F. Hickock, *Laparoscopic Abdominal Surgery*. McGraw-Hill, New York, 1993.

John B. McGinty, Richard B. Caspari, Robert W. Jackson, and Gary G. Poehling, eds., *Operative Arthroscopy*. Raven Press, New York, 1996.

QUESTIONS

Q2.1.   Manufacturers go to great effort and expense to design fiber optic bundles for imaging that have small optical fibers, and the greatest possible number of fibers packed into the imaging bundle. Explain the advantages of having small optical fiber diameters and closely packed optical fibers in an imaging bundle.

Q2.2.   Explain briefly the advantages of coherent (ordered) fiber optic bundles over incoherent (unordered) bundles. Name one application that requires coherent bundles, and one application for which incoherent bundles would suffice.

PROBLEMS

Reflection and refraction

P2.1.   (a) A person shines a flashlight onto a lake. A ray of light from the flashlight travels from air into water with an incident angle of 20°. What is the refracted angle? What is the angle of the reflected ray? Make a sketch that shows the incident, reflected, and refracted rays and their angles as accurately as you can. (b) A scuba diver in the lake shines a flashlight upward. A ray from that flashlight travels from water into air with an incident angle of 5.0°. Again, compute the refracted and reflected angles, and sketch the three rays.

P2.2.   At an interface between an unknown transparent material and water, a ray of light is incident from the water side at an angle of 30.0° to the normal. The refracted ray makes an angle of 25.0° with the normal. What is the index of refraction for the unknown material?

Total internal reflection and fiber optics

P2.3.   (a) What is the critical angle for total internal reflection for the interface described in Problem 2.2? (b) Make a drawing showing the geometry for rays that would undergo total internal reflection at this interface. Label the two media and any angles carefully.

P2.4.   Two medical students, Lynn and Bob, decide to build their own endoscopes. Along the way, they ask themselves some basic questions about the operation of the device. (a) What is the value of critical angle for total internal reflection within the glass fibers if the material that surrounds the fibers has an index of refraction $n_o = 1.5$ and the optical fibers themselves have $n_i = 1.65$ (Figure P2.6)? (b) Bob twists Lynn's scope into a corkscrew shape (Figure P2.4a). She retaliates by tying his scope into a knot (Figure P2.4b). He then disassembles one of the ends of her scope and scrambles the order of the fibers (Figure P2.4c). She does the same for the fiber bundle that transmits his light source. Do any of these four manipulations interfere with the operation of the scopes? Explain why or why not.

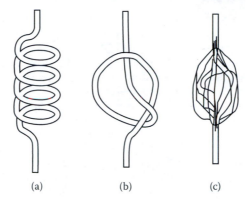

(a)   (b)   (c)

P2.5. Which of the following rays will be totally internally reflected (Figure P2.5)? Explain your reasoning. (See Table 2.1 for values of the index of refraction.)

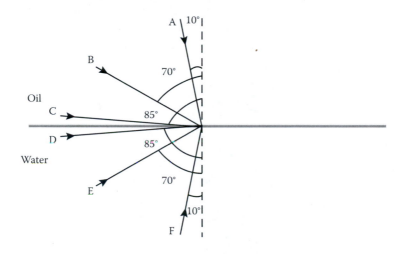

P2.6. What is wrong with this design for an optical fiber cable? A cross-sectional view of the proposed fiber optic cable is shown in Figure P2.6. The optical fibers have an index of refraction equal to 1.55 and the medium surrounding the fibers has an index of refraction equal to 1.60.

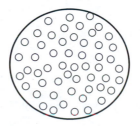

P2.7. For which of the interfaces described below could total internal reflection happen? (See Table 2.1 for values of the index of refraction.)

a. Alcohol/water, light coming from the alcohol side
b. Water/glass, light coming from the water side
c. Air/water, light coming from the air side

P2.8. As mentioned earlier, some biological systems can act like an optical fiber. Below is a drawing which illustrates how this might occur. Imagine you have a long, thin cell surrounded by fluid with index of refraction 1.38. The average index of refraction inside the cell is 1.48. These values are actually quite typical of the actual ones found in some settings in nature.

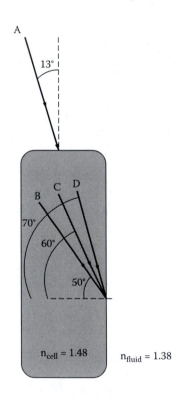

a. Compute the critical angle, θ_{crit}, for total internal reflection for this system. Show all of your computations.
b. What will the angle of refraction be for ray A (shown below) that has an angle of incidence of 13 degrees? Show all of your calculations. Indicate the new ray's direction and its angle of refraction on your drawing. You can draw in the angles approximately.
c. Will rays B, C, or D undergo total internal reflection? Their angles of incidence are shown to be 50, 60, and 70 degrees. (Explain your answer using your value for part (a). If you

cannot finish part (a), assume a value and explain how you would answer using that value.)

d.   Comment on how all this relates to the idea that the rod cells (appropriately named) in our eyes can function as fiber optics.

ADVANCED PROBLEMS

P2.9.   The following equation gives the fraction of light intensity incident on an interface (I_{total}) that is reflected (I_{Refl}) and transmitted as refracted light (I_{trans}) at normal incidence, corresponding to an incident angle of 90°. This equation can be used to compute, e.g., how much of the light is transmitted through a endoscope or how much of a laser's light intensity can be transmitted inside the body through a fiber optic guide.

$$\frac{I_{Re\,fl}}{I_{total}} = \frac{\left(n_1 - n_2\right)^2}{\left(n_1 + n_2\right)^2}$$

$$\frac{I_{Trans}}{I_{total}} = 100\% - \frac{I_{Re\,fl}}{I_{total}}$$

a.   Assuming that the fiber optic has an index of refraction of roughly 1.5, and that the light is entering from air, compute the percentage of the light intensity that is reflected from and transmitted through the front face of an optical fiber in air.

b.   The light encounters a second interface at the exit end of the fiber optic. What fraction of the light incident upon the fiber optic finally *gets out* of the fiber optic?

3 Lasers in medicine
Healing with light

3.1 INTRODUCTION

In Chapter 2 we saw how endoscopes guide light within the body, permitting examinations and surgery in otherwise inaccessible locations. By contrast, lasers use light itself as a tool for surgery and therapy. Laser light can be guided into the body using optical fibers, often in combination with an endoscope. Once inside, the laser light can be focused into tiny intense spots that can burn or blast away tissue cleanly, leaving a bloodless cut. Lasers have become an effective and versatile surgical tool for surgery, where they can be used in place of a scalpel in many applications.

Surgical lasers are used in a wide host of general surgical contexts to make incisions and remove tumors. For example, they are routinely used in such gynecological procedures as the treatment of cervical warts, endometriosis, and infertility. Some conditions can be treated by lasers even without cutting open the body. In dermatology, many popular cosmetic treatments involve using laser beams to treat superficial blemishes such as birthmarks, age spots, and spider veins (Figure 3.1a). Many tattoos can also be removed using laser treatments. We will study how their pure color allows lasers to safely penetrate the skin while destroying the birthmark's pigments or the tattoo's dyes.

Nowhere are the abilities of lasers used more dramatically than in ophthalmology. In eye surgery, laser light can be directed harmlessly into the eye for treating diseases of the retina or glaucoma. Lasers operating at light energies invisible to our eyes can be used to destroy cloudy deposits in the eye following cataract surgery (Figure 3.1b), or to help correct nearsightedness.

An innovative cancer treatment called photodynamic therapy uses laser light to target and kill tumors. In this method, special chemicals called **photosensitizers** are introduced into the body, where they collect in tumor cells. When photosensitizers are irradiated with laser light, they produce toxic chemical species. The ability of this technique to kill tumors specifically, its low toxicity to other parts of the body, and its compatibility with other therapies have made photodynamic therapy a promising new addition to the cancer-fighting arsenal.

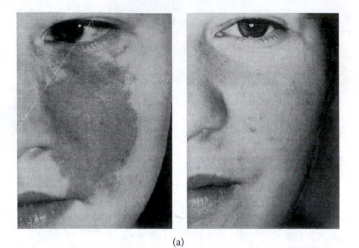

(a)

Figure 3.1 (a) Port wine stain birthmark before (left) and after (right) laser treatment. (Reproduced with permission courtesy of A.N. Chester, S. Martellucci, and A.M. Scheggi, eds., *Laser Systems for Photobiology and Photomedicine*, Plenum Press, New York, 1991.) (b) Cataracts are cloudy regions that form in the lens of the eye, potentially causing blurred vision and eventual blindness. In cataract surgery, the eye's lens is removed and a plastic replacement lens inserted in order to restore clear vision. Sometimes, however, a new opacified region forms after the corrective surgery. The top figure shows a close-up view of the iris and cloudy pupil of an eye in which this has occurred, while the bottom figure shows how an operation called laser posterior capsulotomy can clear away the new obscuring tissue. (Reproduced with permission courtesy of Ian J. Constable and Arthur Siew Ming Lim, *Laser: Its Clinical Uses in Eye Diseases*, Churchill Livingstone, Edinburgh, 1990.)

In this chapter, we first will extend our study of the science of light to understand how lasers work and how light interacts with the human body, then examine in detail how this basic science leads to important medical applications with unique capabilities.

3.2 WHAT IS A LASER?

The word *laser*, used to denote a wide variety of specialized sources of light, is actually an acronym for *light amplification* by *stimulated emission* of *radiation*—a definition we will explore shortly. You may consider lasers exotic and dangerous, but in fact, you routinely encounter them in everyday life. For example, supermarket price scanners utilize tiny red lasers for reading the bar code information from packaging. Compact

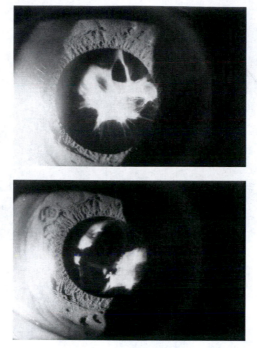

(b)

Figure 3.1 (continued).

discs and DVDs have their audio and video information encoded in a pattern of tiny reflective and nonreflective patches etched on their surfaces. A laser beam is used to detect this pattern, which is converted back into sound and pictures by electronic circuitry. The laser printers used with computers utilize lasers to "write" an image of the page to be printed on a light-sensitive surface to which ink then adheres, and then is transferred to paper. Pen-sized lasers are used as pointers for giving presentations, and laser light shows are a popular entertainment at music concerts and science museums.

Figure 3.2(a) shows an image of the thin pencil of light emitted from a red helium neon laser, called a **laser beam**. Figure 3.2(b) shows an argon laser used in ophthalmological surgery. What you see in this figure is a box containing the optics, electronics circuitry, and power supply needed to generate the laser's light. The laser light itself is inconspicuous in this picture since it is conveyed to an eye examination apparatus in a fiber optic cable. The physician controls the laser light using a foot pedal. Other controls on the laser's front panel allow for changing the laser's power and the time the patient is exposed to the laser beam.

Before we explore lasers further, we first need to understand more about the basic science of light and its interaction with matter.

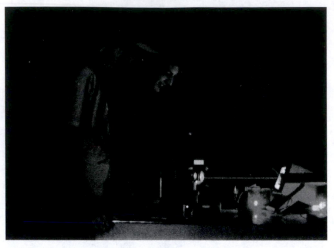

(a)

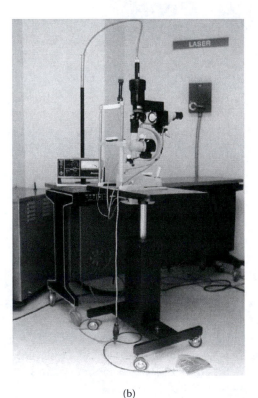

(b)

Figure 3.2 (See color figure following page 78.) (a) A green argon ion laser used in an undergraduate science laboratory. The bright line emerging from the laser unit is the light of its laser beam. (b) Argon ion laser used in ophthalmological surgery. The actual laser and power supply sit on the floor, the laser's light is carried by optical fibers to an apparatus similar to those used for eye examinations. The surgery is performed while the surgeon looks through this apparatus at the inside of the eye.

3.3 MORE ON THE SCIENCE OF LIGHT: BEYOND THE RAINBOW

In the situations discussed in Chapter 2, light travels in straight lines unless reflected or refracted, much as though it consisted of streams of particles shot from a source. On the other hand, when light travels through tiny holes or slits, its behavior can no longer be explained by the rules of geometrical optics. Everyday life holds few instances in which these latter phenomena can be observed, but they become important for understanding laser beams. In fact, light has a dual nature: the behavior of light as it propagates through space is more reminiscent of waves than particles, but the particle picture must be invoked whenever light interacts with matter.

The particle-like aspect of its behavior is described well by treating light as rays that obey the laws of geometrical optics described in Chapter 2. The wave nature is described by saying that light consists of periodical changes in electrical and magnetic forces, sweeping through space and time (Figure 3.3). These forces can act upon molecules to induce chemical changes. If the atoms in a molecule sit at one point in space as light shines upon them, they experience oscillating forces as the wave sweeps by them; this can be thought of as analogous to a floating bottle bobbing up and down in the ocean as a wave of water sweeps past it.

The distance between repeats of the disturbance are called the **wavelength**, denoted by the Greek letter *lambda*, λ. This wavelength is generally a very tiny distance for visible light, only a few thousand times larger than individual atoms, in fact. The energy carried by light is transported

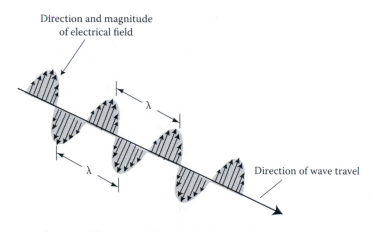

Figure 3.3 Schematic illustration of the electrical forces acting on a molecule due to a wave of light. The electrical forces vary in direction and magnitude in a fashion similar to the forces experienced by a buoy when an ocean wave sweeps past it. The distance between successive wave crests or troughs is called the wavelength of the light.

in packets by individual particles of light called **photons**. The energy of a photon depends upon the wavelength of the light it is associated with. The longer the wavelength of light, the smaller the energy carried by its photons. In fact, the energy varies in inverse proportion to wavelength; that is, doubling the wavelength corresponds to reducing the energy per photon, E, by one-half:

$$E = h\,c/\lambda \tag{3.1}$$

We will measure energy in the metric units of **joules** (**J**). (We will get a feeling for the size of this unit shortly.) Here, h is a constant called **Planck's constant**, equal to 6.63×10^{-34} J s (this unit stands for Joules × seconds), and c is the speed of light in empty space, equal to 3.00×10^8 m/s. This relationship is not obvious from our discussion; rather, it has been established experimentally from measurements of the energy and wavelength of actual light waves. We can also describe the **frequency** with which the fluctuations associated with the light wave move past a fixed point by counting the number of complete cycles of oscillation that pass each second. Frequency is typically measured in **hertz** (abbreviated **Hz**) or cycles/second. If we multiply the number of cycles passing a point each second by the wavelength of each cycle, we have computed the speed of light: how far the light wave travels in a fixed amount of time. The product of frequency and wavelength is therefore equal to the speed of light:

$$f\,\lambda = c \tag{3.2}$$

The frequency of visible light waves is typically about 10^{15} Hz, so the fluctuations happen so quickly that there is no way to observe them directly. We will regularly refer to only wavelength and energy in this chapter, but frequency will become an important issue for waves of sound in Chapter 4.

The most dramatic consequence of the wave nature of light is that a prism splits white light into a rainbow containing every color of the spectrum (Figure 3.4). (This is because the speed of light in the prism is different for different wavelengths of light, and each wavelength is refracted by a slightly different angle as a result. Crystal ornaments use this effect to create rainbows.) What our eyes perceive as white light is actually a mixture of different colors and wavelengths of light. Our eyes associate each range of wavelength between roughly 400 to 700 **nanometers** (or **nm**) with a characteristic color. (A nanometer is equal to one-billionth of a meter: 1 nm = 10^{-9} m.) For example, light with wavelength 630 nm is perceived as red, while 420 nm light appears blue. Table 3.1 gives the association of wavelength with colors of the rainbow. Our eyes are capable of sensing only a limited range of all possible wavelengths, but the spectrum extends to other forms of light that are invisible to humans. The range of wavelengths

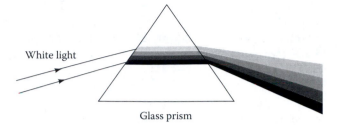

Glass prism

Figure 3.4 White light is spread into a rainbow of colors by a glass prism. This happens because the index of refraction is different for each wavelength of light, and hence the angle of refraction also depends upon wavelength and color. This effect spreads out the colors into the familiar spectrum of a rainbow, arranged from shortest to longest wavelength.

Table 3.1 The electromagnetic spectrum

Type of electromagnetic radiation	Color	Wavelength
Radio		0.1 cm–kilometers
Infrared		700 nm—0.1 cm
	Red	630–700 nm
	Orange	590–630 nm
Visible light	Yellow	530–590 nm
	Green	480–530 nm
	Blue	440–480 nm
	Violet	400–440 nm
Ultraviolet		10–400 nm
X-rays and gamma rays		10 nm and less

extends to **ultraviolet** wavelengths smaller than the shortest visible blue wavelength, while there are also **infrared** wavelengths much longer than the red. (Interestingly, insects can see ultraviolet light, a "color" we cannot perceive, and snakes can detect infrared radiation.)

The total range of available wavelengths is called the **electromagnetic spectrum,** and light is more generally called **electromagnetic radiation** to take into account the regime we cannot see. Microwaves, radio waves, gamma rays, and x-rays are all forms of electromagnetic radiation, differing from visible light only in wavelength, frequency, and energy. Table 3.1 summarizes the various types of electromagnetic radiation present in nature. You have already experienced these other forms of radiation. Heat lamps produce infrared radiation, and tanning lamps emit ultraviolet radiation. Every hour, naturally occurring radioactive materials within the body of a typical adult emit about 20 million gamma rays. We see from Table 3.1 that x-rays have much shorter wavelengths than visible light or microwaves. This results in the various forms of electromagnetic radiation having drastically different energies also, causing them to interact differently with the tissues of the body.

Sample calculation: We will now compute and compare the energies of an x-ray photon, a microwave photon, and a photon of visible light. The x-ray photon has an energy and wavelength in the range of those used to take x-ray images (Chapter 5). We can use Equation 3.1 to find out each of these values. To make our computations meaningful, we will compare our results with the energy of a single chemical bond between two carbon atoms, equal to approximately 6×10^{-19} J.

Using typical values for the wavelengths from Table 3.1, we have $\lambda_{x\text{-ray}} = 0.02\,\text{nm} = 2 \times 10^{-11}\,\text{m}$, $\lambda_{microwave} = 0.1\,\text{cm} = 0.1 \times 10^{-2}\,\text{m} = 0.001\,\text{m}$ and $\lambda_{visible} = 500\,\text{nm} = 500 \times 10^{-9}\,\text{m}$. This gives for the energies:

$$E_{x\text{-ray}} = (6.63 \times 10^{-34}\,\text{J-s}) \times (3.00 \times 10^{8}\,\text{m/s})/\lambda_{x\text{-ray}} \qquad (3.3)$$

$$= (6.63 \times 10^{-34}\,\text{J-s}) \times (3.00 \times 10^{8}\,\text{m/s})/2 \times 10^{-11}\,\text{m}$$

$$= 1 \times 10^{-14}\,\text{J} \gg 6 \times 10^{-19}\,\text{J}$$

$$E_{microwave} = (6.63 \times 10^{-34}\,\text{J-s}) \times (3.00 \times 10^{8}\,\text{m/s})/\lambda_{microwave} \qquad (3.4)$$

$$= (6.63 \times 10^{-34}\,\text{J-s}) \times (3.00 \times 10^{8}\,\text{m/s})/0.1 \times 10^{-2}\,\text{m}$$

$$= 2 \times 10^{-22}\,\text{J} \ll 6 \times 10^{-19}\,\text{J}$$

$$E_{visible} = (6.63 \times 10^{-34}\,\text{J-s}) \times (3.00 \times 10^{8}\,\text{m/s})/\lambda_{visible} \qquad (3.5)$$

$$= (6.63 \times 10^{-34}\,\text{J-s}) \times (3.00 \times 10^{8}\,\text{m/s})/500 \times 10^{-9}\,\text{m}$$

$$= 4 \times 10^{-19}\,\text{J} < 6 \times 10^{-19}\,\text{J}$$

We see from this example that an x-ray photon used in medical imaging can carry over 10,000 times the energy required to break one of the chemical bonds commonly found in body molecules. (Another convenient unit of energy, the **electron-Volt (eV)** is equal to 1.60×10^{-19} Joules, so a chemical bond energy of 6.4×10^{-19} J can be expressed as approximately 4 eV.) By contrast, these chemical bonds are thousands of times as energetic as a microwave photon, and somewhat higher in energy than a photon of visible light. Because microwave and visible light photons have *less* energy than most chemical bonds, their absorption by the body usually does not generate chemical damage directly. This has the highly important practical consequence that microwaves can only damage human tissues by heating them, while gamma rays, x-rays, and even ultraviolet photons have enough energy to actually break chemical bonds. Most chemical damage of this sort is quickly repaired by the body, but changes to molecules of DNA, which carry our body's genetic information, potentially can lead to cancer. Visible and infrared light usually generate damage by heating only, but in special cases they also can be used to cause chemical changes. We will return to this topic in Chapter 7, when we consider the interaction of x-ray photons with matter in radiation therapy.

3.4 HOW LASERS WORK

(Note: This section can be read in sequence or returned to at a later point in the chapter.)

Lasers' striking advantages in medicine rely on two special characteristics: they emit light in a slender high-intensity beam and their light is confined to one color of incredible purity. In this section we will see how these surprising features of lasers come about through the detailed science behind their operation.

To better understand how lasers work, we first will consider the structure of matter at the atomic level. All matter, including all body tissues and fluids, is composed of atoms. Atoms consist of central nuclei surrounded by electrons, tiny particles with a negative electrical charge. The nuclei themselves consist of protons, which have a positive electrical charge, and neutrons, which are electrically neutral. Each atom is electrically neutral overall: its negative and positive electrical charges sum to zero because it has the same number of electrons as protons. (**Ions** are formed when atoms are separated, resulting in electrons and positively or negatively charged nuclei.) Its number of neutrons can vary. By specifying the number of protons in an atom, we also specify which chemical element it corresponds to. Hydrogen has a nucleus with 1 proton, carbon has 6 protons and 6 neutrons, sulfur has 16 protons and 16 neutrons, etc. All of chemistry is determined by the complex repulsions and attractions due to the electrical forces between nuclei and their attendant electrons.

Atoms are sometimes drawn with the electrons shown orbiting around the nucleus, just as the Moon orbits around the Earth. This picture is an oversimplification, however. A better image would be to think of the positions of the electrons as being determined by a diffuse cloud called an **orbital** around the nucleus. Electrons can inhabit many different types of orbitals, and each type has a characteristic energy and shape. We are concerned with the organization of electrons in an atom or molecule because each electron

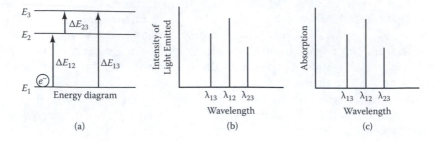

Figure 3.5 (a) Simplified orbital energy diagram for an electron bound to an atom. Transitions the electron can make between different orbital energy levels are illustrated. (b) Sample emission spectrum for the atom whose energy diagram is shown in (a). The atom can emit only light with a wavelength and energy per photon corresponding to possible jumps between energy levels. (c) Similarly, the atom can only absorb light with a wavelength and energy per photon corresponding to these same jumps in energy levels.

has energies characteristic of the orbital it inhabits. These orbitals and their energies depend upon the chemical elements with which the electrons are associated and their organization into molecules.

We can display the values of these electron orbital energies using an **energy level diagram** (Figure 3.5a). The symbol E represents the different values of energy, or **energy levels**, a particular electron can have when bound to an atom in various orbitals. Energy *differences* between orbitals are labeled ΔE (here Δ is the capital Greek letter *delta*.) Electrons can inhabit each of the energy levels drawn here for this atom, but no other values of energy. In particular, energies *in between* those shown are not allowed. This energy level diagram is drawn so that the lowest level, called the **ground state**, represents the lowest energy an electron associated with the atom can have. Higher levels will be filled if electrons are added, or if an electron in the ground state gains additional energy. We will only consider the latter case for now.

The fact that electrons can have only restricted energies means that an electron can only gain or lose energy by steps. These steps, called **quanta** (singular, **quantum**), are determined by the difference, ΔE, between electron energies. The fact that the electron's energy can only change in steps has several consequences. First, the electrons can only exchange energy with their environment by the values of ΔE in Figure 3.5(a). Electrons can absorb energy and be promoted to a higher level, a process called **excitation**. This can happen by the absorption of a photon of light or through collisions with other atoms. The photon must have exactly the right energy, ΔE, and corresponding wavelength to promote the electron to a new energy level, no more and no less. Once excited, the electron eventually will fall back down spontaneously to a lower energy orbital, usually by emitting a second photon also having energy ΔE.

The above system can either absorb or emit photons with energies exactly equal to one of these energy differences. Thus, the electrons belonging to an atom will absorb and emit light at only particular wavelengths. These wavelengths are a fingerprint of the atom's chemical element. If a gas of an element is excited so that it gives off photons by this process, a characteristic color will result (Figure 3.5b). For example, the sodium vapor lamps used in street lights are yellowish because the ΔE values of emitted photons lie in the yellow. For similar reasons, if one shines light of all wavelengths through a gas of sodium atoms, only yellow light of the same wavelengths will be absorbed (Figure 3.5c). Neon lamps emit very pure red light, and neon vapors absorb the same wavelength in the red.

Electrons can be excited to higher energy states by absorbing energy through a number of processes, such as collisions in a gas, the flow of an electrical current, or the absorption of photons. Once an electron reaches an excited state, it eventually gives off a photon and decays to its ground state. This process is called **spontaneous emission** (Figure 3.6a). Ordinary incandescent lightbulbs give off light by spontaneous emission. They emit

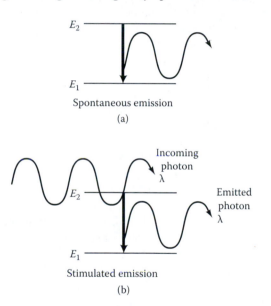

Figure 3.6 An atom can emit photons of light by two different processes. (a) In spontaneous emission, an electron in a higher energy level decays to a lower energy level, emitting a photon with a wavelength determined by the energy (E_2-E_1) equal to the difference between the two levels. (This is the same process already discussed in Figure 3.15.) (b) In stimulated emission, an already-existing photon with energy equal to (E_2-E_1) causes the electron to decay. The emitted photon has the same energy (E_2-E_1) as in the case of spontaneous emission. However, in addition, the emitted photon has exactly the same direction as the first, and it moves in phase with the stimulating photon.

light of many wavelengths because no particular energy spacing is selected for, so electrons are excited into many different energy levels and decay into a variety of lower energy states. As they do so, they emit photons with many different energies and wavelengths. The photons are emitted from the lightbulb uniformly in all directions since no physical limitation confines their directions.

However, spontaneous emission is only one way by which an excited electron can emit light. Another possibility exists: the excited electron can interact with a pre-existing photon that just happens to be passing by. If the photon's energy coincides with the spacing between energy levels in the atom, it induces the electron to decay. Upon decaying, the electron emits a new photon (Figure 3.6b). This process is called **stimulated emission** because the first photon initiated the emission of the second. Stimulated emission occurs only when the first photon has the same energy as the difference between the ground and excited states. Hence, the second photon has the same energy, wavelength, and color as the first photon.

In addition, a more complete physical picture of this process shows that the emitted photon also travels in the same direction and exactly in step with the first photon. Physicists describe this by saying the second photon is **in phase** with the first. This synchronization in energy and time gives rise to **temporal coherence**; among other things, it means that laser light is emitted essentially at a single, extremely pure wavelength.

Both stimulated and spontaneous emission take place all the time in ordinary light sources, but spontaneous emission is more common. Why? An electron in an atom stays excited for very short times, ordinarily. It generally emits a photon before encountering a photon with the right energy for stimulated emission. The atoms in a system are much more likely to absorb a photon (or just ignore it altogether) than to undergo stimulated emission.

For stimulated emission to happen frequently, the atoms and their electrons must be carefully prepared. Many more electrons must be held in an excited state than in the ground state. This ensures that there are few electrons able to absorb the incoming photons, and many ready to be stimulated into releasing a new photon. Only then is there a fighting chance for the less frequent process of stimulated emission to take place. This situation is called a **population inversion**, and it requires a means for keeping electrons stuck in an excited state for a long time.

We call the process by which electrons are pushed into the relatively long-lasting excited state **pumping**. To understand this phenomenon further, let us study the specific case of the red helium neon laser. This laser consists of a glass tube filled with a mixture of gases of the chemical elements helium and neon. The gas is called the **active medium**. The helium and neon gases' atoms are heated by an electrical current. Collisions in the hot gases excite the helium atoms' electrons into many different energy states, most of them short-lived. One state is very long-lived and electrons get stuck there for quite a while. We say this state is **metastable** and cannot easily decay by spontaneous emission of light (Figure 3.7).

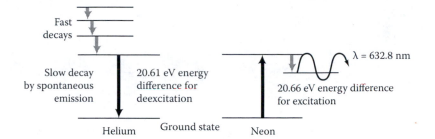

Figure 3.7 Energy diagrams for the two atomic species used in a helium-neon laser. The energy spacing between two energy levels in a helium atom (20.61 eV) is coincidentally very close to that found for a spacing in neon (20.66 eV). As a result, energy can be easily transferred between the two atoms, permitting a population inversion to be established in which many electrons accumulate in the highest energy level shown for neon, many more than are in the intermediate energy level. As a result, more light is emitted at wavelength of 632.8 nm corresponding to this spacing than is absorbed.

These helium atoms' electrons can escape to the ground state by transferring their energy to a neon atom's electrons through a collision. This excites the neon electron from its ground state. This is because, purely by chance, neon has an energy level almost equal to the helium energy level with slow decay. This coincidental agreement is taken advantage of in order to promote the neon atoms' electrons to an excited state.

Now, many electrons bound to neon atoms are pumped into a particular excited energy state, many more than are in the state to which it decays. This represents the desired condition for a population inversion. Eventually an electron belonging to a neon atom spontaneously decays and emits a photon. This event sets off a chain reaction whereby the spontaneously emitted photon can go on to cause the stimulated emission of a second photon. Then both photons can go on to create even more photons through stimulated emission. Soon many identical photons are coursing through the gas, all with the same energy and wavelength.

In order to make a laser out of this situation, the tube containing the gas of helium and neon atoms is placed into a configuration called an **optical resonating cavity**. This can be thought of as two parallel mirrors placed a fixed distance apart (Figure 3.8). Now, each time a photon of light passes through the active medium, it induces more stimulated emissions. These photons travel in the same direction as the first. However, if a photon travels at an angle to the mirrors, it will reflect outside the cavity and fail to return. Only photons traveling straight down the optical resonating cavity can make multiple passes. This restriction maintains the directionality of the lasers and is responsible for their spatial coherence and narrow beam.

Each successful photon enlists many other photons, each with the same energy and phase as the first, each traveling in the same direction. This

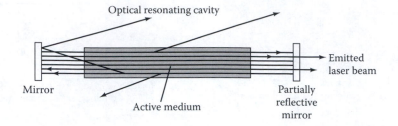

Figure 3.8 Schematic illustration of the inside of a typical laser. The active medium, which contains the atoms or molecules that emit the laser light, is confined between two mirrors that form the optical resonating cavity. While light is emitted by the active medium in all directions, only those photons that are emitted perpendicular to the mirrors will be reflected back into the medium. These photons can cause spontaneous emissions of still more photons, which will also travel in the same direction. After many reflections, a single photon will have enlisted many more photons, all with the same direction, a process called amplification, or gain. Photons emitted in all other directions will escape from the medium and not cause further spontaneous emissions. One of the mirrors is only partially reflective, so it allows a small fraction of the light to escape, producing the laser beam.

mechanism for multiplying the number of photons is called **amplification** or **gain**. A typical value for the gain is 5% more photons for each trip. In 100 passes down the tube, the photons increase their numbers by 130 times and in 200 passes by 17,000 times.

If one of the mirrors is only partially silvered, transmitting only 1% or 2% of the light hitting it, some of this light escapes out the end. This small loss is not enough to stop the process. This escaping light is what you see emerging as the slender, highly parallel laser beam. The laser's light is a single wavelength due to stimulated emission. The light travels in a single direction because of the optically resonating cavity and the tendency of stimulated emission to create photons in phase with one another.

The power lost as the laser's beam escapes from the optical resonating cavity must be replaced by electrical power. In the helium neon laser, an electrical current is used to constantly heat the atoms in the gases, creating a constant supply of newly excited electrons and a steady intensity of laser light. In other systems, a white light, called a **flashlamp**, or even another laser is used to pump the excited electrons. Electrical energy sources power the flashlamp and hence the laser.

The preceding description was given for a red helium neon laser. Other lasers work using similar processes that take place in other gases. For example, the carbon dioxide (infrared), argon ion (green), krypton (red), and helium cadmium (blue) lasers all utilize similar mechanisms taking place in the gases that give them their names. Because each atom or molecule has a different set of energy spacings, each laser also has a

Table 3.2 Some medical lasers and their properties

Laser	Wavelength (nm)	Power (watts)	Sample applications
Excimer	190–350 (UV)	<1–20 watts	Ophthalmological surgery (PRK and LASIK)
Dye	400–800	<1–5 watts	Removal of port wine stains and pigmented lesions
Nd:YAG	1064 (IR), with frequency doubling: 532 (green)/355 (UV)	<1 –> 100 watts	General surgery, ophthalmological surgery; tattoo removal, laser lithotripsy
Argon (CW)	514 (green) and 488 (blue-green)	<1–20 watts	Surgery for glaucoma
Copper vapor	578 (yellow) and 511 (green)	<=1 watt	Ophthalmological surgery
Gold vapor	630 (red)	<=1 watt	Photodynamic therapy, ophthalmological surgery
Helium neon (CW)	632.8 (red)	<1–25 milliwatts	Ophthalmological surgery
Krypton (CW)	676.4 (red)	<=5 watts	Ophthalmological surgery
Ruby (pulsed)	694 (red)		Tattoo removal
Diode lasers	750–1550 (red and near IR)	<=10 watts	Photocoagulation for general surgery, hair removal
Erbium:YAG (pulsed)	1540 (IR)		Hair removal, skin resurfacing
Holmium:YAG (pulsed)	2140 (IR)	≤60 watts	General surgery
Carbon dioxide (CW or pulsed)	10,600 (IR)	<100 watts	General surgery, skin resurfacing

characteristic wavelength and color. Table 3.2 lists various lasers used in medicine.

The active medium need not be a gas. Examples of lasers with solid active media are diode lasers, used in various medical applications, compact disc players, and supermarket scanner devices. Glasses such as neodymium-yttrium-aluminum-garnet (abbreviated Nd:YAG and pronounced "neodymium yag"), erbium:YAG, and holmium:YAG are used to make especially versatile, high-power lasers. The Nd:YAG laser can be operated at one of three wavelengths: the infrared (1064 nm), and—with a special optical element called a frequency-doubling crystal—green (532 nm), and ultraviolet (355 nm) wavelengths.

Dye lasers instead use a liquid active medium, a solution of large organic dye molecules in water, which allow them to emit light at a variety of wavelengths because of the dye's complicated orbital structures. The optics of the resonating cavity can be adjusted to select only one wavelength for operation at any time. The yellow light from dye lasers is extremely useful in dermatology, for example.

Now that we have a brief background for appreciating the special properties of lasers, we will return to an investigation of just how those properties are turned into medical applications.

3.5 HOW LIGHT INTERACTS WITH BODY TISSUES

In this chapter, we are principally interested in how light of various wavelengths interacts with the tissues of the body. This is because laser surgery and light therapy both involve the transfer of energy from light to human tissue through several mechanisms. Figure 3.9 shows five different phenomena that can happen when light interacts with any medium. Reflection from an interface and transmission of refracted light were discussed already in Chapter 2. The transmitted light can also be absorbed by a variety of processes. At each point along its path, the light's intensity is progressively diminished if this happens. Light that gets absorbed also can be re-emitted by a process known as fluorescence.

Light can also be scattered by the medium. In this case, light interacts with the medium and is re-emitted, but with a direction that can differ

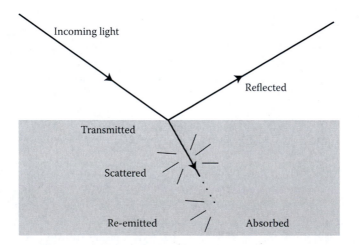

Figure 3.9 A ray of light incident on an interface between two media is partially reflected and partially transmitted or refracted, as was discussed in Chapter 2. In the earlier chapter we only considered transparent media. More generally, the medium can absorb light from the original beam, reducing its intensity, or scattering light.

from the original path. For example, on a foggy night you can see the beam of a car's headlights from the side because the light scatters from suspended water particles in the fog. On a clear, dry night you only see the beam when it is reflected from objects in its path because air does not cause appreciable scattering in the absence of water vapor. Because scattering can be thought of as a collision of photons of light with particles of matter, it constitutes another mechanism by which light can transfer energy to tissue.

The light employed in laser surgery does damage because it transfers energy by absorption or scattering to human tissues. Each photon carries a packet of energy that can be converted from light into other forms of energy, such as chemical bond energy. Although energy can be transformed between different types of energy (kinetic energy—energy of motion— chemical bond energy, light energy, etc.) in this way, energy has never been observed to be lost or created from nothing, a phenomenon referred to as the **conservation of energy**. More commonly, a different form of transfer occurs. Within any material, the atoms are in constant random motion, vibrating in place. The **temperature** of the material characterizes the average energy of this motion. The energy carried by light is most often converted into additional energy of motion of the molecules of the tissue being illuminated; this energy input thus raises the material's temperature. We define **heat** as a transfer of energy resulting in raising the temperature of a material. Thus, the transfer of energy from photons of light can also result in the heating of tissue. For example, heat lamps work by providing infrared radiation that is efficiently absorbed by our tissue as heat. On a clear day this effect is quite evident for the sun's light.

The amount of damage caused by light depends upon the **power** of the light source used. This is because power is a measure of the rate at which energy is transferred by the light—higher power light sources thus transmit energy more rapidly than do lower ones. Since energy must be supplied in order to heat tissue, make incisions, or break chemical bonds, the crucial practical issue in laser surgery is delivering enough energy in the right form to the tissue to be operated on. However, in fact, the lasers used in most applications have fairly low powers. A typical 100-watt incandescent lightbulb emits only a few watts of power in the form of light; the rest of the electrical power it consumes is converted into heat. This is about the same output as many powerful medical lasers! While power is an important feature, more important is the high intensity of laser light: that is, the very high concentration of light power into a small area. How effective a particular source of light is in exchanging energy also depends crucially upon the wavelength of the light. This is because the amount of energy a particular molecule receives is determined both by how much energy each photon carries (given by the wavelength) and by how many photons it encounters. In the following sections, we will see why lasers are especially effective at transferring energy to body molecules.

3.6 LASER BEAMS AND SPATIAL COHERENCE

The phrase **spatial coherence** means that the laser's light is emitted in a very well-defined beam, even more so than the light of a flashlight or a car's headlight. If you turned on a bare lightbulb in the middle of a room, the entire room would be illuminated (Figure 3.10) because the lightbulb's light is emitted in all directions uniformly. By contrast, if you did the same experiment with a laser, a single tiny spot on the wall would be lit up since all of the laser's light is concentrated into a narrow beam (Figure 3.11). If we represented the laser's light using rays, all of the rays would be very nearly parallel and confined to a well-defined pencil of light. That small illuminated spot is extremely bright, since all of the laser's light is confined to that one region. Thus, even if the laser emits much less light than the lightbulb overall, that light nevertheless is confined to one small spot.

Why is this important? Obviously, a well-defined beam of light is easier to aim at the tissue to be operated on. More importantly, the energy carried by lasers can be delivered to only a tiny, bright spot. This funneling of light energy into a small region is required in order to actually destroy or cut tissue. To describe this concentration of light, we need to introduce some new terms that render more concrete our notions of "emitted light," "brightness," etc. The power, P, of light emitted by a light source is equal to the energy emitted per second. The relation between a given amount of emitted energy, E, power, and time, T, is thus:

$$E \text{ [J]} = P \text{ [watts]} \times T \text{ [s]} \tag{3.6a}$$

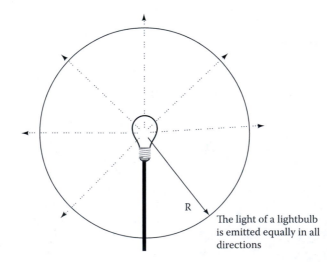

The light of a lightbulb is emitted equally in all directions

Figure 3.10 The rays of light from an ordinary light source, such as a lightbulb, are emitted in all directions. As a result, the lightbulb can illuminate an entire room.

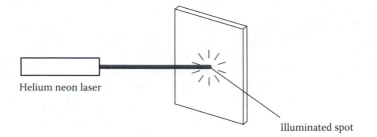

Figure 3.11 The intensity of a laser source is confined to a very narrow beam of light since all of the rays of light are emitted very nearly parallel. As a result, the laser illuminates only a tiny circular spot on a distant object.

In metric units, we measure power in units of J/s or **watts**. For example, to determine the total energy, E, emitted by a lamp delivering 1 watt of light power, P, in a time $T = 10$ s, one would multiply the power by the illumination time:

$$E = P \times T = 1 \text{ watt} \times 10 \text{ s} = 1 \text{ (J/s)} \times 10 \text{ s} = 10 \text{ J} \qquad (3.6b)$$

Because the same amount of power can be spread out into greater or lesser areas, as we have seen above, we define a new quantity, **power density** or **intensity**, the power delivered to a surface *per unit area*. (Laser surgeons prefer the term power density, while physicists generally use intensity.) This quantity has units of watts/cm². As we shall soon see, it is a crucial measure of the usefulness of lasers for surgery. To compute the power density of a laser's spot, for example, one would take the ratio of the power in watts emitted by the laser to the area of the illuminated spot.

$$I\left(\text{watts}/\text{cm}^2\right) = \frac{P_{\text{laser}}\left(\text{watts}\right)}{A\left(\text{cm}^2\right)} \qquad (3.7)$$

where I is the average power density within the spot, A is the spot's area, and P_{laser} is the power of the laser light. For a fixed power laser, smaller spot sizes correspond to greater power densities; naturally, increasing the power for fixed spot size also leads to a greater power density.

A simple calculation using Equation 3.7 (see box) shows that even a laser with a low power of one milliwatt has a power density 400 times higher than that of a typical lightbulb held at arm's length. Since the lasers used for laser surgery have powers ranging up to tens of watts and a typical spot radius of about 1 mm, they have extremely high power densities compared to ordinary lightbulbs.

Sample calculation: Let us compare the power densities of the light-bulb and laser 1 meter away. (There is nothing special about the choice of 1 meter—we will see that moving even farther away would favor the laser still more.) To do so, we consider the total light power emitted by the lightbulb, generously assumed to be 10 watts. This light power is spread evenly over an imaginary sphere surrounding the lightbulb with a radius R of 1 m. (We consider the imaginary sphere only because the lightbulb's light is spread uniformly in almost every direction, so it illuminates this surface uniformly.) The area of the surface of a sphere is given by the formula $A = 4\pi R^2$. Here we have $R = 1$ m = 100 cm, so the power density of the lightbulb at 1 meter from the lightbulb is:

$$I_{\text{lightbulb}} = \frac{P_{\text{lightbulb}}}{A} = \frac{10 \text{ watts}}{4\pi R^2} = \frac{10 \text{ watts}}{4\pi \left(100 \text{ cm}\right)^2} = 8\times10^{-5} \text{ watts/cm}^2 \quad (3.8)$$

(Notice that if computed at a greater distance—hence at larger R and A—this power density would drop even further.) Now let us put this number in context by repeating the computation for a *low* power laser, assuming a very modest power output of 1 milliwatt. Its total power output of 1 milliwatt (10^{-2} watt) is emitted into a circular spot with radius $r = 1$ mm = 0.1 cm. (This is true at a distance of 1 meter, but the spot is very close to this size for a much larger distance as well, so the exact distance at which we compute the power density isn't crucial.) The area of the circular spot is given by $A = \pi r^2$. Its power density is:

$$I_{\text{laser}} = \frac{P_{\text{laser}}}{A} = \frac{10^{-3} \text{ watts}}{\pi r^2} = \frac{10^{-3} \text{ watts}}{\pi \left(0.1 \text{ cm}\right)^2} = 3\times10^{-2} \text{ watts/cm}^2 \quad (3.9)$$

We make sense of these two values by taking their ratio:

$$\frac{I_{\text{laser}}}{I_{\text{lightbulb}}} = \frac{3\times10^{-2} \text{ watts/cm}^2}{8\times10^{-5} \text{ watts/cm}^2} \approx 400 \quad (3.10)$$

The power *density* of the 1 milliwatt laser is about 400 times that of the lightbulb emitting 10,000 times as much power!*

---

* Although we have made the simplification that the laser's power density is uniformly intense across the beam's diameter, we would get similar results if we used a more realistic model that took into account the actual variation in intensity.

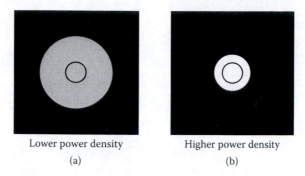

Lower power density   Higher power density

(a)   (b)

Figure 3.12 Illustration of the effects of lower and higher power densities of light on an absorber. An absorber of light, such as the circular region shown, intercepts a smaller fraction of the light's total power for a lower power density (a) than does the same region illuminated by a higher power density in (b).

The power density of a surgical laser determines how much light energy a body cell, for example, would encounter if illuminated by the laser. This in turn determines the laser's effectiveness for surgery or therapy. This is illustrated in Figure 3.12. Two spots of light with the same *power*, but differing power *densities*, illuminate the same region of the body. More photons are intercepted by the region illuminated by the brighter, more intense spot.

In medical applications of lasers, another important concept is the **fluence**, *F*: the total *energy* delivered by the laser beam, divided by the illuminated area. This is given by the product of the power density and exposure time, T_E:

$$F \, [\text{J/cm}^2] = I \, [\text{watts/cm}^2] \times T_E \, [\text{sec}] \tag{3.11}$$

This can be thought of as similar to a dose of light energy delivered to a given region of tissue; note that the higher the power density, the shorter the exposure time required to deliver a specific "dose" of light. In a later section we will see that the high power density of lasers can sometimes make practical a procedure that would otherwise require overly long exposure times to ordinary light sources.

At this point, you may be wondering whether lenses (Chapter 2) can be used to further concentrate the light. In fact, another advantage of spatial coherence is that laser light can be focused down to an extremely small spot, as shown in Figure 3.13. This is because a lens focuses essentially parallel light into a point one focal length, *f*, away from the lens. Actually, at the focal length the light is not concentrated into a true mathematical point, but instead forms a bright spot with a diameter determined by how parallel the incoming rays are, how wide the original beam is, the wavelength of the light, and the focal length of the lens. Focused spot sizes as

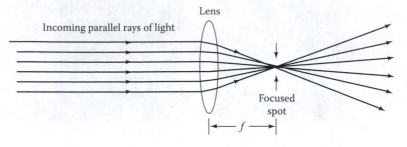

Figure 3.13 Illustration of the effect of a lens on collimated light, such as a laser beam. Collimated (parallel) rays of light are focused down to a very small spot at a distance from the lens equal to the focal length, *f*. (Compare to Figure 2.8 from Chapter 2.) After this point, the rays again diverge and spread.

small as 100 microns to approximately a micron in diameter are readily achievable. Since the laser beam diameters are typically 1 mm to begin with, this additional concentration gives power density increases of 100 to 10,000 times. Since the rays of light diverge once again after the focal spot, lenses can also be used to spread out the laser beam to achieve lower power densities as well.

Spatial coherence also allows one to direct a laser beam into an optical fiber using lenses. This means that fiber optics can be used to deliver very intense laser light to the inside of the body for laparoscopic surgery. Once inside the body, lenses can be used to refocus the laser light as it emerges from the optical fiber.

You can observe the effects of a very high power density by performing a simple experiment with sunlight and an ordinary magnifying glass (Figure 3.14). The power density of the sun's light in the absence of focusing is not great enough to damage most materials. However, when focused by a large lens, such at that of a magnifying glass, the intense focused spot can easily set a piece of paper on fire on a sunny day. The cornea and lens of our eyes also can focus the sun's light down to a tiny spot on the retina, and the resulting power density is high enough to create a burn.

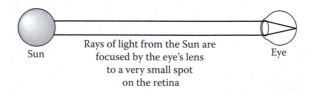

Figure 3.14 Rays from the sun can be focused to a very small point using a lens, such as a magnifying glass or the lens of the eye. In the case of the eye, the focused light produces a very high power density at the retina (lining of the inside of the eyeball), which can cause damage.

Because of its lack of spatial coherence, a lightbulb's light can never be focused down to as small a point as a laser beam. You also can easily see this for yourself with an ordinary magnifying glass. You can indeed focus down the light of a lightbulb. However, the spot is never as intense as that formed by the sun or a laser's beam. Indeed, you can safely put your hand in the spot. In addition, the lens always intercepts and focuses only a fraction of the lightbulb's light. In practice, these trade-offs result in extremely low power densities unless very high power lamps are used.

3.7 COOKING WITH LIGHT: PHOTOCOAGULATION

In laser surgery, energy from a laser's beam gets transferred to blood, body tissue, or bone in the form of heat, in most cases. Consequently, the damage that is done during laser surgery is usually entirely due to heating. Two cases concern us in the present discussion: slow, gradual heating and rapid heating.

What happens when you slowly heat muscle and other tissues—a process known as cooking in the everyday world? Ordinarily, all the molecules in your body are arranged in special highly ordered configurations. Not only is the chemical makeup of these molecules important—how many carbons, how many oxygens, how they are connected, etc.—but the details of their configuration in space determine how the molecules function within the body. One extremely important category of molecules is **proteins**. Proteins form the muscles, connective tissues, and blood vessels; they also transport the oxygen necessary for your metabolism to work. Most major structural and functional chemicals in the body are proteins. Proteins are composed of atoms of carbon, nitrogen, oxygen, and hydrogen linked together by chemical bonds into a very orderly arrangement. These atoms are linked together into larger units called amino acids; proteins consist of chains of amino acids wound into very well-defined configurations.

Figure 3.15(a) shows schematically the complex structure of the oxygen-carrying protein **myoglobin**. At temperatures much higher than body temperature (98.6°F or 37°C), myoglobin and other proteins destabilize, or **denature**; at temperatures over 122°F (50°C), their complex structures begin to uncoil, losing their natural order and forming dense, tangled networks (Figure 3.15b).

This heat-induced disordering of proteins is called **coagulation**; when this effect is achieved by heating tissue with a laser, we call it **photocoagulation**. You likely have seen more common examples of this phenomenon. Egg whites coagulate when cooked, becoming brittle and turning from clear to white. Red meat turns grayish-brown because coagulation during cooking disorders the oxygen-carrying proteins hemoglobin in blood and myoglobin in muscle. They lose both their ability to bind oxygen and their bright red coloring. Structural proteins like collagen become more easily damaged, so it is easier to pull apart coagulated area; in other words,

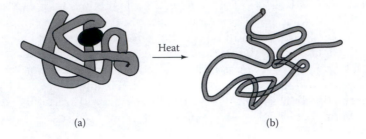

Figure 3.15 (a) Proteins are biologically important molecules made of a strand of repeating units, called amino acids, arranged into very specific configurations. The structure of the oxygen-carrying protein myoglobin is shown here. (b) Upon being heated, proteins lose their specific configurations, turning into random coils; with this loss of structure, they also lose their ability to perform necessary biological functions. This can occur upon heating, in a process called coagulation.

cooking meat usually makes it easier to chew. The coagulated masses also typically shrink in size because water is expelled as the uncoiling occurs.

When lasers are used to photocoagulate tissue during surgery, the tissue essentially becomes cooked. The region heated to high temperatures changes color and loses its mechanical integrity, so it is easier to pull apart and remove. Cells in the photocoagulated region die and a region of dead tissue called a **photocoagulation burn** develops. Photocoagulation burns are used, for example, in destroying tumors and in treating various eye conditions, such as retinal disorders caused by diabetes.

Photocoagulation also accounts for laser surgery's excellent **hemostatic** properties—its ability to stop bleeding. A blood vessel subjected to photocoagulation develops a pinched point due to shrinkage of proteins in the vessel's walls. This coagulated constriction helps seal off the flow, while damaged blood cells initiate clotting. This hemostatic effect allows the bloodless excision of tissue, a major advantage of lasers for performing surgery. By drastically reducing the amount of blood loss during major surgery, lasers can increase the amount of surgery done during a given time and reduce the need for blood transfusions. The prevention of bleeding also keeps the surgeon's field of view clear during the operation, which can improve the precision of the surgery.

3.8 TRADE-OFFS IN PHOTOCOAGULATION: POWER DENSITY AND HEAT FLOW

In 1946, ophthalmologist Gerd Meyer-Schwickerather performed the earliest recorded surgery utilizing light. Using the sun as a source, he was able to treat detached retinas and tumors of the eye. In 1956 he developed a surgical device using a high power xenon arc lamp focused down with lenses,

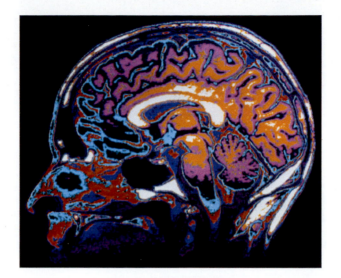

COLOR FIGURE 1.6 Magnetic resonance imaging (MRI) permits detailed studies of the anatomy and physiological functioning of virtually the entire body, including the human brain. In this image, color is used to distinguish the different tissues of the brain and head, seen in cross section. (Reproduced with permission courtesy of Siemens Medical Systems.)

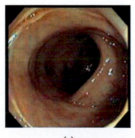

(c)

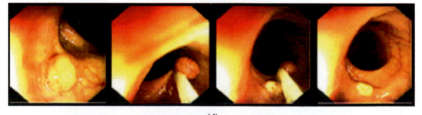

(d)

COLOR FIGURE 2.1 (c) A view of the inside of the colon as it normally appears when viewed through an endoscope. (d) Time sequence showing the removal of a precancerous growth (or polyp). The first image shows, at lower left, a polyp growing within the colon, as seen through an endoscope. In the middle two images, a lasso-like tool called a snare is used to hook and remove the polyp. The final picture shows the site after the removal. Note that no bleeding occurs during the procedure. (Figure 2.1c and d reproduced with permission from http://www.gastro.com/index.htm, courtesy of Drs. Peter W. Gardner and Stuart Waldstreicher. This website contains much useful information about, and interesting images of, common endoscopic procedures.)

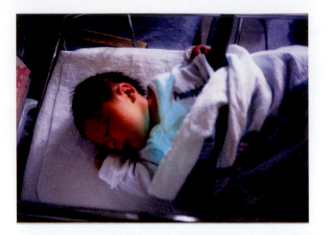

COLOR FIGURE 2.15 Fiber optic blankets can enable parents to treat jaundice at home rather than in the hospital; here a newborn baby rests while receiving phototherapy from the biliblanket swaddling her.

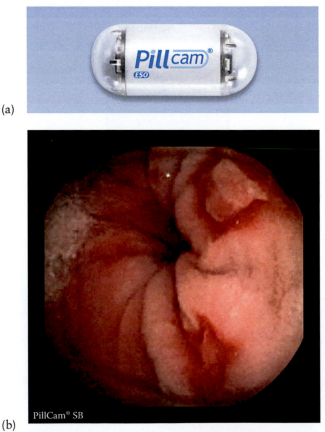

(a)

(b)

COLOR FIGURE 2.19 (a) Video capsule endoscopy. The camera pill (PillCam™) is an alternative to using a flexible endoscope for some examinations of the gastrointestinal tract. (b) Camera pill image of an inflamed esophagus in esophagitis. (Images used with permission courtesy of Given Imaging.)

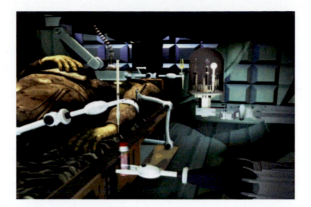

COLOR FIGURE 2.21 Conceptual image of the Trauma Pod, showing an injured soldier lying prone on an operating table while robotic surgery is performed. (Image used with permission courtesy of SRI International.)

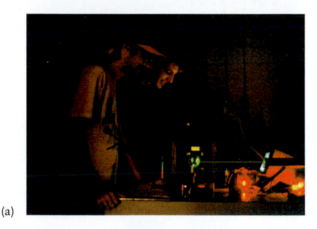

(a)

COLOR FIGURE 3.2 (a) A green argon ion laser used in an undergraduate science laboratory. The bright line emerging from the laser unit is the light of its laser beam.

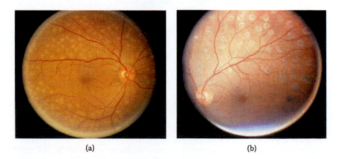

(a)   (b)

COLOR FIGURE 3.30 Photographs illustrating (a) the appearance of fresh photocoagulation burns on the retina, such as those used to treat diabetic retinopathy. Note that the burns are densely peppered about the retina's blood vessels. (b) Scars left by healed burns. After the burns heal, they leave scar tissue that can, for example, seal off leaking blood vessels in diabetic retinopathy, thus preventing further damage to the retina. The burned regions themselves are no longer sensitive to light, but they prevent further degeneration of the retina. (Reproduced with permission courtesy of Ian J. Constable and Arthur Siew Ming Lim, *Laser: Its Clinical Uses in Eye Diseases*, Churchill Livingstone, Edinburgh, 1990.)

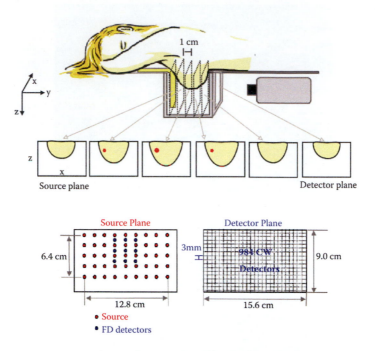

Source plane

Detector plane

Source Plane

Detector Plane

6.4 cm

3mm

984 CW
Detectors

9.0 cm

12.8 cm

15.6 cm

● Source

● FD detectors

COLOR FIGURE 3.33 (a) Schematic of a parallel plate diffuse optical tomography (DOT) instrument for breast imaging. A female subject lies in the prone position on a bed with her breasts inside a chamber surrounded by an index-of-refraction-matching fluid to allow infrared light to enter the breast. Continuous-wave transmission and frequency-dependent remission measurements are performed simultaneously by a CCD camera and nine photodiodes connected by fiber optics on the source plate for 45 source positions at multiple wavelengths.

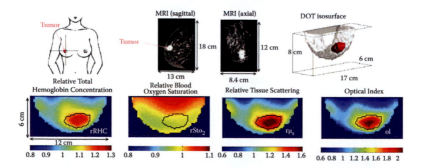

Tumor

MRI (sagittal)

MRI (axial)

DOT isosurface

Tumor

18 cm

12 cm

8 cm

6 cm

13 cm

8.4 cm

17 cm

Relative Total
Hemoglobin Concentration

Relative Blood
Oxygen Saturation

Relative Tissue Scattering

Optical Index

6 cm

rRHC

rSto₂

rμₛ

ol

12 cm

0.8 0.9 1 1.1 1.2 1.3

0.8   0.9   1   1.1

0.6 0.8 1 1.2 1.4 1.6

0.6 0.8 1 1.2 1.4 1.6 1.8 2

COLOR FIGURE 3.33 (b) MR (magnetic resonance) image and DOT image of a 53-year-old woman with a 2.2-cm invasive ductal carcinoma (a form of breast cancer) in her right breast. Top left most frontal-view diagram shows the approximate tumor location with lines indicating the slice positions for the following images. Top middle images are dynamic-contrast-enhanced (DCE) MR images along the vertical (sagittal) and the horizontal (caudal-cranial) lines, respectively. Enhancement of Gd (a contrast medium for MRI)-uptake indicates the malignancy on the MR image. DOT images of relative total hemoglobin concentration, relative blood oxygen saturation, relative tissue scattering at 786 nm and optical index of refraction are shown in the caudal-cranial view with a black line indicating the region identified as a malignant tumor. High tumor-to-normal contrast in total hemoglobin concentration, scattering coefficient, and optical index of refraction are visible within the region. (Image and caption reproduced with permission courtesy of Arjun Yodh and Regine Choe.)

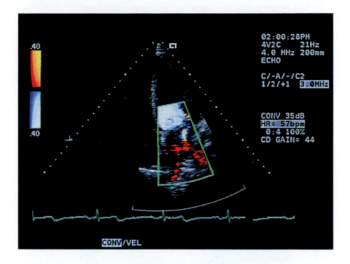

COLOR FIGURE 4.22 Cross-sectional image of the four chambers of the heart and map of the flow of blood within the heart obtained by color-flow ultrasound. The schematic drawing shows the heart's structure. The normal flow of blood from the left atrium through the mitral valve into the left ventricle is indicated in blue. The red regions indicate "regurgitating" blood flowing upward through the defectively closed mitral valve. (Reproduced with permission courtesy of Acuson Corporation.)

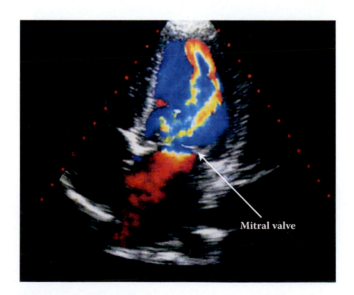

Mitral valve

COLOR PROBLEM P. 4.12

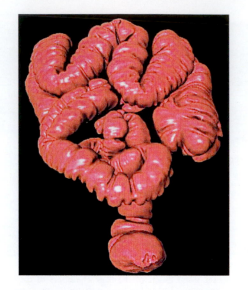

COLOR FIGURE 5.33 Three-dimensional reconstruction of the outside and inside of the colon, made using spiral CT for the purposes of virtual colonoscopy. The sequence of images re-creates a "flight" through the colon similar to what is usually seen during an actual endoscopic exam. (Reproduced with permission courtesy of David J. Vining, "Virtual colonoscopy," *Gastrointestinal Endoscopy Clinics of North America*, Vol. 7(2) (April 1997), pp. 285–291.)

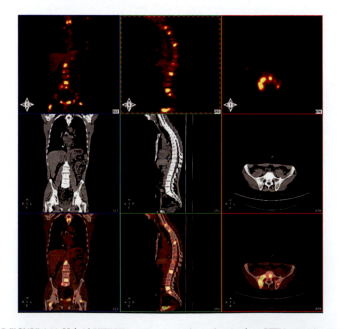

COLOR FIGURE 6.14 Hybrid PET/CT imaging in oncology, showing how PET images (top row) can be combined with CT (middle row) by "coregistering" color maps from PET onto the grayscale CT images (bottom row). These hybrid images allow regions of enhanced contrast in PET to be compared to the anatomical information from CT for enhanced diagnostic accuracy. (Images courtesy of Drs. Daniel Appelbaum and Yonglin Pu, University of Chicago.)

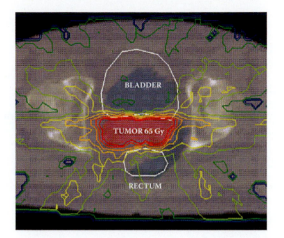

COLOR FIGURE 7.10 (b) In three-dimensional (3D), intensity modulated radiation therapy (IMRT) using stereotactic systems, gamma ray beams converge on a malignant tumor from all possible directions, using information from 3D CT image reconstructions to create a treatment that confines the dose to the contours of the tumor. The image shows a superimposed axial CT scan and radiation dose map from 3D IMRT planning for a case of prostate cancer. To target the prostate tumor, it is desired to confine the radiation dose so as to avoid the bladder and rectum (also shown as outlines.) Contour lines of the radiation dose in Gy indicate that the highest doses are indeed confined to the tumor, with little exposure to bordering normal tissues. (Image reproduced with permission courtesy of Robert Levine, Ph.D., Spectral Sciences, Inc.)

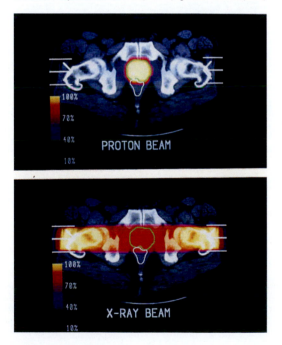

COLOR FIGURE 7.12 (b) CT scan of the hips and prostate tumor, with superimposed color maps indicating radiation dose delivered at various points. The top image indicates the radiation dose (color map) from two proton beams incident from the sides of the body, while the bottom image shows the radiation dose due to two 18 MeV x-ray beams also incident from the sides. These images illustrates how for a fixed beam geometry, the radiation dose due to proton therapy (top) conforms much better to the tumor volume (green contour) than that for photon therapy (bottom). (Reproduced with permission courtesy of the National Association for Proton Therapy.)

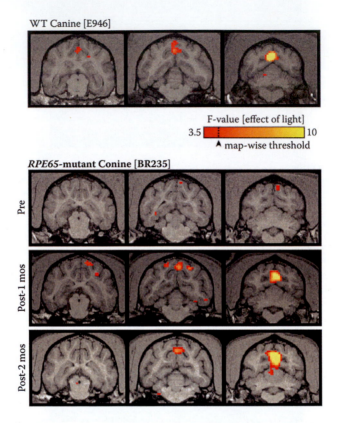

COLOR FIGURE 8.27 Functional MRI scans (fMRI) scans have been used to study whether gene therapy can restore vision to humans and dogs born with a mutation causing blindness. The coronal MRI scans shown here were performed on a dog with normal vision ("WT canine" top row) and the same congenitally blind dog under three different conditions ("RPE65-mutant canine," three lower rows), using fMRI to measure blood oxygenation levels indicative of brain activity. For the blind dog, the top row shows MRI scans before gene therapy, while the bottom-most two rows show results 1 and 2 months post-gene therapy, respectively. The color-mapped signals superimposed on structural MRI scans (in gray scale) indicate increasing levels of brain activity in the visual cortex after gene therapy; the dog with normal vision and congenitally blind dog 2 months post-therapy have similar fMRI levels. These results indicate that gene therapy indeed holds hope of restoring vision in these cases of congenital blindness. (Reproduced with permission from Canine and Human Visual Cortex Intact and Responsive Despite Early Retinal Blindness from RPE65 Mutation, Aguirre GK, Komáromy AM, Cideciyan AV, Brainard DH, Aleman TS, et al. *PLoS Medicine* Vol. 4, No. 6, e230 doi:10.1371/journal.pmed.0040230.)

and utilized it in treating retinal disorders. Why do physicians now use lasers exclusively if cheaper, simpler lamp sources were effective?

Meyer-Schwickerather's device worked by heating up an area of the retina until a localized photocoagulation burn was induced; these lesions were used to tack down the detached retina or to destroy a tumor. However, because of the low power density of this device, each burn required an exposure of 1.5 seconds. During the long exposures, the heat from the light spread into neighboring tissues beyond the actual area to be treated. This made the tissue damage difficult to control, leaving adjacent regions of the eye damaged and causing much pain to the patient. These problems occurred because the heat energy delivered to the targeted tissues had time to flow into adjoining regions.

You can observe this same effect by noticing how hot the handle of an all-metal saucepan becomes, even when only the body of the pan is on a burner. Heat flows from the pan's body to the handle. However, as we saw earlier, heat is a form of energy transfer that changes the temperature of a material. Why, then, does heat flow like a fluid from hot to cold? In the cases we are interested in, temperature corresponds to the average energy of motion of the atoms within a material. In their ceaseless microscopic agitation, these atoms can interact with their neighbors, colliding with them and thus communicating some of their energy of motion. If a hot, energetically moving region is next to a colder, sluggishly moving region, atoms from both regions collide at random with their neighbors, sometimes gaining, sometimes losing energy. *On average*, atoms from the high temperature side transfer energy to their low temperature neighbors, a phenomenon called **heat flow**. This tends to even out the temperature in both regions, lowering the high temperature and raising the low. If a source of energy maintains the high temperature at one end, this flow of heat continues indefinitely.

The **thermal relaxation time**, T_R, is defined as the amount of time required for heat to flow into adjacent regions so as to reduce any temperature increase in the exposed tissue by one-half; it is fixed by the geometry and thermal properties of human tissue. In order to cause a large local increase in temperature, energy must be delivered to the tissue by the laser more rapidly than the heat can flow from the site: in other words, the exposure time, T_E, must be less than T_R. Because T_E is effectively fixed by this argument, we see from Equation 3.11 that this means that a fairly high power density must be employed in order to deliver enough fluence to heat the tissue to the point of coagulation.

Ordinary lamp sources do not cause burns because they have extremely low power densities. This is because, at low power densities, a very long exposure time is required to deliver enough energy to cause a burn. There is then enough time for the heat to flow harmlessly into a large region of surrounding tissue (Table 3.3), resulting only in a modest amount of heating. For laser beams or heat lamps with moderate power densities, the exposure time required is much shorter. The heat then can flow only a short distance during the exposure time, so the added energy is confined to a small region.

Table 3.3 Power density levels used in laser surgery
determine the types of damage done and
hence their surgical applications

Power Density	Result
Low (<10 watts/cm²)	Gentle heating
Moderate (≤10 – 100 watts/cm²)	Photocoagulation
High (>100 watts/cm²)	Photovaporization

Note: Approximate ranges for each biophysical effect are given.

This targeting of heat to only the illuminated tissue causes a photocoagulation burn. When even higher power densities are used, surgeons create a very different type of damage, which we will discuss in the next section.

3.9 CUTTING WITH LIGHT: PHOTOVAPORIZATION

When extremely high power densities are used, instead of moderate heating of the tissue to create a burn, it is possible to quickly heat to temperatures above the boiling point of water, 212°F (100°C). This phenomenon is called **photovaporization.*** In this case, the water within the body's tissues boils. Since most body tissue is almost entirely water, this boiling changes the tissue into a gas. Photovaporization results in the complete removal of the vaporized tissue, making possible either incisions or the delicate removal of thin layers of tissue. Fortunately, coagulation occurs around the edges of a photovaporized region, making it a bloodless procedure as well.

Two conditions must be met for vaporization to occur. First, the tissue must have been heated to at least the boiling point of water, and maintained at that temperature for some time. The amount of time needed for vaporization to occur is controlled by the amount of energy needed to vaporize a given volume of material. This is determined by the energy needed to disrupt all of the associations between neighboring molecules of water to convert them into isolated gas molecules. The amount of energy required for different tissues depends upon their varying water contents. Very short exposure times and high power densities must be used so there is no time for the heat to flow outward before enough energy has been delivered to vaporize the entire targeted region (Table 3.3 and Figure 3.16b). When these conditions have been met, layers of tissue can be vaporized completely, with enough heat flowing to a thin surrounding region to coagulate it. A delicate balance must hold in laser surgery using photovaporization, since unlike a scalpel, the laser beam can cut deeply beyond its apparent extent if too high a power density is used.

---

* This phenomenon is sometimes called photodisruption or photoablation. Since different sources use these terms to mean a variety of effects, I have tried to use the most common meanings, giving preference to definitions that accord well with their origins in physics.

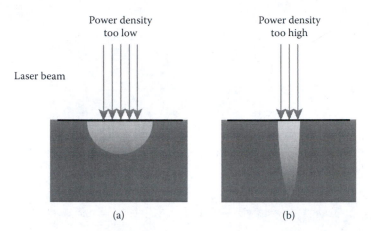

Figure 3.16 Illustration of the effects of differing extremes of power densities upon tissue. (a) For too low a power density, the time required to cause a certain amount of coagulation is so long that heat can flow into surrounding tissues, leading to damage to a larger area than was desired. (b) For too great a power density, the affected region might be deeper than desired, since it is not possible to directly view the extent of damage. Surgeons must determine the correct combination of power density and exposure time for each application.

In practice, for fixed laser intensity, a small spot size is used for precise incisions made by photovaporization, a larger spot size for vaporizing larger areas of tissue, and yet larger spot sizes for photocoagulating tissue. Conversely, by using a fixed spot size, all these effects can be achieved by changing only the intensity of the incoming laser beam. Either method changes the power density appropriately.

The term **photoablation** is also used to describe the use of high laser powers at ultraviolet wavelengths to selectively break chemical bonds in tissue *without* causing local heating. This ability to destroy more localized regions by causing chemical changes with light opens up the possibility of yet another very specific way of performing laser surgery. Lasers also can be used to cut and photocoagulate in what is called contact mode. For example, the Nd:YAG laser is sometimes used with an absorbing sapphire tip at the end of the fiber optic waveguide. This tip heats up to extremely high temperatures when irradiated by the infrared light. When pressed against the tissue to be destroyed, this ultrahot device gives fine cutting and good control.

3.10 MORE POWER: PULSED LASERS

Lasers can operate in one of two modes (Figure 3.17): **continuous wave** (**CW**), where the laser's power is constant over the entire time it operates (Figure 3.17a), and **pulsed**, where the light is emitted in intense bursts, or pulses (Figure 3.17b), with no light emitted in the intervals between pulses.

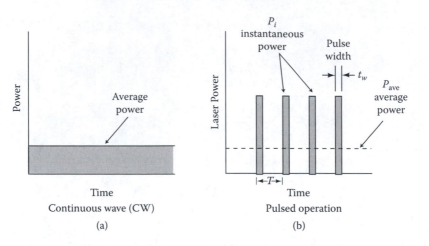

Figure 3.17 (a) The power of a CW laser is emitted continuously, like that of a lightbulb. The same average power is present the entire time the laser is in operation. (b) By contrast, the power of a pulsed laser is emitted in bursts, like that of a flashlight switched rapidly on and off. In general, the instantaneous power during each laser pulse is much greater than the average power of the CW laser. Because no power is emitted between pulses, the average power that results is much lower than the instantaneous power.

The lasing medium determines whether a laser can operate continuously, or needs to rest and be cooled in between pulses. Some types of lasers can be manufactured to operate in either mode. Pulsed lasers are ideally suited for the demands of photovaporization, so we will consider them in more depth here.

In one method for achieving laser pulses, called **Q-switching**, a device called a **Pockel's cell** is inserted inside the lasing medium. The Pockel's cell acts like an electromagnetic switch that prevents lasing from occurring by blocking the passage of light while the population inversion accumulates to very high levels. When the switch is opened, lasing occurs, releasing an enormous amount of energy rapidly. This rapid release of laser energy is what creates the pulses of light in a pulsed laser.

Because pulsed lasers store up energy and emit it in one extremely short pulse, rather than in a continuous beam, this results in extraordinarily high power levels during the brief pulse time. A typical pulse duration, indicated as t_w in Figure 3.17(b), is several **nanoseconds** (**ns** or 10^{-9} s), and a typical pulse carries enough energy (on the order of several J) to vaporize a small volume of tissue. The repetition rate is typically several pulses per second (1 to 10 Hz). This gives huge instantaneous powers during a pulse of over *one million* watts (1 megawatt), with correspondingly high power densities.

Pulsed lasers are a boon in medicine, because they deliver pulses with higher instantaneous power than can continuous wave lasers, making photovaporization or photodisruption possible. The high pulses are necessary to deliver the enormous power densities needed for these processes. (Recall that this is necessary in order to avoid substantial heat flow during the laser irradiation.) However, because the high powers are present only during the brief instant the pulse is on, the tissue is destroyed in a slow, controlled fashion. Examples of pulsed laser systems include pulsed Nd:YAG lasers and the Q-switched ruby laser.

We can determine the equations that govern the behavior of pulsed lasers with the help of some additional quantities. The energy emitted during each pulse, E_{pulse}, is typically given in joules, and the width of each pulse, t_w, is its duration in time. These two values enable us to calculate the instantaneous power, P_i, emitted *during* a single laser pulse:

$$P_i(\text{watts}) = \frac{E_{pulse}(\text{J})}{t_w(\text{s})} \tag{3.12}$$

Sample calculation: The instantaneous power during a 1 milliJoule laser pulse that lasts 1 nanosecond can be computed using:

$$P_i(\text{watts}) = \frac{E_{pulse}(\text{J})}{t_w(\text{s})} = \frac{1 \text{ milliJ}}{1 \text{ ns}} = \frac{10^{-3} \text{ J}}{10^{-9} \text{s}} = 10^6 \text{ watts} \tag{3.13}$$

In fact, pulsed lasers deliver values of total energy per pulse and power density ideal for photovaporization. This extraordinarily high power is only available while the pulse is present. In between pulses, no laser power is delivered, so unwanted photocoagulation is not a problem. As a result, the **average power** delivered by a pulsed laser is much lower than the instantaneous power. To define the average power, we first introduce the **pulse repetition rate, R,** the number of pulses emitted per second, which is measured in Hz. This is related to the period, T, the time from the end of one pulse to the beginning of the next, by the equation $R = 1/T$. The average power is then determined by multiplying the energy per pulse by the number of pulses per second:

$$P_{ave}(\text{watts}) = E_{pulse}(\text{J}) \times R(\text{Hz}) \tag{3.14}$$

This average power properly takes into account the time in between pulses, when the power is zero. From this equation we see that if either the energy per pulse, or the pulse repetition rate is increased, the power delivered for laser surgery also increases.

> **Sample calculation:** If pulses with the same energy, 1 milliJ = 10^{-3} J, described above are emitted at a pulse repetition rate of 5 Hz, then the average power emitted is:
>
> $$P_{ave}\left(\text{watts}\right) = E_{pulse}\left(\text{J}\right) \times R\left(\text{Hz}\right) = 10^{-3}\,\text{J} \times 5\text{ Hz} = 5 \times 10^{-3}\,\text{watts} \qquad (3.15)$$

This result—that even a very high instantaneous power can average out to a fairly low average power—can be seen graphically in Figure 3.17. In that plot, the laser power levels during each pulse are plotted as a function of time. For a CW laser, the power is a constant for all times. For the pulsed laser, a very high power is plotted during each pulse, and zero power in between pulses (solid lines and shaded bars). The shaded area for each pulse is given by the product of its width and its power, a quantity equal to the energy per pulse (compare with Equation 3.12). By contrast, the dashed line in the same plot gives the average power, as computed by Equation 3.14. This dashed line is found by spreading the shaded area under each pulse (energy per pulse) over a time equal to the period. Since the period is much longer than the pulse width, this average power is lower than the instantaneous power.

Which power—the average or instantaneous value—is the one that matters for laser surgery? *Both* are relevant. The instantaneous power (Equation 3.2) describes the power present briefly during each pulse, which determines the pulse's power density for photovaporization. The average power (Equation 3.14) would be used to describe how much energy gets deposited in a region of tissue over a longer period of time. This would determine the fluence and hence how much total tissue gets vaporized during an incision.

One use of the extremely rapid photovaporization made possible by pulsed lasers is a technique called **photodisruption**. Photodisruption effectively generates a small-scale explosion at the laser beam, sending forth shock waves that tear tissues apart and break up hard deposits. In **laser lithotripsy**, this effect is used to break up gallstones and stones in the urinary tract. The small pieces of the shattered stones can then either be passed by the patient or removed laparoscopically.

3.11 LASERS AND COLOR

In order for lasers to cause the types of tissue damage discussed above, the laser's light must first be absorbed. However, everyday experience indicates that water is transparent to light. Since human tissue is primarily made of water, how can it absorb light energy? We will now explore how an understanding of the origins of color—the rich red of blood, the brown tint of

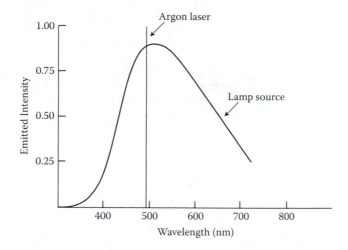

Figure 3.18 Comparison of the emission spectra of an ordinary lightbulb (tungsten lamp) and an argon laser, which emits only green light. Note that the lightbulb emits light at wide range of wavelengths, with a peak in the visible region of the spectrum. The argon laser's emission spectrum has all of its intensity confined to a very narrow peak at one wavelength in the green.

skin pigments, the black of the eye's pupil, and the clarity of water—will allow us to see how to harness laser light for surgery.

An ordinary lightbulb emits white light, which a prism can break into an entire spectrum of colors. What happens when one does the same for a laser? A spectrum with only one line appears, because the laser's light is emitted at a single wavelength; this is the property of **temporal coherence**. Various medical lasers emit light at a specific wavelength, which can range from just under 200 nm (in the ultraviolet) to somewhat over 10 microns (in the infrared). We can compare lasers and ordinary sources of light using a plot that displays the light power emitted at various wavelengths. Such a plot is called an **emission spectrum**. The emission spectrum in Figure 3.18 shows the amount of light emitted at various wavelengths for two sources: a lightbulb (tungsten lamp) and a green argon laser. The laser's spectrum has a much narrower peak because all of its intensity is confined to essentially one wavelength, and hence one color. Thus, in order for a laser to effectively transfer its energy to tissue, that tissue must efficiently absorb light with the laser's wavelength.

Indeed, parts of the body and other objects have particular colors because their absorption of light depends upon wavelength. For example, shiny metallic objects reflect most of the light falling on their surfaces. If these surfaces are smooth, the angles of the reflected rays preserve the angles of the incoming light. This is why we can see images reflected from a shiny metallic surface. White objects also reflect most of the light from

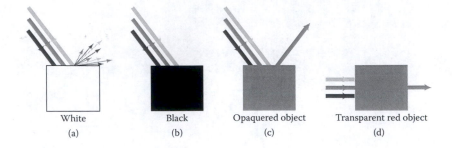

| White | Black | Opaquered object | Transparent red object |
| (a) | (b) | (c) | (d) |

Figure 3.19 The color we perceive an object to have depends upon its ability to reflect and transmit visible light. A white object (a) reflects light of all wavelengths without preferentially absorbing any specific color. (b) By contrast, a black object strongly absorbs all visible wavelengths without preference. (c) A colored reflective object does selectively absorb visible light. For the case of the red object shown here, red light is much less strongly absorbed than that of other wavelengths corresponding to green, blue, etc. (d) A similar rule holds for a transparent red object, except that red light is preferentially transmitted, rather than reflected.

their surfaces (Figure 3.19a), but their surfaces are rough, causing light to reflect off in random directions. For example, the white of the eye simply irregularly reflects all wavelengths in this way. Black objects absorb nearly all the light falling on them, and hence reflect little light for our eyes to sense (Figure 3.19b). This is why the pupil of the eye appears a deep black; almost all of the light entering the eye is absorbed inside the eyeball, and virtually none exits the pupil.

Most things in nature are not white, black, or metallically reflective. Many materials instead have characteristic colors because they absorb some wavelengths more than others. The wavelengths transmitted (for transparent objects) or reflected (for opaque ones) give them their characteristic color; conversely, this means that the wavelengths that get absorbed are the ones we *do not* see. For example, a red object is one for which the green, blue, yellow, etc. wavelengths primarily are absorbed and only the red light is strongly reflected (Figure 3.19c) or transmitted (Figure 3.19d). A similar rule holds for radiant sources of light, such as lasers and lightbulbs: a red light emits red wavelengths of light preferentially. Knowing which wavelengths get absorbed tells us the color of a particular material. We will now examine how many biological materials have absorption properties that depend strongly on wavelength, giving them their characteristic colors and also determining which color laser light they will absorb.*

---

* For a full understanding of our perception of color, you would need to study the physiology of color vision. A good basic discussion can be found in Harriet Rossotti's *Colour: Why the World Isn't Grey*, Princeton University Press, Princeton, NJ, 1983.

3.12 THE ATOMIC ORIGINS OF ABSORPTION

As we have seen above, the way in which materials absorb light is governed by the properties of their electronic orbitals. For isolated atoms, the energy differences between orbital levels can fall in the x-ray, the ultraviolet, or the visible, depending upon the chemical element. Molecules are made when two or more atoms share electrons, while crystalline solids involve enormous numbers of atoms associated with one another. The molecule or crystal will have a new energy level diagram that can accommodate all of the electrons of its component atoms. This new energy level diagram is consequently more complicated than that of a single atom. Usually, forming a larger system will stabilize the electrons, making transitions between the ground state and higher levels cost more energy. This shifts the absorption and emission of light to higher energies and hence shorter wavelengths.

For example, when sodium binds to chlorine, it forms sodium chloride—table salt. In the salt, the electrons are stabilized and their energies shifted from the yellowish sodium lines to the ultraviolet for sodium chloride salt. The compound only absorbs light in the ultraviolet. Since our eyes cannot discern this absorption of ultraviolet light, we perceive table salt to be white.

In some molecules, the new splitting between energy levels will still be small, in some cases, small enough to permit transitions that still absorb or emit visible light. This often occurs with heavy metals such as iron and lead, and in certain organic pigments where the electrons are loosely held. Artists' paints utilize the rich colors generated by heavy metal compounds; paint pigments consequently go by names such as cadmium red, chrome yellow, and cobalt blue. Many biological pigments have evolved chemical mechanisms to absorb light in the visible range, where the sun's light is most intense. Examples include the incorporation of metals such as iron in the oxygen-carrying hemoglobin found in blood, and magnesium in the photosynthetic pigment chlorophyll in plants, and complexes containing loosely bound electrons such as in carotene, a form of vitamin A, or in retinol, a visual pigment found in the retina.

How do we measure and describe the absorption of light by a material of interest? Figure 3.20 shows the operation of a device called a **spectrophotometer**. This device selects particular wavelengths one at a time, shines each one through a dilute sample of the material, then measures how much of the light at that wavelength is transmitted, and hence how much has been absorbed instead. The fraction of the incident light that has been absorbed is used to compute a quantity called the **extinction coefficient**, which characterizes the probability of absorption for a standard-sized dilute sample of standard concentration. This quantity is then plotted vs. wavelength in the resulting **absorption spectrum**. A large value of absorption at a particular wavelength means that light is absorbed efficiently at that wavelength, while a small number means that not much is absorbed.

In addition to the inherent absorption properties of each molecule, the concentration of molecules present affects the absorption of a material.

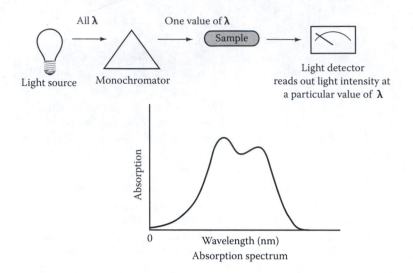

Figure 3.20 The absorption properties of a material can be described by measuring its absorption spectrum using a spectrophotometer. The operation of such a device is indicated schematically in (a). Radiation from a source that emits a broad range of wavelengths is passed through a device called a monochromator, which selects out only one wavelength. This radiation is then transmitted through the sample of interest, such as a solution of protein in water. A detector then measures what fraction of the original beam was transmitted, and uses this to compute the fraction that was absorbed. Using information about the sample's dimensions and the concentration of the molecule of interest, a standardized measure of absorption, such as the extinction coefficient, can be computed. A new wavelength is then selected, and the entire procedure is repeated. A plot of, for example, extinction coefficient versus wavelength then constitutes the absorption spectrum.

For instance, a pint of blood appears dark red, while a small drop of blood diluted into a pint of water appears essentially clear. The blood's pigments have the same tendency to transmit red, and to absorb green and blue wavelengths, in either case, but the different concentrations result in a greater or lesser actual absorption.

Biological molecules have very complex absorption spectra because of the many different excitations that can occur in a large molecule. Instead of many different separate absorption lines, what we actually measure is a smooth curve that represents the smearing together of many absorption lines (Figure 3.21).

Figure 3.22 shows absorption spectra characteristic of the blood's oxygen-carrying protein, hemoglobin. Hemoglobin has a chemical group, called a **heme**, a complex of iron and other atoms with loosely bound electrons, which absorbs visible light. This heme group is responsible both for

Absorption Spectrum for a Complex Molecule

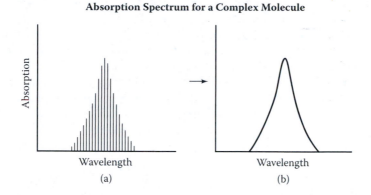

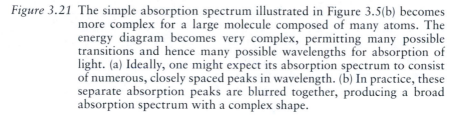

(a)   (b)

Figure 3.21 The simple absorption spectrum illustrated in Figure 3.5(b) becomes more complex for a large molecule composed of many atoms. The energy diagram becomes very complex, permitting many possible transitions and hence many possible wavelengths for absorption of light. (a) Ideally, one might expect its absorption spectrum to consist of numerous, closely spaced peaks in wavelength. (b) In practice, these separate absorption peaks are blurred together, producing a broad absorption spectrum with a complex shape.

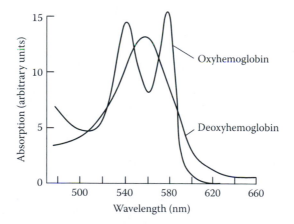

Figure 3.22 Absorption spectrum of hemoglobin, the protein responsible for transporting oxygen in blood. The two lines correspond to the absorption spectrum of hemoglobin bound to oxygen (oxyhemoglobin), and not bound to oxygen (deoxyhemoglobin). Both forms absorb long wavelengths weakly, giving blood its red color. Note that the absorption in the shorter wavelength region of the spectrum is weaker for deoxyhemoglobin, such as the oxygen-depleted hemoglobin found in the veins, leading to the bluish cast of venous blood.

the molecule's color and for its ability to bind oxygen. The heme group has different absorption spectra depending on whether or not it is bound to oxygen. When bound to oxygen (oxyhemoglobin), hemoglobin appears red, because short wavelengths are heavily absorbed, the blues less strongly than the greens and yellows, and longer, red ones hardly at all. (You can see this from Figure 3.22, which has low extinction coefficient values for wavelengths over 600 nm [the red], larger values throughout the yellow and green [590 to 520 nm], and intermediate values for less than 520 nm [the blue-green and blue].) Hemoglobin not bound to oxygen (deoxyhemoglobin) absorbs light with wavelengths in the blue range less strongly than when it is oxygenated (Figure 3.22). Hence appreciable amounts of both red and blue light get transmitted. This is why oxygen-rich arterial blood is deep red and oxygen-poor venous blood has a purplish tint.

There are a variety of biological molecules with notable absorption spectra in the visible, infrared, and ultraviolet, including hemoglobin, myoglobin, bilirubin (a pigment found in bile), and the visual receptor pigments mentioned above. Figure 3.23 shows the absorption spectrum of melanin, a brown pigment found in the skin and iris of the eye. Melanin absorbs some light at all wavelengths, as would a black object. However, its absorption is strongest at short (blue and green) visible wavelengths, so it preferentially transmits yellow and red light, resulting in a brownish tint. The selectivity with which wavelengths of light are absorbed and transmitted by many of the body's molecules (and the ways in which this can be altered by body chemistry) provides a handle for laser surgery and photodynamic therapy.

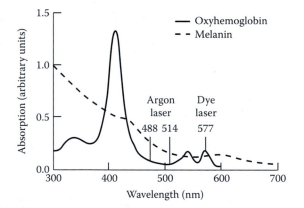

Figure 3.23 Absorption spectra for oxyhemoglobin and melanin, showing the emission spectra for an argon laser, which emits light in the green at 488 nm and in the blue-green at 514 nm, and a dye laser, which emits light at 577 nm. These laser wavelengths are chosen for surgery because they correspond to visible wavelengths at which the absorption of hemoglobin and melanin is appreciable. (It is difficult to make high-power lasers that operate in the blue region of the spectrum, at wavelengths around 400 nm, even though these wavelengths would correspond to even better absorption by these pigments.)

The notion that the chemistry of biological molecules changes their absorption spectra also has many applications in clinical testing. For example, the level of oxygen in the blood can be determined by measuring the absorption spectrum of hemoglobin in the blood at several wavelengths. The degree to which its absorption properties resemble those of oxyhemoglobin or deoxyhemoglobin can then be determined and used to compute the oxygen level by a device called an **oximeter**. Small home testing devices used by diabetics to monitor their blood sugar levels work in a similar fashion.

3.13 HOW SELECTIVE ABSORPTION IS USED IN LASER SURGERY

We can see from the following discussion that the absorption properties of molecules within the body's tissues provide a handle for laser surgery if a laser can be found that operates at wavelengths absorbed by the tissue of interest. In general, the soft tissues of the body consist of over 70% water and varying concentrations of biological molecules that absorb light strongly in the infrared, visible, or ultraviolet. The combination of these two factors gives each specific body tissue its own peculiar absorption properties. Although water is transparent to visible wavelengths, it strongly absorbs both ultraviolet light below 300 nm and infrared wavelengths over 1300 nm (Figure 3.24). Proteins generically absorb much more strongly in the ultraviolet than in the visible. Thus, even though not all tissue has special pigments, some wavelength can always be found at which absorption is significant. Tissues that contain blood have visible absorption spectra dominated by hemoglobin, and the brown pigment melanin is present in varying amounts in many parts of the body. The net effect is that most

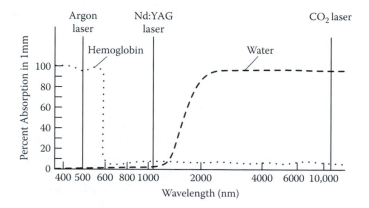

Figure 3.24 Percentage absorption of light of various wavelengths in 1 mm of water, and 1 mm of hemoglobin; the wavelengths of emission for CO_2, Nd:YAG, and argon lasers are shown for comparison.

soft tissues tend to highly absorb UV and blue and green light, but most transmit red light and near infrared relatively well.

Infrared lasers such as the Nd:YAG and carbon dioxide lasers offer high powers and are popular choices for general purpose photovaporization. The Nd:YAG operating in the infrared at 1064 nm is not absorbed strongly by blood, water, or tissue (Figure 3.24). However, it still transfers energy effectively to most tissues through strong scattering, which is not as specific to wavelength. The carbon dioxide laser also operates in the infrared at a wavelength of 10,600 nm. Unlike visible light, this wavelength is strongly absorbed by water. In fact, over 99% of the beam is absorbed within 50 microns of water. This makes the carbon dioxide laser a general purpose laser for many procedures where no pigment is available to selectively absorb the laser light. The infrared light of the erbium:YAG is both powerful and strongly absorbed. Because its wavelength is shorter than the carbon dioxide laser, it can be focused down to smaller spot sizes, allowing it to drill bone and dental enamel.

In addition, surgeons can use lasers to cause damage selectively to only tissues containing a particular molecule with interesting absorption properties. For example, a surgeon can select a laser that emits only a green wavelength readily absorbed by the hemoglobin in blood. Figure 3.23 shows the absorption spectrum of hemoglobin over a wider range of wavelengths than shown in Figure 3.22. The lines indicate that the argon laser's blue-green light at either 512 or 484 nm is absorbed by hemoglobin. (The ND:YAG's green 532 nm is used in similar applications. An even better match is provided by a dye laser emitting 577 nm, which coincides with an absorption peak. High power lasers operating in the blue are difficult to construct, so the optimal absorptions at shorter wavelengths are not easy to take advantage of.) Conversely, the red 632.8 nm light of a helium neon laser would be poorly absorbed by the blood, as indicated by the very low values of the absorption spectrum for wavelengths over 600 nm.

This specificity in absorption makes possible very precise surgery. For example, the retina, the inside lining of the eyeball, has many different layers, each with a different assortment of pigments: visual receptor molecules, blood, melanin, etc. Figure 3.25 shows schematically how the light from two types of lasers is absorbed differently in different parts of the retina, shown in cross section. Ophthalmological surgeons could choose to use the red light of a krypton laser, which is absorbed much more strongly by melanin granules in the pigment epithelium than by blood. Consequently, in that case the pigment epithelium layer of the retina will be damaged more significantly than the layers covering and surrounding it. By contrast, the green light of an argon ion laser would be absorbed by blood, leading to photocoagulation over more of the retina's entire thickness.

How much of the laser's light is absorbed by a particular tissue? In general, as light travels through tissue, its intensity diminishes by an amount that depends upon distance. In addition, we would expect that the

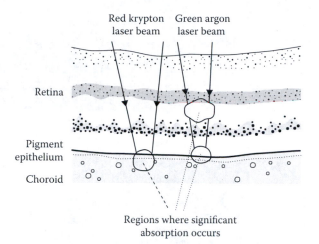

Figure 3.25 Laser surgery can take advantage of the very different absorption properties of different parts of the body. One example is illustrated here, that of the differing absorption of layers in the retina, the lining layer of the inside of the eyeball. This cross section of the retina shows the different absorption properties of two different types of lasers used in eye surgery. The red laser light of a krypton laser (at left) is preferentially absorbed in the pigment epithelium and choroid layer of the retina, after harmlessly passing through outer layers of the retina. The green light of an argon laser (at right) is absorbed in several regions of the retina; its green light is more generically absorbed by any tissue containing blood, so its absorption properties are less tissue specific.

absorption of light should depend upon the concentration of the absorbing medium; for example, we noted earlier that blood absorbs much more light when concentrated than when diluted in water. The degree to which light is absorbed in tissue should also depend upon wavelength as described by the absorption spectrum. All of these dependences are summarized using a quantity called the **penetration depth**, L, defined as the thickness of tissue over which absorption has reduced the light intensity to roughly one-third of its starting value. If the penetration depth for a particular tissue is 1 mm, then after 1 mm the intensity has dropped to approximately 37% of its starting value, after 2 mm to approximately (37%) × (37%) or about 14%—reduced by another factor of 37%—and after 3 mm to (37%) × (37%) × (37%), or about 5%. This decrease in intensity by a fixed fraction for every penetration depth is termed **exponential falloff**. (Later, we will see this same falloff occurs in ultrasound imaging and the time decay of radioactivity.) This falloff in intensity is plotted and shown schematically in Figure 3.26.

Table 3.4 summarizes several approximate penetration depths for some common medical lasers in water and in blood. Note in particular how

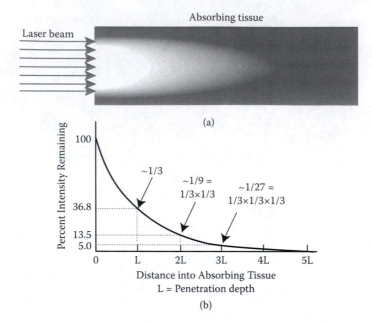

Figure 3.26 A laser beam is not abruptly absorbed in a well-defined thickness of tissue. Rather, as the laser beam penetrates into the tissue, its intensity is gradually absorbed, leading to a falloff in the light intensity with the characteristic shape shown in the plot in (b). This falloff is called an exponential decay, and it is characterized by a distance called the penetration depth, in which the intensity falls off to approximately one-third of its original value.

Table 3.4 Some approximate penetration depths for common surgical lasers

Laser	Wavelength (nm)	Penetration depth in water (cm)	Penetration depth in blood (cm)
Argon ion	514	>1000 cm	0.03 cm
ND:YAG	1064	<6 cm	0.25 cm
Carbon dioxide	10,600	0.004 cm	<0.004 cm

dramatically short the penetration depth is for the carbon dioxide infrared light, and how much the presence of hemoglobin in blood shortens the penetration depth for the argon ion green line.

The penetration depth is determined by the extinction coefficient and concentration of the absorbing molecules by the equation:

$$L = 1/(\varepsilon c) \tag{3.16}$$

where ε is the extinction coefficient and c is concentration. This means that the more absorbers present along a given pathway, the shorter the distance light travels before being absorbed—higher concentrations lead to shorter penetration depths. Similarly, the penetration depth is shorter if the extinction coefficient of the material is greater; both depend on wavelength. For example, for green light, blood-filled tissue absorbs light in a shorter distance than tissue containing little blood. Similarly, the lens of the eye has a long penetration depth for visible light. By contrast, visible wavelengths have short penetration depths in the retina, which has a high concentration of strongly absorbing visual pigments.

3.14 LASERS IN DERMATOLOGY

Now that we have some background in the concepts necessary to understand medical applications, we will review some specifics of how lasers are used in various procedures. Lasers can be used in virtually any type of routine dermatological surgery that can be accomplished as effectively and less expensively by traditional methods, such as scalpels, freeze burns, and electrocauteries. However, for some applications, surgical lasers, such as the pulsed carbon dioxide laser, have proven superior tools. For example, skin cancers can be excised by laser surgery because of the clear visibility and good precision of tissue removal afforded by this technique. Presently, laser surgery is also favored for some types of cosmetic surgery involving skin resurfacing. There, lasers are used to remove extremely fine layers of skin (roughly 0.1 mm thick) to reduce fine wrinkles, sun damage, or scarring. Other infrared pulsed lasers such as the erbium:YAG have been employed for hair removal and other cosmetic procedures.

These infrared lasers take advantage of the presence of water in the skin to provide an ability to remove skin and body tissues in general. However, the absorption specificity of lasers operating in the visible has opened new possibilities in dermatology not available with conventional techniques. In particular, lasers can eradicate certain blemishes otherwise resistant to removal. This is especially true of port-wine stains, a type of birthmark often covering extensive regions of the body. The fine mesh of blood capillaries that makes up the port-wine stain is not dangerous, but many people wish to have them removed for cosmetic reasons (Figure 3.1a). In the past, the principal treatment for this condition was a thick layer of concealing makeup. Now a favored treatment for removing port-wine stains is the use of a pulsed dye laser operating at a yellow wavelength of 585 nm. This corresponds to a peak in the absorption of hemoglobin (Figure 3.23), giving good destruction of the blood vessels, and fading the port-wine stains by 80% to 90%. The more transparent surrounding skin absorbs much less of the laser light, and hence there is no scarring. The same laser can also be used for treating unsightly superficial capillaries on the legs, often called spider veins.

Similarly, tattoos can now be removed by using a variety of lasers whose wavelengths coincide with the absorption of the dyes used, while sparing

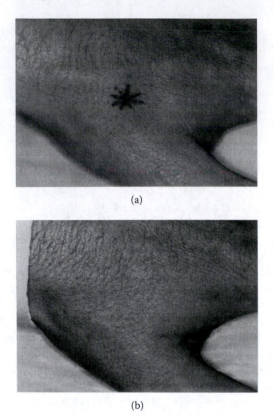

(a)

(b)

Figure 3.27   Laser removal of tattoo before (a) and after (b) treatment. (Reproduced
with permission courtesy of A.N. Chester, S. Martellucci, and A.M.
Scheggi, eds., *Laser Systems for Photobiology and Photomedicine*,
Plenum Press, New York, 1991.)

surrounding skin. This is because many tattoo inks have broad absorption
appreciable for wavelengths greater than 600 nm, where the absorption of
hemoglobin and melanin has dropped off to relatively low levels. Pulsed
lasers such as the Nd:YAG laser at 532 nm or the ruby laser at 694 nm can
be used to fade blue and black tattoo pigments without scarring and bleach-
ing the overlying skin (Figure 3.27). Inks that have absorption properties
overlapping those of hemoglobin and melanin are harder to fade without
skin damage. Melanin-pigmented blemishes such as café au lait spots, len-
tigos, or dark areas under the eye, can be bleached using wavelengths (such
as the argon ion 488 nm or ruby 694 nm light) where melanin absorbs more
strongly than hemoglobin.

Most of these procedures can be performed with minimal local anesthesia on an outpatient basis. The sensation felt when a laser is used to
remove blemishes is often compared to the snapping of a rubber band on

the skin. Surgical lasers can be wielded through an optical fiber ending in a hand piece for the surgeon. This system allows precise delivery of the beam to the affected region of skin. Often, the exact exposure time and intensity for a particular procedure are metered out by computer-controlled systems, making procedures both safer and more precise. The popularity of these procedures—and their high payoff—has led to a constant technological evolution in the variety of lasers available for all surgical applications, with new wavelengths and laser properties constantly coming available.

3.15 LASER SURGERY ON THE EYE

Lasers are widely used in ophthalmology, both because they can make incisions without cutting open the eye, and because their precision and selectivity of damage are ideal for operating on such a tiny organ. The surgery is performed with the laser light either beamed into the eye directly, or endoscopically transmitted using optical fibers inserted through tiny incisions. Most laser eye surgery is performed relatively quickly on an outpatient basis, using sedation rather than general anesthesia.

The anatomy of the eye is shown in Figure 3.28(a). The white of the eye is called the **sclera**. Light enters the eye through the **cornea** and the **pupil**, the opening of the iris. It then passes through the lens and the **vitreous humor**, a jellylike substance that fills the eyeball, and falls upon the inner lining of the eyeball, called the **retina**. Both the cornea and the lens refract entering rays of light in such a way as to project tiny images of the outside world onto the retina, which plays a role analogous to the film in a camera. The retina is a complex structure consisting of many specialized layers, including the **pigment epithelium**, which contains specialized cells for sensing light, and **choroid**, which contains blood vessels and dark blue pigments to absorb stray light. Some layers hold the rod and cone cells that actually sense light, some provide circulation and support. In the regions of the retina known as the **fovea** and the **macula**, or yellow spot, visual acuity is highest because of a high concentration of light-sensing cells. The optic disc, or blind spot, is where the optic nerve enters the retina. Preserving the functioning of these regions is of especial concern during laser surgery.

What happens when laser light with a visible wavelength enters the eye (Figure 3.28b)? Since the lens and cornea of the eye are both transparent to these wavelengths, visible laser light can pass through them to the inside of the eye without being significantly absorbed, and hence without damaging either structure. The vitreous humor also transmits visible light. Because the eye is adapted to utilize as much light as possible, the retina strongly absorbs the visible laser light. Hence, for surgery on the retina, visible laser light can be shown directly into the eye without incisions, using external lenses plus the lens and cornea of the eye itself for focusing. For ultraviolet

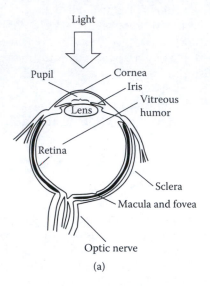

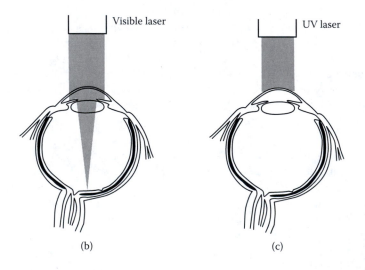

Figure 3.28 (a) Cross-sectional drawing of the eye, showing the anatomy relevant for laser surgery. (b) Lasers enter the eye through the cornea and lens, which are transparent to visible light (left). The lens of the eye focuses visible laser light to a small spot on the retina. This focused spot has very high power density compared to the original unfocused beam. Hence, the retina experiences a much higher power density than does the cornea or lens. However, for ultraviolet (UV) light (right) from an excimer laser, absorption occurs at the cornea, and the laser light is not transmitted into the eye.

wavelength light, such as that emitted by the excimer laser, laser light is strongly absorbed by the cornea and lens, permitting laser surgery on these areas as well (Figure 3.28c).

In Figure 3.28(b), the power density of the visible laser beam is low as the laser travels through the cornea, lens, and vitreous humour, because the beam is still quite wide. Only at the focal point is the beam concentrated to power densities high enough to cause damage. If focused by an external lens, visible lasers can be used to operate on opaque parts of the eye, including the iris (which contains visible-light-absorbing pigments such as melanin). For example, in **glaucoma**, excessive pressure builds up inside the eyeball, threatening damage to the optic nerve. A common operation for this condition involves using an argon laser to create drainage holes for the excess aqueous humor, thereby relieving the pressure, by making incisions in the trabecular network (the eye's drainage network) or iris.

Lasers are also used for removing eye tumors and in treating retinal disorders. For example, Figure 3.29 shows how photocoagulation burns can be used to help repair tears in the retina. These tears can occur because of trauma to the head or eye, and threaten vision loss because of subsequent fluid buildup behind the retina (Figure 3.29a). In repairing retinal tears that threaten to turn into a detached retina, surgeons can use small photocoagulation burns to tack down the ripped area; these burned areas then heal onto their proper base against the back of the eye (Figure 3.29b).

Another condition that can be treated with photocoagulation is **diabetic retinopathy**, the second most common cause of blindness in the U.S. High blood sugar levels in the disease **diabetes mellitus**, which affects an estimated 20.8 million in the U.S., can cause circulatory problems, often resulting in inadequate blood supply to the retina. In an attempt to restore better circulation, the body sends new blood vessels into the retina, but these new vessels can leak and cause swelling and inflammation, leading to a progressive loss of vision.

To treat this condition, small photocoagulation burns by a green argon or diode laser can be peppered over the retina to cover regions damaged by leaking blood vessels. Figure 3.30 depicts the back of the retina, showing

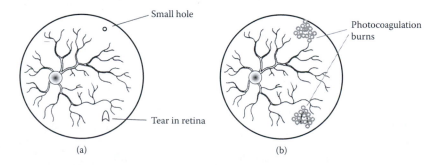

Figure 3.29 (a) Drawing of a circular region of the retina, showing blood vessels radiating out from the blind spot, and a small hole and tear in the retina that are to be repaired. (b) Small photocoagulation burns produced by a laser are used around the tear. After healing, these burns lead to scar tissue that prevents the tear from further growth.

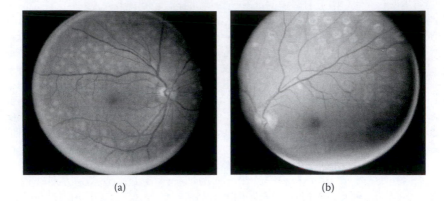

(a)   (b)

Figure 3.30 (See color figure following page 78.) Photographs illustrating (a) the
     appearance of fresh photocoagulation burns on the retina, such as
     those used to treat diabetic retinopathy. Note that the burns are
     densely peppered about the retina's blood vessels. (b) Scars left by
     healed burns. After the burns heal, they leave scar tissue that can, for
     example, seal off leaking blood vessels in diabetic retinopathy, thus
     preventing further damage to the retina. The burned regions them-
     selves are no longer sensitive to light, but they prevent further degen-
     eration of the retina. (Reproduced with permission courtesy of Ian J.
     Constable and Arthur Siew Ming Lim, *Laser: Its Clinical Uses in Eye
     Diseases*, Churchill Livingstone, Edinburgh, 1990.)

how many burns with diameters of several hundred microns are applied
over a wide region of the retina, targeting the troublesome blood vessels and
sparing normal ones. Each burn takes approximately one-tenth of a second,
and hundreds are applied. While laser surgery for diabetic retinopathy cannot correct deterioration that has already occurred, it is frequently effective in preventing future losses. Several large studies of photocoagulation's
effectiveness have shown that persons treated in this way are much less
likely to suffer from severe vision loss. Even more dramatic improvements
are seen in treating some cases of a related retinal disease, **macular degeneration**, with photocoagulation.

Many people develop **cataracts**—milky structures in the lens of the
eye—as they age, leading to a gradual loss of vision. These can be easily corrected through surgery to remove the cataract, often using intense
ultrasound to break up the entire lens, and suction to remove the resulting debris. A plastic substitute lens is inserted at the same time to restore
vision. This technique is extremely successful at restoring good vision to
people who would otherwise grow progressively blind. However, around
25% of the time, new opaque regions reform around the new lens. In a
procedure called **posterior capsulotomy**, surgeons can use YAG lasers to
vaporize these opacifications, producing debris that can be absorbed by the
eye (Figure 3.1b).

Excimer lasers produce ultraviolet wavelengths that are absorbed well in general by water and proteins. This means their power can be absorbed by the transparent structures of the eye, allowing surgery on the lens and cornea. One of the newer uses of lasers involves sculpting the cornea to correct problems in vision. The most common example is **myopia** (or nearsightedness), in which a steeply curved cornea results in images being focused in front of, rather than on, the retina itself. In one form of this operation, called **photorefractive keratectomy** (PRK), an excimer laser is used to directly remove material from the surface of the cornea to flatten it out. A different technique, called **LASIK** (for **laser-assisted in-situ keratomileusis**), uses a thin knife called a microkeratome (or sometimes another laser) to slice a flap off the top of the cornea first, after which an excimer laser is used to reshape and flatten the cornea. The flap is replaced, and a flatter cornea overall results after healing. While these procedures are typically used to correct nearsightedness, in some cases they can also be used to correct for farsightedness due to an overly flat cornea. In wavefront-guided LASIK, the excimer laser is used to sculpt the cornea to attempt to correct subtler visual errors. While many have benefited greatly from PRK and LASIK, the utility of laser surgery for refractive corrections remains limited. Not everyone is a good candidate for LASIK, and ophthalmologists now assess potential recipients for various risk factors, such as a rapidly changing refractive error, overly thin corneas and a tendency toward dry eyes. In a small percentage of cases, patients report serious side effects from LASIK, such as light sensitivity, glare, dry eyes, and problems with night vision.

3.16 NEW DIRECTIONS: LASERS IN DENTISTRY

Yet another surgical application of lasers is only gradually emerging: lasers for surgery on the soft tissues of the mouth and jaw. Dentists can also drill out cavities, bleach, and reshape teeth with laser light, as well as perform many other forms of oral surgery. In addition to the advantages described earlier in this chapter, lasers may present a less intimidating option for the person frightened of dental drills and standard procedures. Another reason driving dentists' interest: patients report a reduced need for pain medication with these procedures.

For soft tissue procedures, dental lasers perform essentially the same functions as those used for other types of surgery. For example, they can be used to remove tumors, ulcers, or other lesions, to sculpt troublesome excess tissue on the gums or tongue, to relieve temperature sensitivity, and to staunch bleeding. Just as in other surgical applications, the generally useful carbon dioxide, Nd:YAG, Holmium:YAG, and argon ion lasers are adequate for most needs. Possible lasers for hard-tissue surgery include the carbon dioxide, Nd:YAG, and Erbium:YAG lasers, now being investigated for removing dental plaque and for cutting the hard, mineralized dentin and enamel of the tooth. The excimer laser, able to vaporize tissue without heating, also promises to make hard-tissue surgery more feasible.

If you have had a cavity treated recently, you may have noticed your dentist shining a bright light in your mouth after preparing the filling. This light induces chemical reactions within the resin composite that makes up the filling, causing it to cure, harden, and bond to the tooth. Used in the place of ordinary curing lamps, argon lasers promise to reduce the time required for such procedures, while yielding fillings with superior mechanical properties.

3.17 ADVANTAGES AND DRAWBACKS OF LASERS FOR MEDICINE

As you may have figured out by now, *any* method of delivering heat rapidly would be equally effective in causing the various effects described above. The main advantage of lasers for excising tissue lies with their versatility and ability to stop bleeding: they can cut to varying depths while keeping the surgical site clear. Extremely fine cuts and deep incisions are possible with the same tool. In combination with endoscopic techniques, lasers can reduce the invasiveness, blood loss, and risk of infection associated with an operation. The selectivity of absorption that results from temporal coherence allows extremely precise targeting of specific tissues. Finally, lasers can penetrate some organs, such as the eye or the skin, *without* incisions.

For many applications, surgeons still choose scalpels or electrocauteries over lasers. Some studies actually have shown that healing proceeds more quickly for scalpel cuts because they involve less damage to neighboring tissue. Both traditional techniques are cheaper and have been in use for many years with satisfactory results. Both represent a trivial expense compared with medical lasers costing up to tens of thousands of dollars per system. As shown in the preceding section, multiple types of lasers are often required for different operations, increasing the expense yet further. Since lasers must be located near the operating room or physician's office, these systems cannot be shared among many different sites. Even in their most successful applications, surgical lasers have probably added to the overall healthcare bill.

As laser surgery has become increasingly popular, surgeons accustomed to traditional surgical techniques have had to learn new skills using a very complex and sophisticated instrument. This includes determining by trial and error the way in which damage occurs during surgery on specific tissues. Surgeons train and practice surgical techniques using lasers on test animals, fresh meat, and fruit (which has roughly the same water content as much of the human body).

Some controllable risks associated with laser surgery include the potential for igniting materials in the operating room, such as hair or surgical draperies, and damaging the eyes of the operating room staff. Since many laser wavelengths used in surgery are invisible, the presence of the beam is not always apparent. These dangers are avoided by taking standard precautions for working with lasers, such as providing protective eye goggles for the patient and operating room staff, avoiding the use of lasers near flammable gases, and wetting surgical drapes and gauze to prevent their accidental ignition. In unskilled hands, lasers can also lead to dangerous wounds on the patient. For example, as Figure 3.16 shows, deeply penetrating burns can easily be produced if too high an intensity beam is used for too long an exposure time. This could be especially dangerous in cases where a hollow organ or major blood vessel could be punctured. Because they are by definition invisible, infrared lasers require the use of a low-power helium neon red laser directed along the infrared beam. This red laser beam enables the surgeon to see where the laser is aimed.

Some physicians have raised concerns that the genetic material of viruses in vaporized tissues might remain viable and lodge in a new location. This has now been proven for the papilloma virus associated with warts. Since this possibility represents a serious concern, adequate ventilation and careful suctioning of photovaporized tissue is routinely provided for during surgery.

3.18 NEW DIRECTIONS: PHOTODYNAMIC THERAPY— KILLING TUMORS WITH LIGHT

Lasers can be employed in therapy by using them as agents for causing highly specific chemical changes. One such application, **photodynamic therapy,** uses light to target and destroy the cells in the cancer therapy and other applications. In this technique, a light-activated chemical called a **photosensitizer** is introduced into the body. One such chemical is a naturally occurring blood component, called **hematoporphyrin derivative (HpD)**, one member of a family of chemicals called porphyrins. This substance is introduced orally or injected in high concentrations into the bloodstream of a person with cancer. After the initial dose, the HpD accumulates in cells of the body. While it clears from normal, noncancerous cells in roughly 72 hours, malignant cells retain the HpD longer (Figure 3.31).

One advantage of this fact is that tumor cells can be more readily visualized after they have been treated. Since the HpD luminesces in the red when exposed to ultraviolet light, areas where HpD is concentrated glow red. Thus, physicians can use this idea to locate and determine the extent of a tumor. Since tumor cells are only subtly different from those found in normal tissues, this is a useful tool for determining the extent of their spread.

The photosensitizer can destroy tumors as well. The absorption spectrum of HpD is shown in Figure 3.32, along with that for the hemoglobin of blood. At long wavelengths, between roughly 600 and 650 nm, there exists a peak of absorption for HpD. At that wavelength, the absorption of hemoglobin has fallen to a small value. If the tumor and its surrounding

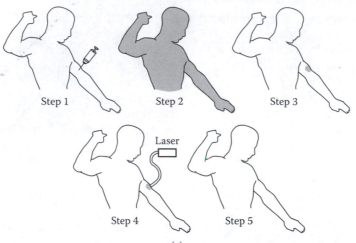

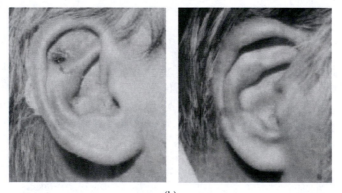

Figure 3.31 (a) Schematic illustration of the events in photodynamic therapy: A photosensitizer molecule is injected into the body of a person with a cancerous tumor (step 1). The photosensitizer enters all of the cells of the body, shown schematically in step 2, but eventually clears most rapidly from normal cells, leaving a high concentration in tumor cells (step 3). Laser light is used to activate the toxic properties of the photosensitizer (step 4). If the therapy is successful, this kills the tumor cells (step 5). (b) Photographs of a case of skin cancer before (left) and after (right) treatment by photodynamic therapy; there were no reoccurrences of the cancer after four years in this case. (Reproduced with permission courtesy of James S. McCaughan, M.D., Laser Medical Research Foundation, Columbus, OH.)

normal region are illuminated with red or orange light in this wavelength interval, the HpD will absorb light, while relatively little will be absorbed by hemoglobin. Thus, tumor cells will preferentially absorb the light. HpD chemically disintegrates when irradiated with light of wavelength 630 nm.

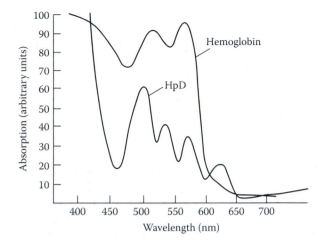

Figure 3.32 Absorption spectra of the photosensitizer HpD, and hemoglobin.

In doing so, it produces a toxic form of oxygen, called **singlet oxygen,** which travels throughout the tumor cell, causing widespread chemical damage. Because this chemical damage within the tumor cells occurs with only an insignificant rise in temperature, the surrounding normal tissue is unaffected. Since it is light activated, turning off the laser also stops the cell-killing activity.

Similar ideas hold with other proposed uses of PDT in dermatology, to treat skin conditions such as psoriasis, actinic keratosis, and acne, while in ophthalmology PDT can be used to treat macular degeneration.

Light with the proper wavelength for PDT with these photosensitizers can be produced by a red gold vapor laser, a diode laser, or a dye laser operating at 630 nm, or by an intense LED (light emitting diode) source that emits light in this wavelength range. The laser beam can be defocused to form a large, lower-power density spot to prevent normal tissue from being photocoagulated. While the extremely high-power densities used for photocoagulation are not needed for PDT, light sources for PDT must still have high intensity so they can achieve high fluences in reasonable treatment times.

Several synthetic photosensitizers either have been approved by the FDA for use in photo-dynamic therapy or are being tested in clinical trials of photodynamic therapy with promising results. A modified version of HpD called porfimer sodium (Photofrin®) has been approved for use by the FDA in treating esophageal and certain types of lung cancer in the U.S. Phototodynamic therapy is being investigated for treating basal and squamous cell carcinoma, common forms of skin cancer. In various countries it is being studied as an additional therapy for skin, bladder, stomach, cervix, and gastrointestinal cancer, among other conditions. Photodynamic therapy is limited to cases where the tumors are small, well confined, and accessible by light, for example, tumors on hollow organs, the skin, and the lungs. This restriction results mostly because the red light used can only penetrate approximately 3 cm (slightly over one and one-eighth inches) into the body because of absorption. However, endoscopic techniques can be used to introduce light into many otherwise inaccessible regions of the body. To improve the penetration of light, the laser light also can be delivered through optical fibers inserted directly into the tumor.

This technique offers new hope for treating many inoperable cancers or those that do not respond to chemotherapy or radiation therapy, but its effectiveness is still under study worldwide. One problem that researchers are trying to address is the time required for the photosensitizer to clear from the body altogether, which presently can be as high as two months. This determines the amount of time during which a treated person needs to avoid direct sunlight. Newer compounds have improved times for clearing the body, with the same good distinction between normal and diseased tissue. Another issue is better partitioning of the photosensitizer into only tumor tissues, since HpD also accumulates in the skin and liver. Photodynamic therapy has already earned a place as a highly promising tool in the struggle against cancer, and progress in photosensitizer development may dramatically broaden its scope in the near future.

3.19 NEW DIRECTIONS: DIFFUSIVE OPTICAL IMAGING

One novel application of these ideas from optics in medicine involves the use of infrared radiation, not for therapy, but for imaging inside the body. It may seem surprising that light can be used to image inside the body, since the body seems opaque to radiation near the visible. However, everyone has likely had the experience of shining a flashlight through a cupped hand and noticing that some reddish light shines through one's fingers. However, this light is diffuse—it has been scattered so many times that its original direction is entirely corrupted. A similar effect occurs in milk or frosted glass, either of which can transmit a glow from a light source even though neither is transparent. However, a new technique called **diffusive optical imaging** uses this diffuse light to diagnose breast cancer and other diseases (Figure 3.33). The idea is simple: in the infrared, the absorption of water and many body tissues is small compared that for visible wavelengths, so light can travel a significant distance without being absorbed. If the light's wavelength is chosen to coincide with values differentially absorbed by, for example, oxy- or deoxyhemoglobin, then the light will be absorbed preferentially by tissues with differing patterns of blood oxygenation, such as tumors or brain tissue affected by a stroke; similar results can be gotten by a wise choice of chemical tags with interesting optical properties. Scattering is still a problem, however, since it prevents one from simply using a lens to form an image from light transmitted from these regions. How can this diffuse light be used to create an image? If the infrared light

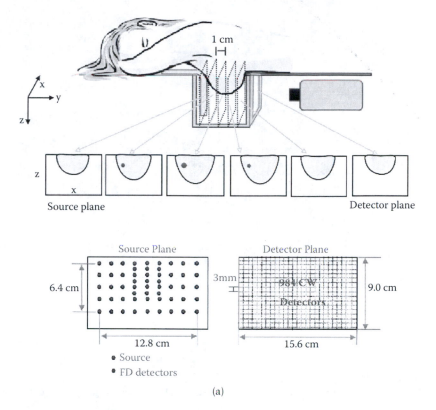

Figure 3.33 (*See color figure following page 78.*) (a) Schematic of a parallel plate diffuse optical tomography (DOT) instrument for breast imaging. A female subject lies in the prone position on a bed with her breasts inside a chamber surrounded by an index-of-refraction-matching fluid to allow infrared light to enter the breast. Continuous-wave transmission and frequency-dependent remission measurements are performed simultaneously by a CCD camera and nine photodiodes connected by fiber optics on the source plate for 45 source positions at multiple wavelengths. (b) MR (magnetic resonance) image and DOT image of a 53-year-old woman with a 2.2-cm invasive ductal carcinoma (a form of breast cancer) in her right breast. Top left-most frontal-view diagram shows the approximate tumor location with lines indicating the slice positions for the following images. Top middle images are dynamic-contrast-enhanced (DCE) MR images along the vertical (sagittal) and the horizontal (caudal-cranial) lines, respectively. Enhancement of Gd (a contrast medium for MRI)-uptake indicates the malignancy on the MR image. DOT images of relative total hemoglobin concentration, relative blood oxygen saturation, relative tissue scattering at 786 nm, and optical index of refraction are shown in the caudal-cranial view with a black line indicating the region identified as a malignant tumor. High tumor-to-normal contrast in total hemoglobin concentration, scattering coefficient, and optical index of refraction are visible within the region. (Image and caption reproduced with permission courtesy of Arjun Yodh and Regine Choe.)

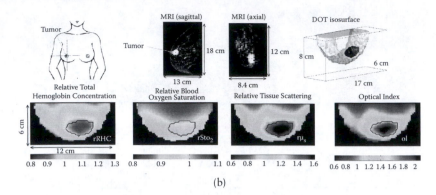

Figure 3.33 (continued).

is shone into the body at a well-defined time and location using an optical fiber, and then detected at a different location and time using a second optical fiber, its path inside the body can be inferred using mathematical techniques established to model the flow of diffusive light. These methods are being explored in research settings, establishing the feasibility of imaging with typical millisecond time resolution and several mm spatial resolution. These techniques are being investigated in combination with other imaging modalities, which can provide anatomical information to use in constructing the basic mathematical models, and with new biochemical techniques designed to provide tracers for interesting body functions and disease processes.

SUGGESTED READING

Other descriptions of medical lasers for general audiences

Michael W. Berns, "Laser surgery," *Sci. Am.* (June 1991), pp. 84–90.
Abraham Katzir, "Lasers and optical fibers in medicine," *Opt. Photonics*, Vol. 2 (1991), pp. 18–22.
Abraham Katzir, *Lasers and Optical Fibers in Medicine*. Academic Press, San Diego, 1993.

Ophthalmology

D.J. D'Amico, "Medical progress: diseases of the retina," *New Engl. J. Med.*, Vol. 33(2) (1994), pp. 95–106.

Dermatology

Tina S. Alster and David B. Apfelberg, eds., *Cosmetic Laser Surgery*. John Wiley & Sons, New York, 1995.
Randall K. Roenigk, "Laser: When it is helpful, unequivocal or simply a marketing tool?" *Cutis*, Vol. 53(4) (1994), pp. 201–210.

Angioplasty

Lawrence I. Deckelbaum, "Coronary Laser Angioplasty," *Lasers Surg. Med.*, Vol. 14 (1994), pp. 101–110.

Dentistry

Articles in a special issue of the *Journal of the American Dental Association*, Vol. 124 (Feb. 1993): Marilyn Miller, "Lasers in dentistry: an overview," pp. 32–35; Robert M. Pick, "Using lasers in clinical dental practice," pp. 37–47; V. Kim Kutsch, "Lasers in dentistry: comparing wavelengths," pp. 49–54.
JGM Associates, Inc., *Dental Applications of Advanced Lasers*, Burlington, MA.
Leo Miserendino and Robert Pick, *Lasers in Dentistry*. Quintessence Publishing Co., Inc., Carol Stream, IL, 1995.

Photodynamic therapy

Ivan Amato, "Hope for a magic bullet that moves at the speed of light," *Science*, Vol. 262 (1994), pp. 32–33.

Laser safety

C. Nezhat, W. Winer, F. Nezhat et al., "Smoke from laser surgery: Is there a hazard?" *Lasers Surg. Med.*, Vol. 7 (1987), p. 376.
J. Garden, K. O'Banion, L. Sheltnitz et al., "Papillomavirus in the vapor of carbon dioxide laser-treated verrucae," *J. Am. Med. Assoc.*, Vol. 259 (1988), p. 1199.

QUESTIONS

Q3.1. Figure 3.23 in Chapter 3 shows the absorption spectrum of the pigment melanin found in skin, the iris of the eye, and other parts of the body. Comment briefly on how the absorption spectrum of melanin would influence the choice of a laser for surgery performed on human skin.

Q3.2. What absorption characteristics would tissue need to have for an argon ion laser with wavelength 514.5 nm to be the appropriate choice for laser surgery? Would you expect blood to have such properties? The lens of the eye? The iris of a brown eye?

Q3.3. Explain why a dentist who is using a laser to remove tooth enamel would first mark the tooth's surface with a black dye.

Q3.4. Why isn't it necessary for the CO_2 laser to have an exact match of its wavelength to the absorption spectrum of tissue for laser surgery?

Q3.5. A surgeon will be performing an operation to remove abnormal growths in a case of endometriosis. A great deal of tissue must be removed over a fairly large area during this operation, and the chief pigment present in the tissues will be blood. Which of the lasers mentioned in the text would be appropriate choices? Discuss the possible use of at least two lasers, one that would be appropriate, one that would not.

Q3.6. Explain in detail the essential differences between the types of damage done to tissue during photocoagulation and during photovaporization. Give one example of an application in which each is the appropriate surgical technique to use.

Q3.7. (a) What do you need to know about a laser to predict its performance as a surgical tool? Give at least four factors and explain the significance of each in detail. (b) What do you need to know about the tissue being operated on? Make your answer as complete as possible.

Q3.8. Explain why the use of a pulsed laser is sometimes preferable to a continuous wave (CW) laser in medicine. Name one such application.

Q3.9. Explain briefly why excimer lasers are used in photorefractive keratectomy, in which the front of the cornea is sculpted to correct nearsightedness. Why is the argon ion laser not a good choice for this operation? Why is the reverse true for laser surgical procedures performed on the retina?

PROBLEMS

P3.1. (a) Compute the energies (in joules) of a photon of light produced by: a carbon dioxide laser with wavelength 10,600 nm; a Nd:YAG laser with wavelength 1064 nm; an argon ion laser with wavelength 512 nm; and an excimer laser with wavelength 200 nm. Which laser produces the most energetic photon? The least energetic photon? (b) What type of electromagnetic radiation does each of these wavelengths correspond to? If the answer is visible light, what is its color? (c) Which of these lasers produce photons of light with energy sufficient to break a chemical bond of energy 6×10^{-19} J?

P3.2. A Nd:YAG laser operates in pulsed mode, with an energy of 100 millijoules per pulse, and a pulse repetition rate of 10 Hz (i.e., 10 pulses per second). Its light can be emitted at one of the following wavelengths: 1065 nm, 532 nm, or 355 nm.

a. Each pulse lasts for 1 nsec, and in between pulses, no light is emitted. What is the instantaneous laser power *during each pulse*?

b. The total energy deposited depends upon the average power per pulse. What is the average power output of this laser?

c. Compute a crude estimate for the exposure time for depositing 10 J (approximately enough energy to vaporize a spot of tissue 1 cm in diameter to a depth of 0.05 mm) assuming 100% of the laser light is absorbed by this volume.

P3.3. Compute the power densities for the medically realistic situations described below.

    a. Photocoagulation of the retina using 500-m-diameter spots and a laser power of 200 milliwatts.

    b. Photovaporization of opacities within the eye using 50 μ diameter spots and a laser power setting of 2 watts.

    c. Compare these two power densities by computing the ratio between them, and explain why your answer makes physical sense given the uses to which the lasers are applied.

P3.4. The spot size is clearly extremely important in determining the power density of a focused laser beam, an important determinant of how it may be used in surgery. However, there is a basic limitation on how small a spot one can achieve with a given wavelength laser beam, λ; a given diameter laser beam (D); and a lens with focal length, f. This smallest spot size is given by:

$$d = \frac{2\,\lambda\,f}{\pi\,D}$$

where d is the diameter of the focused laser beam at the focal point of the lens (Figure P3.4). This equation can be derived using the wave theory of light, but we will not examine the mathematics of this derivation.

    a. Use the above formula for the spot size, d, and a wavelength of 514.5 nm for an argon laser, to estimate the spot size of the laser inside the eye after the laser has passed through the lens of the eye. The eye's focal length is approximately $f = 2$ cm (the approximate distance from the lens to the retina). Explain why ophthalmological surgeons would use a lens to defocus (spread out) the laser beam before it enters the eye when performing photocoagulation.

    b. Find an equation for the ratio of the power densities of two lasers with different wavelengths, λ_1 and λ_2, but with the same power, P, and the same initial beam diameter, D. Assume the power density is given by $I = P/\pi(d/2)^2$. Assume each laser beam has been focused by a lens with the same focal length, f. (In fact, most laser beams used in medicine start out with a diameter close to $D = 1$ mm, so this is a realistic assumption.) Which laser beam is focused to the higher power spot—the one with the shorter or the one with the longer wavelength?

    c. Next, use your answer from part b to compare quantitatively the different power densities that result in the following cases:

        i. The three different wavelengths at which the Nd:YAG laser operates (1065 nm, 532 nm, or 355 nm; assume the same power is emitted at each wavelength).

ii. The CO_2 (carbon dioxide gas) laser's wavelength 10,600 nm. (Again, assume the same power is emitted at each wavelength.) (To compare these values, compute the ratio of the power densities for two different wavelengths.)

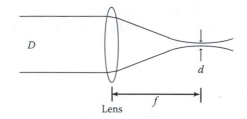

P3.5. All of the ideas you have learned about regarding laser surgery apply equally well to the therapeutic technique called photodynamic therapy (PDT). In PDT, the patient is first fed a light-sensitive chemical (or photosensitizer), which tends to segregate naturally into tumors, but which is poorly retained in normal tissues. Light is then delivered to the tumor through a fiber optic guide. A chemical reaction initiated by absorption of the light by the light-sensitive chemical sets off a chain of cell-killing processes, killing off tumor cells without disturbing even nearby normal cells.

A photosensitizer dye called phthalocyanine has been considered for use in photodynamic therapy (PDT). Assume that this photosensitizer can be concentrated in a malignant tumor, and that a physician wishes to irradiate the tumor with laser light that would be selectively absorbed by phthalocyanine, but not well absorbed by blood or melanin. The absorption spectra of hemoglobin, melanin, and phthalocyanine are shown in Figures P3.5 and 3.23 in the text.

a. One source gives typical values of power densities used in laser PDT in the range of 80 milliwatts/cm². What spot size would you use to achieve this power density for a laser with a continuous wave (CW) power of 1 watt? (Assume you can either focus or spread out the laser beam using some unspecified configuration of lenses.)

b. The total fluence (light energy deposited per square centimeter) of tissue for this procedure was in the range 100 to 120 joules/cm². How long must the exposure time be to deposit this much energy? (Assume you only need to irradiate a region the size of the laser spot size you computed above, and assume that the light is 100% absorbed to get this estimate.) Is this reasonable for a therapeutic procedure?

c. Which of the lasers described in Chapter 3 would be appropriate for treating someone using PDT with phthalocyanine as the light-sensitive chemical? Assume that you want to both maximize absorption by phthalocyanine and minimize absorption by hemoglobin molecules in nearby normal cells. Explain your reasoning.

d. Why do you think lasers are preferred to ordinary lamp sources for this technique? Be as complete as possible in answering.

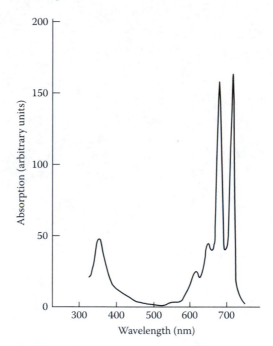

4 Seeing with sound
Diagnostic ultrasound imaging

4.1 INTRODUCTION

You know from experience that sound travels through human tissue because you can hear a heartbeat simply by placing your ear against another person's chest. Medical diagnostic ultrasound imaging uses the body's transparency to sound to "see" within. Because of its safety, diagnostic ultrasound is the only imaging technology favored for routine use in obstetrics, where it provides physicians and parents with images of the fetus within the womb. Figure 4.1(a) shows such an ultrasound image (or **sonogram**) taken of a fetus. Before discussing the science behind this technology, let us first explore some of its most frequent applications.

Let us assume that your physician has ordered an abdominal ultrasound examination. What is this experience like? Ultrasound is an outpatient procedure requiring little preparation, which means you do not have to be admitted to the hospital. Exams are usually administered in the hospital's radiology or imaging department in a small, specially equipped room, or, sometimes, a doctor's office. The ultrasound scanner itself resembles a personal computer (Figure 4.1b). During the exam, you recline on an examination table while a physician or medical technician (called a **sonographer**) applies a gel-coated **transducer**, an ultrasound loudspeaker and microphone in one, roughly the size of an electric razor. The exam is generally painless, the only sensations being due to the gel and the smooth head of the transducer pressed against the skin.

During the exam, the sonographer places the transducer at various positions on your abdomen or back. An image appears on the instrument's television screen, allowing the sonographer to visualize your internal anatomy. The length of the exam depends on many factors, but fifteen minutes to half an hour suffices for many needs. When the exam is finished, the gel is wiped off and you are ready to leave. The images can be forwarded to a radiologist and other physicians for additional analysis.

What, exactly, is the ultrasound instrument doing to produce the images? The transducer's operation is quite simple: it emits a chirp of sound with a pitch so high that it falls outside our range of hearing, hence the term **ultrasound**. This pulse of sound travels through the body, encountering blood

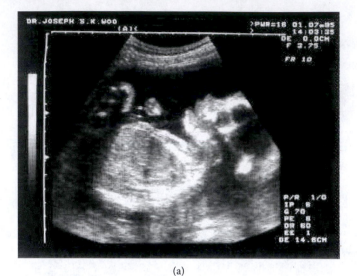

(a)

Figure 4.1 (a) Fetal ultrasound image: cross-sectional view of the head of a fetus at 18 weeks' gestation. (Many other interesting and up-to-date ultrasound images from obstetrics can be found at Dr. Joseph Woo's excellent website located at http://home.hkstar.com/~joewoo/joewoo2.html.) (Used with permission courtesy of Dr. Woo.) (b) Obstetrical ultrasound examination in progress. (Used with permission courtesy of ATL.) (c) Ultrasound image showing the four chambers of the heart in cross section. The atria are at the top of the image and the ventricles at the bottom. (Used with permission courtesy of Acuson Corporation.)

vessels, organ walls, etc. Many of these structures will reflect an echo back in the original direction. The transducer then "listens" for these echoes and keeps track of the time it takes for echoes to return. These echo return times are then used to determine the location of the structure that generated them; this information is used to compile an image of a cross section of the body. The sonar methods used by ships and dolphins to detect underwater obstacles utilize the same idea, and bats have evolved a version of this system (echolocation) to navigate in the dark.

The images formed by an ultrasound scanner are displayed as white-on-black images on a television monitor (Figure 4.1c). They can be preserved on videotape and printed for later review.

Common applications for ultrasound include:

- Obstetrical uses, to monitor the progress of a pregnancy, visualize the fetus within the womb, and enable other forms of prenatal testing for birth defects
- Cardiovascular ultrasound, to see the structure of the heart (Figure 4.1c) and circulatory system

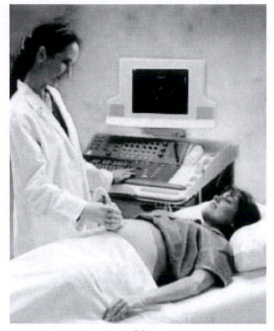

(b)

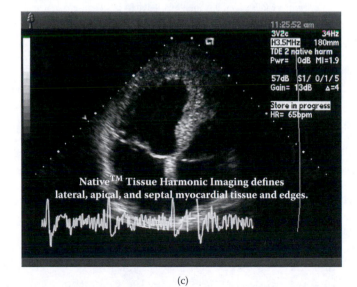

(c)

Figure 4.1 (continued).

- Gynecological ultrasound, to see the structure of the ovaries, uterus, and surrounding regions, and to detect cysts and tumors
- Prostate examinations for tumors

- Ultrasound exams of the breast, to determine whether lumps are cancerous or merely benign cysts
- Abdominal ultrasound, to see the structure of organs such as the bladder, pancreas, spleen, stomach and bowel, and liver
- Renal ultrasound, for imaging the kidneys
- Thyroid examinations, for tumors and cysts
- Ophthalmological ultrasound, for visualizing structures hidden behind the retina or for seeing past opaque obstacles. Eye tumors, retinal detachments, foreign bodies, or hemorrhages can all be imaged
- Interventional ultrasound—ultrasound imaging used as guidance during a surgical procedure, including tumor biopsies, the draining of cysts, treatments for infertility, etc.

An important ultrasound technique called **Doppler**, or **color flow** ultrasound, allows the ultrasound imaging device to measure the speed with which blood flows in the body. This method utilizes the Doppler effect, a physical principle that also underlies the operation of radar speed detectors. Color flow ultrasound allows cardiologists to visualize the beating heart along with a color-coded map of the flow of blood within its chambers. In many cases, this technique can often replace more invasive and dangerous methods for determining blood flow by inserting catheters into the heart and injecting dyes into the circulation.

We will explore the basic concepts behind the generation of ultrasound images shortly. First, however, it is important to pause and understand the basic physics of sound from which these techniques derive. We will also consider how the risks of ultrasound imaging are assessed, and how physicians establish safety guidelines. Two important and common applications—obstetrical ultrasound and cardiac ultrasound—round off the chapter.

4.2 SOUND WAVES

Consider for a moment how humans produce sound. Making a sound always entails a vibration: the vocal cords, a violin's strings, a loudspeaker's diaphragm, or a drumhead all must vibrate to make noise. Vibrations are also necessary for us to detect sounds. The sound generated by the vibrating drumhead, for example, is transmitted through the air, and finally enters our ears, where it is communicated to tiny hairs. When we hear a sound, our nerves are actually responding to the corresponding vibration of these slender hairs. How are these vibrations communicated to the air and hence to our ears? How are they able to travel through so tenuous a medium?

Sound is a wave that occurs when vibrations travel throughout a medium, such as air, blood, or body tissues. It is more difficult to imagine waves of sound than to understand the motions in more readily visualized waves, such

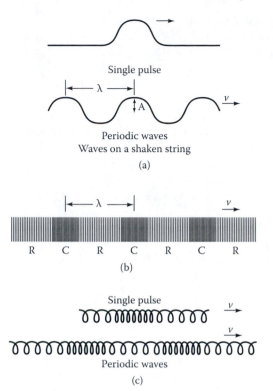

Figure 4.2 (a) Waves on a string, showing a pulse and periodic transverse wave. The wavelength, λ, velocity, *v*, in the direction of travel, and amplitude, A, are indicated. (b) Schematic drawing of the changes in a medium during the passage of a longitudinal sound wave. As the wave travels by, the medium is bunched closer together in some regions (compressions, indicated by C) and spread further apart in others (rarefactions, indicated by R). (c) Longitudinal waves on a spring show similar regions of compression and rarefaction.

as water waves or waves traveling along a shaken string (Figure 4.2a). This is because the **transverse** waves excited by shaking a string consist of movements *perpendicular to* the direction of the wave's movement. Let us consider only these types of waves for the moment. The peaks of the waves we will refer to as **crests**, while the lowest values will be called **troughs**, by analogy with the terms used for ocean waves. The wave moves with a given speed, *v*. The **wavelength**, λ, of the wave is the distance between successive disturbances, while the **frequency**, *f*, is the number of wave crests passing per second (Figure 4.2a). The frequency is related to the **period**, *T*, the time it takes for one complete cycle of the wave to pass a fixed point, by $f = 1/T$: if a complete oscillation of a wave moves entirely past a fixed point in half a second, then two wave oscillations will pass that point in a second (1/0.5 second = 2 per second). We will learn shortly how these three quantities are interrelated.

Molecules in the air move back and forth when a sound wave passes, just as the string moves up and down when the wave passes along it. However, sound waves do not result in the transverse movement of air molecules. Rather, as the source of sound vibrates, it causes the nearby air molecules to first bunch up and subsequently become spread out *along* the direction in which the waves move (Figure 4.2b), forming what is called a **longitudinal** wave. These alternating patterns of bunched-up air molecules (**compressions**) and spread-out air molecules (**rarefactions**) are repeated each time the sound source vibrates. Notice that the air molecules themselves are not streaming around. Just as with the shaken string, they stay put *on average*, but vibrate about their average position when the wave comes by. A commonly used analogy is a shaken spring (Figure 4.2c), in which the waves occur when bunched up or spread out regions of coils move along the spring.

A single disturbance, called a **pulse**, will occur if the source of sound vibrates briefly (Figure 4.2a–c). If the source continues to vibrate regularly, it generates a **periodic wave**, one that repeats itself many times over. Periodic sound waves are characterized by their wavelength, frequency, and speed, just as are waves on a string, or the electromagnetic waves discussed earlier, in Chapter 3. The wavelength is still the length characterizing one disturbance, in this case, the distance between either successive rarefactions or compressions. The frequency is given by the number of compressions or rarefactions passing a point every second.

The **speed of sound** waves in a particular material, v_s, is fixed by the properties of that material. Because the speed of sound describes how far a compression in the wave will move in a given time, it also determines a relationship between the wave's frequency and wavelength. The frequency, f, measures *how often* successive compressions pass a particular point, and successive compressions are always one wavelength, λ, apart. Therefore, the product of frequency and wavelength will give the total distance moved by the wave every second—in other words, the speed.

$$v_s = f \lambda \tag{4.1}$$

As an example, consider a case where we have a frequency of 2 oscillations per second and a wavelength of 1 cm. We use units of hertz or Hz for frequency, where 1 Hz corresponds to one vibration per second, so this is a frequency $f = 2$ Hz. Then, a wavefront moves a distance equal to 2 cm every second: the speed $v_s = (2 \text{ Hz}) \times (1 \text{ cm}) = 2$ cm/s.

Because the speed of sound is a *constant* for a particular material—it does not depend on either f on λ—this means that once f is known, λ is then determined. Conversely, knowledge of λ determines f. We will often convert between frequency and wavelength of sound in a material using the relevant value of v_s.

4.3 WHAT IS ULTRASOUND?

The wavelengths of audible sound waves are appreciable, ranging from centimeters to meters. The speed of sound is also typically quite large, for example, around 344 m/s for air at room temperature. What values of frequency are associated with sound waves? Ordinary, audible sound covers the frequency range 20 Hz to 20,000 Hz (also expressed as 20 kilohertz, or kHz). For example, familiar musical notes have the frequencies 261.7 Hz for middle C, 349.2 for middle F, 440 Hz for middle A, and so on. We experience frequency as pitch in music, and identify high frequencies with the treble and lower frequencies with the bass. Sounds with frequencies greater and lower than the audible range can be generated, even though we cannot hear them. **Ultrasound** has frequencies higher than 20 kHz, while **infrasound** vibrations are extremely low frequency (less than 20 Hz). However, apart from its high frequency, ultrasound is exactly the same phenomenon as ordinary sound.

Ultrasound waves are generated in many commonly used consumer appliances, including ultrasonic cleaning baths, cool mist humidifiers, and antipest devices. Although we are insensible to ultrasound, many animals can hear into the ultrasound regime. Ultrasound is absorbed more strongly in air than ordinary sound, so that rodents using ultrasonic squeaks to communicate with their fellows nearby in a burrow may be undetected by more distant predators. Most notably, bats use ultrasound ranging systems with typical frequencies of tens of kHz to hunt for insects and to avoid obstacles as they fly in the dark.

Sound waves travel within the body by the same mechanisms described for sound traveling through air, although with a very different speed. Table 4.2 gives speeds of sound characteristic of materials found in the body; for example, sound waves travel over twice as fast in bone (3500 m/s) as in soft tissues such as muscle (1570 m/s).

A wide range of values for frequency and corresponding wavelengths of sound in soft body tissues, such as blood, fat, and muscle, are given in Table 4.1. The frequencies useful for imaging body tissues lie in the

Table 4.1 Frequency and wavelength for sound waves in soft tissue

Frequency (Hz)	Wavelength
100	15.4 m
1000	1.54 m
10,000	15.4 cm
100,000	1.54 cm
1,000,000 = 1 MHz	1.54 mm
10,000,000 = 10 MHz	0.154 mm

Table 4.2 Some approximate values for speed
of sound and acoustic impedances
of different media

Material	Speed of sound, v_s (m/s)	Acoustic impedance, z [kg/(m²-s)]
Air	344	400
Fat	1440	1,300,000
Water	1500	1,500,000
Muscle	1570	1,650,000
Bone	3500	7,800,000

ultrasound—ranging roughly from 2 to 15 MHz—much higher than the audible frequency range.

Why these values of frequency and wavelength? The size of an object that can deflect a sound wave depends on the wavelength. If an object is smaller than one wavelength of the sound wave, it will not effectively reflect or bend the sound wave, while larger objects will be effective reflectors. This is one simple way that the wavelength of sound sets the spatial resolution of this technique. Thus, to use sound to detect the detailed shape of organs, a wavelength with dimensions equal to a few millimeters or smaller is called for. Note that the last two values of frequency in Table 4.1, 1 and 10 MHz, which roughly bracket the range of medical ultrasound frequencies, correspond to wavelengths small enough to reflect off features of an organ 1 millimeter or less in extent.

Sample calculation: For the case that interests us most here, v_s = 1540 m/s, an average value for soft tissue. (Note that this is a high speed, close to one mile per second.) Now we can compute the wavelengths that correspond to various frequencies in soft tissue. For example, for the ultrasound frequency of 2.0 MHz = 2.0 × 10⁶ Hz, what is the wavelength of sound in soft tissue? We first re-express Equation 4.1 to solve for wavelength:

$$\lambda = \frac{v_s}{f}$$

$$= \frac{1540 \text{ m/s}}{2.0 \times 10^6 \text{ Hz}} \tag{4.2}$$

$$= 7.7 \times 10^{-4} \text{ m} = 0.77 \text{ mm}$$

Sample calculation: What frequency of ultrasound must be used to image features 0.3 mm across? Assuming for now a spatial resolution set approximately by the wavelength, $\lambda = 0.30$ mm and the speed of sound for soft tissue in the body, we can solve Equation 4.1 for the frequency needed:

$$f = \frac{v_s}{\lambda}$$

$$= \frac{1540 \text{ m/s}}{0.30 \text{ mm}} \tag{4.3}$$

$$= 5.1 \times 10^6 = 5.1 \text{ MHz}$$

Thus, the frequency of ultrasound used should be equal to or exceed 5 MHz if features this small are to be imaged.

Speed of sound in different media: Why does the speed of sound vary from material to material? The exact value of v_s varies with density according to:

$$v_s = \sqrt{\frac{K}{\rho}} \tag{4.4}$$

where ρ stands for the **density** of the material, in units of kilograms per cubic meter, kg/m^3, and K is a number called the **elastic modulus,** which characterizes the stiffness of a material. This equation implies that sound travels at different speeds in media with different densities and stiffnesses. You might think that air and water are not stiff at all since you cannot bend or pull on them. In what sense do they have an elastic modulus? The stiffness referred to here is resistance to **compression.** For example, in the experiment shown in Figure 4.3, you would encounter stiffness while pushing against, or compressing, a column of gas or fluid with a piston.

An analogy with waves on a string may help at this point. A passing wave will move a dense string more slowly than a lighter one, and indeed waves travel more slowly on a denser string and a denser medium with greater ρ. Conversely, the more tightly the string is held, the more rapidly the disturbance will travel; the tension in the string

(continued on next page)

is analogous to K, the elastic modulus or stiffness of a material. Both of these effects are used in tuning string instruments. There, the overall length of the string is fixed, which fixes the wavelength of its vibrations. The speed of wavelike vibrations on the string, and hence their frequency, can then be varied by tightening the string, or by using heavier strings for the lower notes.

For similar reasons, different tissues with different densities and stiffnesses will also have different speeds of sound, as shown in Table 4.2. These changes in the speed of sound are one of the effects that allow different types of tissues to be distinguished in ultrasound imaging.

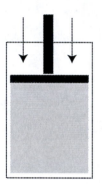

Figure 4.3 The elastic modulus, a measure of rigidity, can be defined even for materials such as gases or liquids by describing how much the volume changes when it is compressed by a piston at a constant pressure without letting the material flow out the sides.

4.4 ULTRASOUND AND ENERGY

Sound waves of all frequencies transport energy. However, unlike the situation for light waves (Chapter 3), the energy carried by the sound wave is not determined by the frequency of the sound wave. Instead, the energy of the wave is determined by *how far* about their average position the molecules vibrate. The maximum movement of the molecules is called the **amplitude** of the sound wave; it is analogous to the amplitude, A, of the wave on the shaken string (Figure 4.2a–b). This makes intuitive sense: more strongly vibrating molecules should have more energy than weakly vibrating ones.

Because the sound wave transports energy as it moves along, the waves also have an associated power. For example, a stereo's speakers are described by giving their power rating in watts. Since all of this power is seldom entirely intercepted, a more relevant measure is how much power is actually received by a particular listener. That is, a stereo may sound very loud close up, but soft very far away because your ears intercept less of the total power at greater distances. To characterize this loudness physically, we use the **intensity** of the sound, the power carried across a given area. (Note that this is identical to the concept of intensity or power density defined for light in Chapter 3.) Sound intensity is measured in units of watts/m².

Because the energy contained in a sound wave is determined by its amplitude, and not its frequency, ultrasound is inherently no more dangerous than ordinary sound. In both cases, the important consideration is the sound's intensity. The intensities of ultrasound waves used in imaging are much smaller than those encountered for laser surgery in Chapter 3. We will consider some typical values of intensity used in ultrasound imaging later in the chapter.

4.5 HOW ECHOES ARE FORMED

Medical ultrasound forms images by detecting echoes reflected from an interface between two body tissues. What properties of the two tissues determine the strength of the reflection? Changes in a new quantity called the **acoustic impedance** determine what fraction of a sound wave is reflected from an interface. The acoustic impedance, denoted by z, is the product of the medium's density, ρ, and the speed of sound in the medium.

$$z = \rho \times v_s \tag{4.5}$$

Acoustic impedance is measured in units of kg/(m²-sec) (also called a **rayle**). Table 4.2 gives values for the acoustic impedance for a variety of body tissues. Note the similarity of acoustic impedance values of all soft tissues, such as fat, water, and muscle, when compared to air and bone. Thus, the quantity that determines whether a sound wave is reflected depends upon not just the speed of sound (as was the case of light waves) but its product with the density as well.

For medical ultrasound imaging, we are primarily interested in the case of sound waves traveling perpendicular to an interface between tissues with acoustic impedances z_1 and z_2 (Figure 4.4a); for example, this situation would describe the reflection of ultrasound traveling from muscle into fat. The wave is partially reflected in exactly the opposite direction (in other words, it will return an echo), and is partially transmitted in the original direction. Let's define I_{total} as the sound intensity striking the interface, I_{refl} as the intensity of sound reflected from the interface, and I_{trans} as the intensity transmitted through the interface. Then, the fraction of the sound's intensity that is reflected is equal to the ratio between these intensities, I_{refl}/I_{total}, and the fraction that is transmitted is I_{trans}/I_{total}. Both of these fractions are determined by the difference between the two acoustic impedances by the following equations:

$$\frac{I_{refl}}{I_{total}} = \frac{\left(z_1 - z_2\right)^2}{\left(z_1 + z_2\right)^2}$$

$$\tag{4.6}$$

$$\frac{I_{trans}}{I_{total}} = 100\% - \frac{I_{refl}}{I_{total}}$$

The fraction of the sound's intensity that is reflected, and the fraction that is transmitted, are determined by the difference between the two acoustic impedances, but also by their sum. While the derivation of these equations is not intuitive, you can see how our statements above are embedded in the math. The amounts reflected and transmitted depend *only* on the fact that two different acoustic impedances are present on either side of the interface. If the acoustic impedances are equal ($z_1 = z_2$), *even if* the materials are different tissues, then no sound is reflected and the entire wave's intensity travels through to the other side of the interface. The larger the difference in acoustic impedances, the greater the reflected intensity.

Sample calculation: In medical ultrasound imaging, how much of the sound is reflected from a typical interface within the body? To determine this, we use the values shown in Table 4.2 to compute how much of the incident intensity is reflected from the interface between water and fat.

From Table 4.2, we have z_{fat} = 1,300,000 kg/(m²-sec) and z_{water} = 1,500,000 kg/(m²-sec). Because the direction the sound travels across the interface does not affect the amount of the sound reflected, it does not matter which acoustic impedance we call z_1 or z_2. Using Equation 4.6, we have:

$$\frac{I_{refl}}{I_{total}} = \frac{\left(z_1 - z_2\right)^2}{\left(z_1 + z_2\right)^2}$$

$$= \frac{\left(1,500,000 - 1,300,000\right)^2}{\left(1,500,000 + 1,300,000\right)^2} \tag{4.7}$$

$$= 0.51\%$$

$$\frac{I_{trans}}{I_{total}} = 100\% - \frac{I_{refl}}{I_{total}} = 99.49\%$$

Only 0.51% of the original intensity is reflected; 99.49% is transmitted.

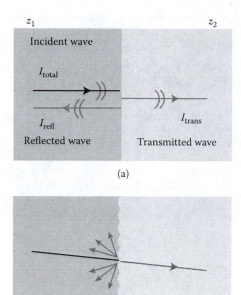

(a)

(b)

Figure 4.4 (a) Reflection of sound at an interface between materials with acoustic impedances z_1 and z_2. Part of the original sound wave incident on the interface is transmitted, and part is reflected, in analogy with the transmission and reflection of light waves discussed in Chapter 2. I_{total} is the total sound intensity incident upon the interface; I_{refl} is the intensity of sound reflected from the interface (the echo intensity); and I_{trans} is the intensity transmitted through the interface. The relationship between these intensities can be computed using the acoustic impedances and Equation 4.6. (b) Interfaces that are rough with irregularities on the scale of the wavelength of sound will produce scattered sound waves as well as specular reflections. (c) High-resolution ultrasound image of a breast lump, shown in cross section as the darker region at the upper left. The uniformly black region at left shows the appearance of a cyst (C), but the grainy region at right is solid (S). Distinctions such as these can be used to discriminate between solid tumors that could be cancerous and benign, fluid-filled cysts. (Used with permission courtesy of Steven Harms, M.D.)

Fortunately, the weak echoes that reflect off most body interfaces can be measured by diagnostic ultrasound imaging devices. Since different types of body liquids and soft tissues have very similar acoustic impedances, most of an ultrasound wave introduced into the body is transmitted, not reflected. This means that ultrasound waves can penetrate far enough within the body to generate echoes from interfaces between many different features.

This basic effect can be observed readily in a simple experiment. Join together two ropes of dissimilar thicknesses to represent a mismatch in

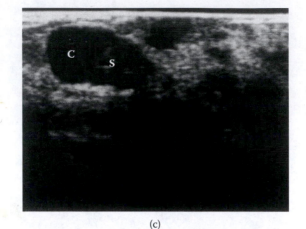

(c)

Figure 4.4 (continued).

acoustic impedance. Notice that when you shake one rope to create a wave pulse, the wave is reflected from the "interface" at the point where the two ropes meet. Stronger reflections result from greater mismatches, while if you join together two ropes of similar properties, the reflection is weaker.

Although the situation described above is the easiest to describe, in fact most interfaces within the body will be rough and irregular, giving rise to scattering at many angles, rather than one clear well-defined reflection (Figure 4.4b). In medical imaging, it is this effect that generates most of the echoes that are intercepted to form the ultrasound image, even if the interfaces are not oriented perpendicular to the original beam. Since the scattered reflections will be spread out in angles, the actual structure of the interfaces encountered will play a role in determining echo intensity; this reflector scattering strength is referred to as **echogenicity**. This means that calculations involving only the acoustic impedance serve merely as a useful estimate of the relative strengths of echoes due to two different interfaces. Structures that produce echoes with intensities *greater* than those from surrounding tissues are called **hyperechoic**, while those generating *weaker* echoes are called **hypoechoic**.

With this much information, we now can understand how physicians use ultrasound to distinguish between a solid tumor and a fluid-filled cyst (Figure 4.4c). The fluid filling a cyst has no irregularities to produce echoes within its structure, so sound travels through without reflection; we say such a region is **anechoic**. As a result, only the cyst's outer edges produce reflections. By contrast, a solid tumor consisting of solid tissues with varying densities will generate multiple echoes. The difference can be due to small reflections within the tumor such as those from tiny mineralized deposits called microcalcifications. By detecting the additional reflections from the tumor, diagnostic ultrasound can distinguish between harmless cysts and potentially dangerous solid tumors in the breasts and abdomen.

4.6 HOW TO PRODUCE ULTRASOUND

How is sound ordinarily generated? The method for producing sound always involves setting up a vibration in an object, called a transducer. A transducer is a device that changes one form of energy into another; a transducer for sound converts electrical energy into sound energy and vice versa. Vibrations set up in a sound transducer in turn induce compressions and rarefactions in the surrounding medium, through which the sound then travels.

You have already encountered a transducer that converts electrical energy into sound in the form of a stereo speaker (Figure 4.5a). In such a loudspeaker, a flexible cone-shaped diaphragm vibrates to create the sound waves you eventually hear as music. The diaphragm's center is attached to a coil of wire through which an electrical current flows. This coil surrounds a permanent magnet fixed to a support; whenever current flows through the coil, it moves because it experiences a force due to the interaction between the magnetic field and the electric current in the wire. Through this means, a fluctuating electric current can cause the attached diaphragm to deflect by varying amounts. A stereo system supplies to the coil an electrical current that varies with strength as a function of time, in a way that is determined by the signals recorded on the medium being played (a compact disc, radio station signal, etc.). The resulting vibrations of the diaphragm are communicated to the air, which conveys the sound waves corresponding to the music to your ears. In a microphone, the reverse process takes place: a delicate diaphragm vibrates in response to sound waves, moving a magnet whose motion induces an electrical current in the coil. This process converts sound into a time-varying electrical signal, which can be subsequently recorded on a tape or compact disc.

Ordinary loudspeakers cannot be induced to vibrate efficiently at ultrasound frequencies. Instead, the transducers used to generate ultrasound are constructed of ceramic discs. One type of material used to construct transducers, **piezoelectrics**, can be made to contract and expand by applying an electrical voltage across the opposing sides of a block of the ceramic. A related class of materials, called **magnetostrictives**, undergo the same changes when a magnetic field is applied. The ultrasound transducer operates in a fashion similar to the loudspeaker when a time-varying voltage or magnetic field is applied, vibrating in response and generating sound at its surfaces (Figure 4.5b). These systems can also be used in the reverse mode as sound detectors: when a sound wave causes the material to expand and contract, it responds by generating its own voltage or magnetic field. This signal can be measured and used to describe the sound received.

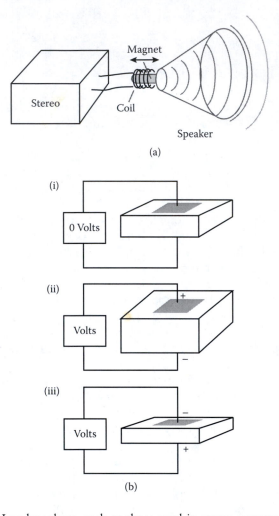

Figure 4.5 (a) Loudspeakers, such as those used in stereo systems, are a form of
transducer that converts electrical voltages into audible sound. A flexible conical diaphragm is connected to a magnet, which is surrounded
by a coil of wire. A time-varying electrical current through this wire
will result in a varying force being applied to the magnet. This force
causes the magnet and its attached diaphragm to vibrate, setting up
sound waves in the surrounding air. (b) One way of making a transducer that converts electrical signals into ultrasound waves is to use a
piezoelectric crystal. An electrical voltage is applied across the faces of
the piezoelectric crystal using metal electrodes. For zero applied voltage, the crystal is undeformed (i). Opposite polarity voltages cause the
crystal to either expand (ii) or contract (iii). When a time-varying voltage of alternating polarities is applied across it, piezoelectric crystal
will vibrate in response. The vibration of its surfaces are communicated
to the medium surrounding it, generating sound waves.

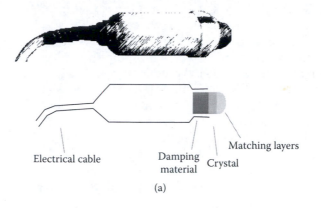

Electrical cable   Damping material   Crystal   Matching layers

(a)

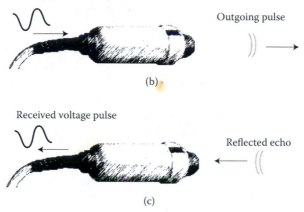

Voltage pulse transmitted

Outgoing pulse

(b)

Received voltage pulse

Reflected echo

(c)

Figure 4.6 (a) Schematic illustration of the design of an ultrasound transducer for medical imaging. A piezoelectric or magnetostrictive transducer, such as that discussed in Figure 4.5(b), vibrates to produce ultrasound waves. Matching layers between the crystal and the transducer's surface provide a transition to the acoustic impedance of skin. The transducer is designed so that a damping material quickly reduces the intensity of the ultrasound wave, resulting in only a short ultrasound pulse being emitted (b) or detected (c). An electrical cable conveys power to the transducer and provides electrical signals that determine the frequency and the intensity of transmitted pulses, as well as conveying to a computer the received electrical signals due to echoes.

The basic design for an ultrasound transducer used in imaging is shown in Figure 4.6(a). The vibrations of the transducer are communicated to the body through a fluid-filled head that is pressed against the skin. An electrical cable both supplies power to the device and collects signals from the transducer. The transducer device is backed with a material that damps out (absorbs) the vibrations after a short interval of time. As a result, when a signal is applied to the transducer to generate sound, the vibration only lasts for a short time and a short pulse of sound is produced (Figure 4.6b). Alternatively, when sound is received by the transducer, it vibrates for a brief interval of time, then is brought to rest by the damping material, turning a received pulse of sound into an electrical pulse (Figure 4.6c). Because the time between emitting and receiving echoes is long compared to this damping time, the same device can both emit an ultrasound pulse and detect returning echoes. Research into advanced materials has resulted in the creation of increasingly better transducers, including modern versions that make use of sophisticated composites (sandwiches of materials with different properties) to enable the transducer to operate at a selectable frequency.

4.7 IMAGES FROM ECHOES

Ultrasound imaging uses a method called the **pulse–echo** technique. The same basic idea is also employed in sonar systems, like the one used by some types of bats. To see how this works, consider the bat and its prey, a moth, located a distance, D, apart (Figure 4.7). The bat emits an ultrasound click, with frequencies in the tens of kHz, and this sound wave travels until it hits the moth. Upon hitting the moth, the sound wave reflects an echo, which travels back to the bat.

Both the original and echo sound waves travel at a speed of v_s on both legs of the trip. The total round-trip distance, $2D$, traveled by the echo equals the product of v_s and t, the time between the sending of the original click and the bat's hearing the echo.

$$2 \times D = v_s \times t \tag{4.8a}$$

$$D = \frac{v_s \times t}{2} \tag{4.8b}$$

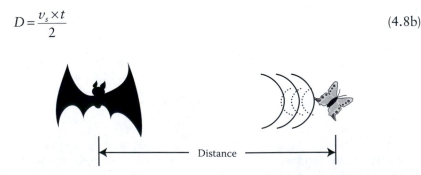

Figure 4.7 Bats use an ultrasound pulse–echo (sonar) system to detect the presence of their prey and to sense obstacles for navigational purposes. They accomplish this by emitting a loud burst of ultrasound, then waiting to hear the echo from a reflecting insect. The elapsed time is proportional to the distance to the insect, and can be computed using Equation 4.8.

In air, the value of v_s used in this computation would correspond to 344 m/s. (This is the same as saying, if you travel by car at 60 miles per hour for 2 hours, you know you have traveled 120 miles.) Thus, by knowing the echo's travel time, t, the bat can pinpoint how far away the insect is.

The same simple pulse–echo idea is used in medical ultrasound imaging (Figure 4.8). An ultrasound transducer generates a brief pulse of ultrasound, which is communicated into the patient's skin and continues onward into the body. Every time the pulse encounters an interface between tissues with two different acoustic impedances, an echo is reflected back to the transducer, which detects it a time, t, later. This time, t, is measured

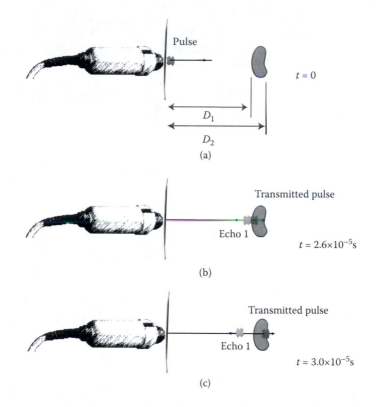

Figure 4.8 Schematic illustration of how an ultrasound transducer detects distances within the body using the pulse–echo technique. The transducer emits an ultrasound pulse (a) and detects returning echoes (b)–(f). Echoes are generated whenever the pulse travels across an interface between materials of different acoustic impedances (b) and (c); for example, the solid organ shown will generate echoes at the entrance and exit points. If we measure all times starting from emission of the pulse from the transducer, then the first echo is generated at a time 2.6×10^{-5} s (b) and the transducer detects this echo at a time $2 \times (2.6 \times 10^{-5}$ s) = 5.2×10^{-5} s (e). The second echo is generated at a time 3.0×10^{-5} s (c) after the pulse was emitted, and detected at 6.0×10^{-5} s (f).

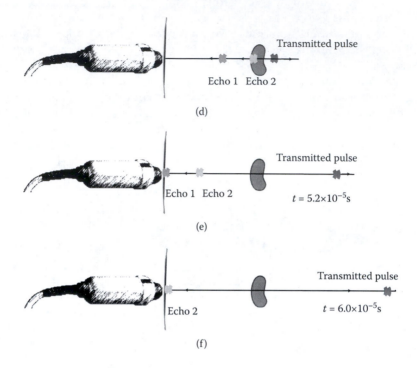

Figure 4.8 (continued).

and used to determine the distance from the transducer to the reflecting interface. For most purposes, a good distance estimate is obtained by using the average value of the speed of sound in soft tissue of 1540 m/s. For Figure 4.8, the main obstacles encountered by the ultrasound pulse are the interfaces between the solid kidney-shaped organ and the surrounding tissue. Echoes are generated when the pulse enters and exits the organ, because the ultrasound encounters a boundary between different acoustic impedances there.

Sample calculation: Assume ultrasound echoes are received from two interfaces of an organ in the path of the ultrasound pulse. The time between sending the original pulse and receiving the echoes are 4.0 $\times 10^{-5}$ s and 8.0 $\times 10^{-5}$ s (see Figure 4.9a). Assume that the speed of sound is 1540 m/s on average along the pathway. How far from the transducer are the interfaces? How wide across is the organ at this point?

(continued on next page)

We use Equation 4.8(b) to compute the distances:

$$D = \frac{v_s \times t}{2} \tag{4.9a}$$

$$D_1 = (1540 \text{ m/s} \times 4.0 \times 10^{-5} \text{ s})/2 = 0.031 \text{ m} = 3.1 \text{ cm} \tag{4.9b}$$

$$D_2 = (1540 \text{ m/s} \times 8.0 \times 10^{-5} \text{ s})/2 = 0.062 \text{ m} = 6.2 \text{ cm} \tag{4.9c}$$

These are the distances to the front and rear interfaces of the organ. The difference between these two numbers gives the dimension along the ultrasound pulse's path: 6.2 cm – 3.1 cm = 3.1 cm. The organ is 3.1 cm wide along this direction.

Sample calculation: Ultrasound imaging machines send out pulses constantly at what is called the **pulse repetition rate, R_{rep}**; this value must be chosen so that the returning echoes from one pulse do not overlap with the next outgoing pulse. For example, a pulse repetition rate of 1 kHz would give the pulses time to travel a distance given by:

$$T = 1/R_{rep} = 1/1 \text{ kHz} = 1/10^{-3} \text{ Hz} = 10^{-3} \text{ s}$$

$$D = v_s T/2 = 1540 \text{ m/s} \times 10^{-3} \text{ s}/2 = 0.77 \text{ m}$$

This is much greater than any distances within the body realistically accessible by ultrasound, so this pulse repetition rate would be slow enough to keep echoes separate.

The intensity of the echo returned is determined in part by how much of a difference in acoustic impedances the wave encountered at the interface. Since typical contrasts between soft tissue give an echo that is at most only a few percent of the original beam, most of the sound continues to travel deeper within the body. As discussed earlier, even these weak echoes can be detected by the transducer while the transmitted beam continues to encounter further interfaces and send back still more echoes, which are used to determine the distances and echo intensities. (In operation, the intensity of the original ultrasound pulse diminishes due to two other effects: absorption of the ultrasound by body tissue and the spreading of the pulse at large distances. These topics, and how the scanner compensates for them, are treated in a later section of this chapter.)

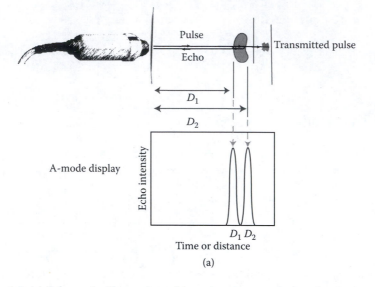

Figure 4.9 (a) Schematic illustration of how images are produced using an ultrasound scanner. The transducer produces an ultrasound pulse that travels in a well-defined beam deep into the body. Echoes are generated
whenever an interface with a different acoustic impedance is encountered. In the simple case shown, this happens when the pulse enters
and exits an organ with an acoustic impedance that differs from its
surroundings. The reflected echoes then travel back to the transducer,
which registers the time elapsed since the original pulse. This travel
time information is used to compute D_1 and D_2, the distances to the
front and back edges of the organ, using Equation 4.8, and the average speed of sound in soft tissues. An A-scan displays the results of an
ultrasound measurement for a single pulse pathway. In an A-scan, the
intensity of the echoes is plotted along the Y-axis as a function of the
distance to the interfaces generating each echo (the X-axis). This gives
the location of the interfaces within the body generating echoes, but
only along one line. (b) A B-scan constructs a picture of the inside of the
body by combining the results of many A-scans into one image. Each
line of the B-scan video image corresponds to one of the pulse paths
shown in (a). The image is generated by plotting a point on the monitor at positions proportional to the pulse echo times, with a brightness
determined by the echo intensity.

There are several ways of displaying the data from an ultrasound scanner, only two of which we will discuss here. An **A-scan** is a simple plot of
echo intensity versus distance made from the echoes received as a pulse
of ultrasound travels along one direction (Figure 4.9a). While the A-scan
directly displays the locations of interfaces creating echoes along one
direction, it does not give a clear picture of spatial structure within the
body. A more informative way of displaying this information, called the
B-scan (Figure 4.9b), instead uses a television monitor to plot both distance
and echo intensity everywhere within a cross-sectional region. A B-scan

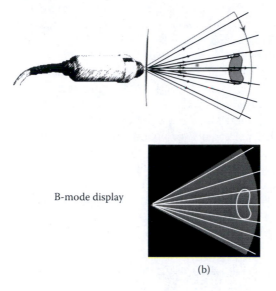

B-mode display

(b)

Figure 4.9 (continued).

compiles a two-dimensional image that resembles a cross-sectional slice of the body. Each line in a B-scan corresponds to a path traveled by an ultrasound pulse within the body. Echo-ranging is used to determine the locations of interfaces within the body, just as in the A-scan. However, the echo intensity received from each interface is used to determine the *brightness* of the monitor along this direction. For example, an interface between soft tissue and cartilage (with very different acoustic impedances, and hence large echo intensities) would appear as a very bright region, while a similar interface between fat and muscle (with very similar acoustic impedances, generating weaker echoes) would be lighter gray. This mapping of some measured quantity—in this case, echo intensity—into displayed brightness levels is called a **gray-scale image**.

As described so far, the B-scan only provides a single line of information about one path. After one pathway has been scanned and plotted, the direction of the ultrasound pulse is changed, and the entire process repeated. Multiple adjacent beam paths are scanned in sequence and the resulting distances and echo intensities are displayed side by side to gradually compile a cross-sectional image. After the full scan is complete, the B-scan will show bright spots that delineate the entire outline of the organ (Figure 4.9b). One can think of the cross-sectional image's relation to the entire body as similar to that of a single slice taken from a loaf of bread. At present, with most ultrasound scanners, one sees only a single "slice" of the body at a time. The exact orientation of the slice depends upon how the transducer is oriented. The plane swept out by the ultrasound pulse is the plane in which the cross-sectional image is generated.

The time to send and receive pulses is fairly short—less than a millisecond in practice. This makes it possible to collect ultrasound images as quickly as a television camera does, then rapidly play them back in sequence, like the frames of a motion picture. This means that motions of the body can be imaged in real-time, and that many different views can be examined during a single session. The images can be stored or printed as stills on film, in addition to being examined by the radiologist or other physician. The brain has the ability to retain an image for an instant after it has disappeared, an effect called persistence of vision. In practice, this means that the images reproduced in texts seem lower in quality than what the physician sees on the monitor, just as the freeze-frame option on a VCR usually has poorer picture quality than a live picture.

Figure 4.10 shows various commercial diagnostic ultrasound apparatuses. The basic components are interchangeable transducer units, a television monitor for viewing the images, electronics for producing and

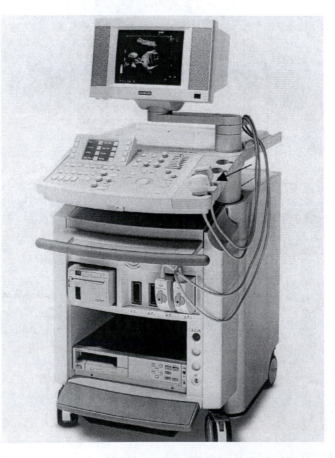

Figure 4.10 Typical commercial diagnostic ultrasound imaging device. Various transducers are indicated by the arrow. (Reproduced with permission courtesy of Siemens Medical Group.)

analyzing the pulses, a computer for manipulating images and controlling the scanner, a videocassette recorder, and a video printer. The entire assembly is usually mounted on a cart to enable it to be easily wheeled about to the patient's bedside. An intermediate buffering layer of gel smeared between the skin and transducer head helps to reduce reflections at the surface of the skin by reducing the change in acoustic impedance between the skin, any intervening air, and the transducer head.

4.8 ULTRASOUND SCANNER DESIGN

Ultrasound scanners offer a variety of formats for producing scans, depending on the exact transducer design employed. The shape of the actual scan produced depends upon which of several methods are employed for scanning the ultrasound pulse's direction (Figure 4.11a–c). Some transducers have a crystal (or crystals), which is mechanically oscillated or rotated so the ultrasound beam sweeps out an arc-shaped path within the body (Figure 4.11a); the resulting pie-shaped scans are referred to as **sector scans**. Others consist of multiple individual transducer elements that can be independently activated to produce or receive ultrasound. A rectangular array of such elements arranged in a straight line is called a **linear array** and produces a rectangular-shaped scan (Figure 4.11b), while a similar arrangement with the elements laid out in a curved geometry is called a **curvilinear array** transducer (Figure 4.11c). The resulting scans cover a wider, arc-shaped field of view than linear arrays. Both linear and curvilinear arrays work by the same basic principle: starting at one end, a small set of adjacent array elements (e.g., 1–4) are activated to transmit a beam of ultrasound and receive echoes along a well-defined direction (Figure 4.12a). After the echoes have all returned, a second set of elements is activated, but this set is shifted over relative to the first set (2–5) (Figure 4.12a). The scan proceeds with the ultrasound beam being gradually swept in direction from side to side to allow the compilation of a B-scan image.

No single method of scanning is superior, so scanners are equipped with a variety of interchangeable transducers to suit varying applications. For example, sector and curvilinear scans may be desirable in applications where the ultrasound beam must pass through a narrow window (e.g., in cardiology, the sound must pass between the ribs to reach the heart); on the other hand, these scanners produce a narrow field of view near the surface, which would be undesirable in scanning structures located just beneath the skin.

A second way in which ultrasound arrays are utilized involves the need to focus ultrasound. When sound is generated by a small vibrating object, it spreads in concentric spheres, instead of a straight line (Figure 4.12b), analogous to the water waves produced when you drop a pebble into water. The water waves will spread out in a circle from the pebble's splash; similarly, when you speak, people on all sides of you can hear, because the sound waves also spread out in almost every direction. However, this has

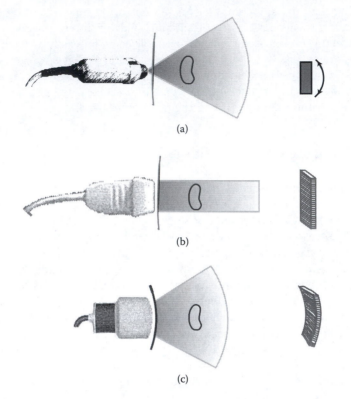

Figure 4.11 Examples of some of the different types of ultrasound scan formats. (a) Sector scans result when the transducer produces ultrasound pulses whose paths are swept out into a fan-shaped region, by either rotating or oscillating the transducer element. (b) Linear scans result from the transducer producing ultrasound pulses that travel along pathways that are scanned in parallel by a linear array (right) across a region of the body. This yields a rectangular image. (c) An arc-shaped arrangement of array elements (right) results in a curvilinear scan format.

the disadvantage of spreading the energy of the sound wave out over larger and larger areas.

To avoid this problem, a focused beam of sound can be achieved in one of two ways: either by using an acoustic lens to focus the sound into a well-defined beam or by using a special configuration of transducers called a **phased array**. The last method is a powerful idea that emerged from similar applications in radioastronomy (the study of the universe by detecting radio waves.) Advances in this field continue to yield unexpected benefits for medical ultrasound. To understand how a phased array works, first think of what happens when a single transducer produces a pulse. Each individual transducer by itself emits a spherical ultrasound wave in the absence of focusing (Figure 4.12b). If two elements in an array fire and produce waves, when their two waves overlap, the disturbances caused by each wave add to form a summed wave, a phenomenon called **superposition**

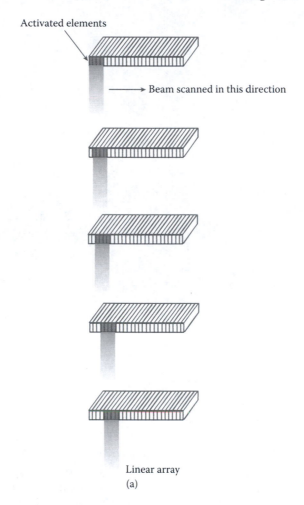

Activated elements

Beam scanned in this direction

Linear array

(a)

Figure 4.12 (a) Illustration of how a linear array produces a scan. Segments of array elements are activated in turn, producing a beam of ultrasound that travels into the body. After all echoes from this direction have been received, a new set of elements is activated at a different location along the array. By this means, the beam's pathway is swept from side to side to create the entire B-scan.

(Figure 4.12c–d). When the waves' crests overlap, they reinforce to form a wave with an amplitude equal to their summed amplitudes (Figure 4.12c); this effect is referred to as **constructive interference**. By contrast, when a wave crest overlaps a wave trough, the two cancel out, leaving no disturbance (Figure 4.12d); this is called **destructive interference**.

In a phased array, several transducers are individually fired at a slightly different time, each producing an ultrasound pulse that leaves the transducer at varying times (Figure 4.12e). This is represented by the circular waves spreading from the transducers, where the larger circles were emitted

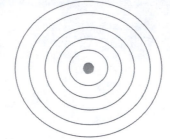

Circular waves on surface of water due to dropped pebble

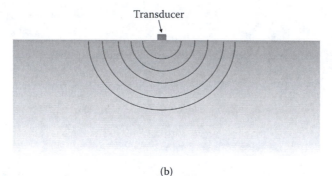

Transducer

(b)

Figure 4.12 (continued) (b) When a pebble is dropped into water, circular waves
spread out in all directions from the point of impact. Similarly, a single
ultrasound transducer would produce waves that spread out uniformly
in all directions.

by the first transducers to fire and the smaller circles emitted later. (This
is true because the waves emitted first have had longer for their crests to
reach the greater distances shown.) The net result of this constructive and
destructive interference is to create a new wavefront with a crest represented by the black arc, which is focused as shown (Figure 4.12e). The
curvature of the new wavefront is due to the fact that the summed waves
have their crests coinciding along the circle indicated. These new circular
patterns of crests and troughs can be made to converge and focus once
again before spreading out by careful choice of the timing between pulses
of each transducer element. The net effect is a beam of focused ultrasound
(Figures 4.12f–g and 4.13b–d).

Phased arrays can either be made from a linear array of transducers
(Figure 4.12g) or a set of concentric rings of transducers energized in turn.
The latter arrangement is called an **annular phased array** (Figure 4.12f). It
has the advantage that the beam can be focused in two directions, while linear arrays can only accomplish focusing in one dimension. A phased array
can form a well-defined, focused beam of sound and even automatically
sweep its direction. Phased arrays can either give linear scans (for linear
arrays) or sector-shaped scans (for annular arrays). Much of the progress

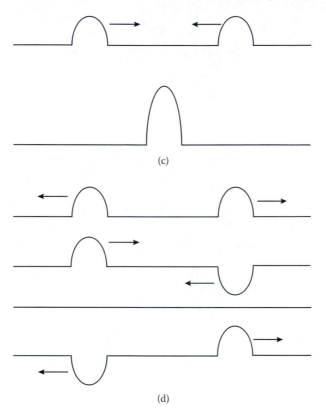

(c)

(d)

Figure 4.12 (continued) (c) When two wave crests overlap, they reinforce to form a wave with an amplitude equal to their summed amplitudes, an effect called **constructive interference**. (d) When a wave crest overlaps a wave trough, a situation called **destructive interference**, the two cancel out, leaving no disturbance.

in modern diagnostic instrument design has arisen from better designs for focusing phased array scanners to give better spatial resolution through more tightly focused beams.

4.9 ULTRASOUND IS ABSORBED BY THE BODY

The energy carried by an ultrasound beam is absorbed gradually by the body tissues encountered along its pathway. This is important for two reasons: (1) for a given pulse intensity, absorption will eventually make the pulses too weak to return detectable echoes, limiting the depth within the body to which ultrasound images can be formed; and (2) since energy is conserved, the lost energy must be accounted for to ensure it does not result in damage to the body, an issue addressed in the next section.

Fortunately, the absorption of sound in the body is reasonably weak over the distances of interest; the *exact* degree to which ultrasound is absorbed

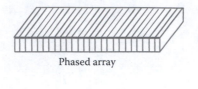

Phased array

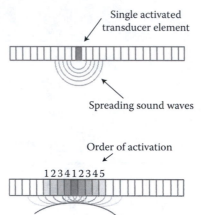

Single activated
transducer element

Spreading sound waves

Order of activation

1 2 3 4 1 2 3 4 5

Focused summed wavefront

(e)

Figure 4.12 (continued) (e) When an array of transducers produce ultrasound
waves, their individual waves sum to produce a new wave by the superposition phenomena described in (c) and (d). The shape of this new
wave is determined by the relationship between when each transducer
fired to produce its wave. In a phased array, several transducers are
fired at slightly different times, each producing an ultrasound pulse that
leaves the transducer at varying times. This is represented by the circular waves spreading from the transducers, where the larger circles were
emitted by the first transducers to fire and the smaller circles emitted
later. The new, focused wavefront is shown as the darker circle.

depends strongly on its frequency. Table 4.3 compares the absorption of
sound by soft tissue at various frequencies by comparing the depth at which
half of the sound's original intensity will have been absorbed, a quantity
termed the **half-intensity depth,** $L_{1/2}$. A long half-intensity depth means the
sound can travel a long way, a short one means it gets absorbed within a
very short distance. Note that *lower* frequencies get absorbed *less* readily,
higher frequencies *more* readily.[*]

   In fact, the half-intensity depth is inversely proportional to frequency.
That is, the ultrasound frequency 5 MHz has a half-intensity depth, $L_{1/2}$,

---

[*] This has been dubbed the "disco moron effect," because when your next door neighbor's
stereo is booming at 2 a.m., you can hear the bass (low frequencies) quite clearly, but the
treble (high frequencies) get absorbed by the walls before reaching you.

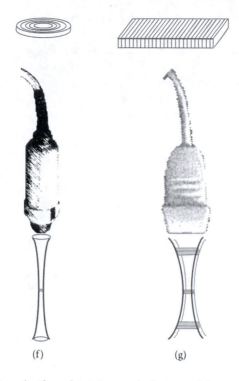

(f)   (g)

Figure 4.12 (continued) (f) and (g) Focused ultrasound beams resulting from an (f) annular or (g) linear-phased array transducer.

Table 4.3 Absorption of ultrasound in human soft tissue

Frequency (MHz)	Wavelength (mm)	Half-intensity depth, $L_{1/2}$ (cm)
1.00	1.54	6.0
5.00	0.31	1.2
10.0	0.154	0.6

Source: Frederick W. Kremkau, *Diagnostic Ultrasound: Principles, Instruments, and Exercises*, W.B. Saunders, Philadelphia, 1993.

of 1.2 cm, but *twice* that frequency, 10 MHz, has an $L_{1/2}$, of only 0.6 cm, *one-half* that of 5 MHz. Thus, an ultrasound pulse with frequency 10 MHz can travel only half as far as a pulse with frequency 5 MHz before suffering the same amount of absorption. We can express this mathematical relationship between ultrasound frequency and half-intensity depth, $L_{1/2}$, using the following equation:

$$L_{1/2} = \frac{C}{f} \tag{4.10}$$

The constant, C (which has no special name), has a value that depends only on the medium in which the sound is traveling. For a given material, and hence a particular value of C, choosing the frequency also determines how far the sound will be able to travel. The values of frequency and half-intensity depth in Table 4.3 allow us to determine how far within the body any ultrasound frequency can travel before being absorbed by any fraction. Figure 4.14(a) shows this mathematical relationship graphically for two ultrasound frequencies of interest.

Sample calculation: Abdominal ultrasound imaging can be performed at a frequency of 3 MHz. From Table 4.3, we can solve for the value of C for soft tissue and use it to compute the half-intensity depth for 3 MHz.

$$C = L_{\frac{1}{2}} f \tag{4.11}$$

$$= 6.0 \text{ cm} \times 1 \text{ MHz}$$

Although this calculation used the value of half-intensity depth corresponding to 1 MHz, the same value of C would have resulted from any of the other entries. Now we can use this value for C to find $L_{1/2}$ for the 3 MHz sound:

$$C = 6.0 \text{ cm} \times 1 \text{ MHz}$$

$$= L_{1/2} f \tag{4.12}$$

$$= L_{1/2} \times 3 \text{ MHz}$$

$$L_{1/2} = \frac{6.0 \text{ cm} \times 1 \text{ MHz}}{3 \text{ MHz}} \tag{4.13}$$

$$= 2 \text{ cm}$$

So the half-intensity depth for 3 MHz sound is 2 cm. Because for every 2 cm that the pulse travels, its intensity diminishes by 1/2, we can also compute that its intensity is reduced to 25% of the original in 4 cm: ($1/2 \times 1/2 = 25\%$), about 13% in 6 cm: ($1/2 \times 1/2 \times 1/2 = 0.125 \approx 13\%$) and about 3% in 10 cm: $(1/2)^5 \approx 0.03 = 3\%$ (Figure 4.14a).

A diagnostic ultrasound instrument can compensate for the absorption of ultrasound by the body, thus giving a more accurate image of tissue deep within the body. However, the relation between frequency and absorption effectively limits how high a frequency can be used without being absorbed within a centimeter or so of the skin. We can see this more clearly by examining Figure 4.13, which shows simple test objects imaged with varying ultrasound frequencies. The smallest discernible spatial details are sharpest

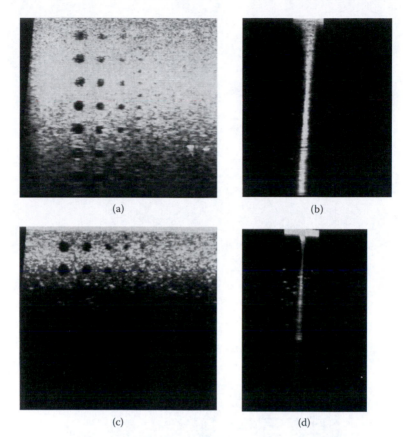

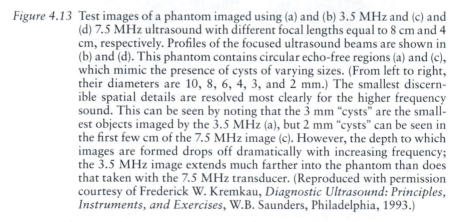

Figure 4.13 Test images of a phantom imaged using (a) and (b) 3.5 MHz and (c) and (d) 7.5 MHz ultrasound with different focal lengths equal to 8 cm and 4 cm, respectively. Profiles of the focused ultrasound beams are shown in (b) and (d). This phantom contains circular echo-free regions (a) and (c), which mimic the presence of cysts of varying sizes. (From left to right, their diameters are 10, 8, 6, 4, 3, and 2 mm.) The smallest discernible spatial details are resolved most clearly for the higher frequency sound. This can be seen by noting that the 3 mm "cysts" are the smallest objects imaged by the 3.5 MHz (a), but 2 mm "cysts" can be seen in the first few cm of the 7.5 MHz image (c). However, the depth to which images are formed drops off dramatically with increasing frequency; the 3.5 MHz image extends much farther into the phantom than does that taken with the 7.5 MHz transducer. (Reproduced with permission courtesy of Frederick W. Kremkau, *Diagnostic Ultrasound: Principles, Instruments, and Exercises*, W.B. Saunders, Philadelphia, 1993.)

for the higher frequency sound, but the depth to which these images are formed drops off dramatically for the higher frequency images. This is shown by the shallow image formed by 7.5 MHz ultrasound pulses in Figure 4.13(c) and (d) compared to the deeper images in Figure 4.13(a) and (b) obtained with 3.5 MHz ultrasound.

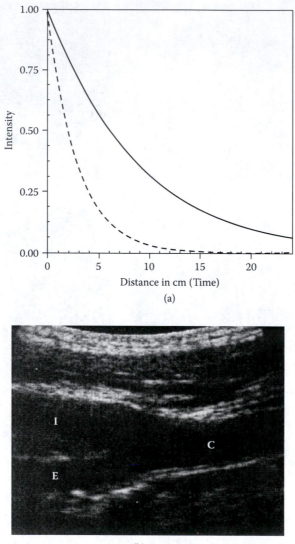

(a)

(b)

Figure 4.14 Illustration of how attenuation and spatial resolution depend on ultrasound frequency. (a) Plot of ultrasound intensity as a function of distance
into the absorber, illustrating the exponential falloff. The intensity of
ultrasound diminishes by a factor of one-half after each half-intensity
depth, $L_{1/2}$. Ultrasound is more strongly absorbed by higher frequency
ultrasound, as indicated by the more rapid attenuation of 3 MHz (dashed
line) when compared with 1 MHz (solid line) intensities. (b) Image of
a normal carotid artery, shown in cross section along its length. The
carotid arteries provide blood to the head; in the neck, their relatively
superficial location allows ultrasound imaging with high resolution
transducers. (Reproduced with permission, Hylton B. Meire and Pat
Farrant, *Basic Ultrasound*. John Wiley & Sons, New York, 1995.)

The smallest feature discernible using ultrasound defines its spatial resolution. The spatial resolution of an ultrasound measurement is most fundamentally limited by the wavelength of the sound being used. However, we now see from the preceding discussion that one cannot use arbitrarily small wavelengths to see finer details because eventually the high frequencies required will be absorbed before reaching the region of interest. This means that two concerns must be balanced in selecting a frequency for ultrasound imaging: the depth to which the image will be formed and the spatial resolution of the image. Consequently, a lower frequency (longer wavelength) is used to see deep within the abdomen, while at higher frequencies (shorter wavelengths) finer details can be resolved, but only close to the surface. Consequently, a frequency higher than that used for abdominal imaging (roughly 3 MHz) can be used for breast ultrasound (7.5 to 10 MHz) because much shallower regions of the body must be imaged in the latter procedure. The higher spatial resolution made possible with higher frequencies can also be taken advantage of if the transducer can be introduced into the body. Thus, probes designed for use in the esophagus, vagina, and rectum are more invasive and less pleasant for the patient, but they do overcome the problems of absorption simply by being located near the region of interest.

Sample calculation: A physician wishes to see the internal structure of the carotid arteries, located relatively superficially below the skin of the neck (Figure 4.14b). Abdominal ultrasound imaging can be performed with ultrasound of frequency 3 MHz, which allows imaging to a depth of somewhat over 10 cm. If similar conditions are used in imaging one of the carotid arteries, which of the following frequencies would be the most appropriate: (a) 1 MHz, (b) 5 MHz, (c) 10 MHz, (d) 15 MHz? What is the best spatial resolution available in this situation?

Ultrasound with frequency 3 MHz allows one to see to a depth of at least 10 cm within the body, when combined with commonly used pulse characteristics. For the carotid one would wish to have the ultrasound penetrate only a few cm, say roughly 2 cm, before undergoing the same amount of absorption. This allows the use of a higher frequency, which also can resolve more of the fine spatial details in a small structure, such as one of the carotid arteries. Equation 4.10 indicates that if we wish to see only one-fifth as deeply into the body, we can use a frequency up to five times as high: 5×3 MHz = 15 MHz. We see from Table 4.3 that 15 MHz corresponds to a wavelength of roughly 0.1 mm. (Other limits on the spatial resolution can emerge from constraints mentioned later in this chapter.) This frequency is small enough to allow the resolution of detailed anatomy and blood flow within the carotid arteries. Such imaging is important in diagnosing the obstruction of these blood vessels by fatty deposits called plaque.

In addition to the falloff of sound intensity due to the absorption of ultrasound by the body, ultrasound scanners need to compensate for the eventual spreading of the sound waves with distance, which also causes the intensity to drop. We can see how the falloff in intensity of ultrasound waves with distance can be modeled and compensated for in a simple case. We will assume that a transducer produces ultrasound pulses that travel in all directions, like the light from a lightbulb. (Compare Figures 4.12b and 3.10.) We assume the ultrasound wave is spread out uniformly at a distance, R, from the transducer, and compute by how much its intensity is diminished as a result. The entire starting intensity of the transducer is spread out over an area equal to a sphere with radius, R; think of this as a large imaginary balloon surrounding the transducer, through which the ultrasound must pass before continuing on its way. The ultrasound waves will be less concentrated the larger we draw the balloon. We can treat the resulting falloff of intensity mathematically by noting that the initial power, P, in the ultrasound wave is fixed, but the area over which it is spread increases as the area, A, of the spherical balloon increases, according to the formula $4\pi R^2$. Since the power is uniformly distributed over this area, the intensity falls off by 1 over the area, or $1/R^2$.

$$I = \frac{P}{A} = \frac{P}{4\pi R^2} \propto \frac{1}{R^2} \tag{4.14}$$

This formula can be used to compensate for the intensity falloff due to the spread of the beam alone. The nature of this falloff of intensity with distance is identical to that derived in Chapter 3 for the incoherent, unfocused light source as well. In general, *any* source of waves will follow this same geometrical rule. Calculations also can be used to compute the more complex decrease in intensity due to focused ultrasound beams.

How "loud" is ultrasound? To explain the intensity of an ultrasound wave, we need to first define several features of the pulses and how often they are emitted. Since ultrasound for imaging purposes is emitted in pulses, one can either define intensities that describe the intensity *during a pulse*, or the intensity *averaged over several pulses*, which takes into account the time between pulses during which no ultrasound is present. (This distinction is similar to that defined in Chapter 3 for pulsed versus continuous wave lasers.) The average intensities used in medical ultrasound imaging range from roughly 0.00001 watt/cm^2 to roughly 0.7 watt/cm^2. (Note that these are very small values compared to those used in laser surgery, as explained in Chapter 3. For comparison, a typical conversation at arm's length would be 3×10^{-10} watts/cm^2, while long-term exposure to *audible*

(continued on next page)

sounds with intensities over 10^{-4} watts/cm^2 can damage the human ear. Since the ear does not respond to ultrasound waves, ultrasound intensities used for imaging are not detected by the human ear and do not damage that organ.) These numbers are only averages, however, during pulses, the intensity can be much higher. On the other hand, the inevitable absorption and spreading of the sound waves causes the intensity to vary, and in general diminish, as the pulses travel into the body. Researchers have conducted extensive safety studies, discussed in a later section of this chapter, to establish that the absorption of relatively intense ultrasound by the body does not result in enough energy being absorbed to cause harm.

4.10 LIMITATIONS OF ULTRASOUND: IMAGE QUALITY AND ARTIFACTS

Many effects can distort the image formed by a diagnostic ultrasound instrument, leading to poor spatial resolution or even images of nonexistent structures. In many clinical situations, confidence in the accuracy of the dimensions of the ultrasound image is essential. Fortunately, many of these distortions and artifacts can be explained, or avoided, by understanding more about how sound waves travel through tissue.

The attenuation of sound waves as they travel through the body results in echoes with decreasing intensity with increasing depth. To offset this, ultrasound scanners compensate for attenuation by a fixed formula that increases the brightness of images with distance using the half-intensity depth relationship. However, this means that any deviation from the expected absorption will introduce errors in brightness. This can result in **acoustic shadowing** if a very absorbing (or very reflective) region effectively prevents the ultrasound pulses from traveling farther into the body, creating a dark region (the "shadow") where no reflections were detected. Conversely, **acoustic enhancement** of the image brightness will occur if a less absorbing region is present, and the scanner overcompensates for its actual attenuation. Since transducers also focus the ultrasound beam, scanners must compensate mathematically for the variation in beam intensity due to the focused beam, or else brightness artifacts will result.

The **lateral resolution** (the resolution perpendicular to the direction of travel) of an ultrasound image is determined by the ultrasound beam's diameter at each point. This can be seen from Figure 4.15(a) and (b), which illustrates how interfaces must be separated by a distance greater than the beam diameter to return distinct echoes in a scan. The lateral resolution can change with distance into the body for a focused beam (Figure 4.13). The beam is focused to improve the spatial resolution within a region of tissue, but the resulting beam is not as nearly parallel as a beam of laser light. Instead, the ultrasound wave converges near the focal point, and

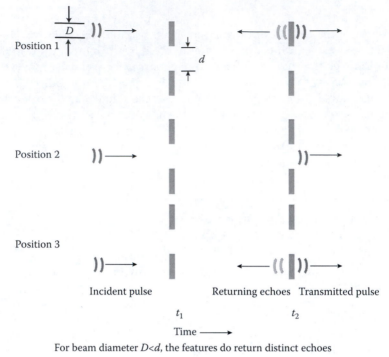

For beam diameter $D<d$, the features do return distinct echoes

(a)

Figure 4.15 Illustration of how lateral resolution depends on beam diameter. An ultrasound pulse with diameter, D, is incident upon two reflectors a distance, d, apart. (a) If $D < d$, then the reflected ultrasound intensity drops to zero as the beam is scanned, and the separation between the two interfaces can be resolved. (b) If $D > d$, then there is no beam position for which the reflected intensity goes to zero, and the two interfaces do not appear as distinct on the resulting image.

then diverges before and after that point. This means that the width of the beam, hence the lateral resolution, varies throughout the body; as a result, details that could be seen clearly near the focus can become blurred in the region where the beam has widened appreciably. For example, breast tissue directly beneath a transducer will not receive the most tightly focused beam so it will be imaged at lower resolution. To ensure that the region of interest in the body corresponds to the region of best resolution, impedance-matching **gel standoff pads** can be used in between the transducer and the body as a spacer. This enables the focused region to extend throughout a structure such as the breast, rather than lying deep within the body. In addition, the representation of the ultrasound pulses as forming a single focused beam may be inaccurate, as the pulse's energy may be spread out in angle into weaker beams called "side lobes." In this case, the ultrasound scanner can misinterpret additional echoes resulting from the side lobes reflecting off neighboring structures. These are indistinguishable from echoes arising

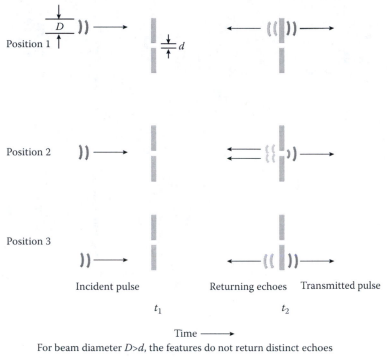

Position 1

Position 2

Position 3

Incident pulse   Returning echoes   Transmitted pulse

t_1 t_2

Time ⟶

For beam diameter $D>d$, the features do not return distinct echoes

(b)

Figure 4.15 (continued).

from reflections along the main beam's pathway, so the image formed can contain artifacts in the form of structures displaced from their true positions.

The length of the pulse, L, along its direction of travel also places an additional limit on the **axial resolution** of an image (the resolution along the pulse's travel). To see this, we ask what is the smallest separation, d, between two reflective objects that can be detected by a pulse of length, L (Figure 4.16). For objects far apart compared to the pulse length, there is no overlap between the two echoes and the distances to each can be clearly measured ($d > L/2$, Figure 4.16a). However, for objects less than $L/2$ apart, the echoes will overlap and no distinction between the two objects' positions is possible ($d < L/2$, Figure 4.16b). In other words, shorter pulses (hence, smaller L) give higher axial resolution; this means that very short ultrasound pulses, equal to only one or several wavelengths, are used in imaging applications. For this case, the axial resolution is then determined by:

$$d = n\lambda/2 \qquad (4.15)$$

where n is the number of wavelengths per pulse. While the exact values of the axial and lateral resolution depend on many factors, including frequency,

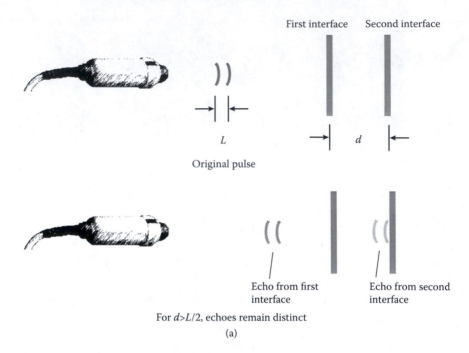

Figure 4.16 The axial resolution is the ability of an ultrasound scanner to distinguish structures along the direction of the pulse's pathway. This is
limited by the length, L, of the original pulse. (a) Distinct echoes result
for two interfaces a distance d apart if $d > L/2$. (b) The interfaces will
generate overlapping echoes if $d < L/2$

pulse length, and transducer design, in general the axial resolution will be
equal to or better than that in the lateral direction. This dependence of
spatial resolution on ultrasound frequency via Equation 4.15 can be seen
in Figure 4.13, where the higher frequency 7.5 MHz scan in Figure 4.13(a)
resolves smaller reflectors than does a scan performed at a lower frequency
(3.5 MHz, Figure 4.13c).

Several problems in ultrasound imaging result from effects easy to understand as applications of simple ideas from geometrical optics. For example,
we have not considered echoes that form along a returning echo's pathway,
because a second echo formed from a first echo is generally too weak to be
significant. However, when two *strongly* reflecting interfaces are located
near each other, the ultrasound beam indeed can bounce multiple times
between the two, creating spurious multiple high-intensity reflections called
reverberations, which show up as bands on the ultrasound image. This can
occur, for example, when the bowels are filled with gas, creating highly
reflective nearby interfaces.

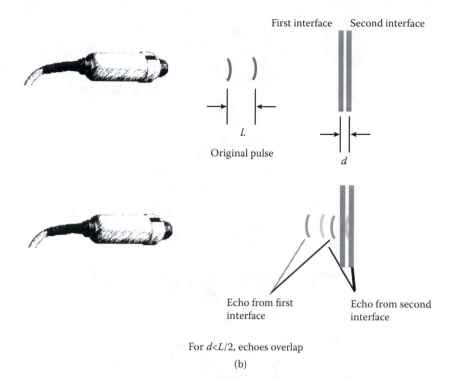

First interface   Second interface

L

Original pulse

d

Echo from first
interface

Echo from second
interface

For $d<L/2$, echoes overlap

(b)

Figure 4.16 (continued).

Another unintended effect arises if an interface between regions with differing speeds of sound is not oriented perpendicular to the incident ultrasound pulse's pathway (Figure 4.17a). In such a case, the transmitted ultrasound is **refracted**—that is, it travels in a direction different from the incoming pulse. This occurs for the same reason that a ray of light is refracted at an interface between two materials with different indices of refraction (Chapter 2). The net effect is to have the transmitted ultrasound travel *displaced* from its expected path through the body. Echoes resulting from this displaced beam can result in artifacts in the creation of ultrasound images, for example, shifting the apparent position of other structures encountered after the refracting interface. This can result in double images being formed of many interfaces in scans of the pelvic region (Figure 4.17b).

Other problems include a simple miscalibration of the speed of sound in tissue, which will tend to make the picture look compressed (the instrument's setting for v_s is too low compared to the value actually encountered) or too expanded (the instrument's setting for v_s is too high), as illustrated in Figure 4.18. This and many other potential problems can be corrected for by using test samples, or **phantoms**, provided for calibrating the ultrasound

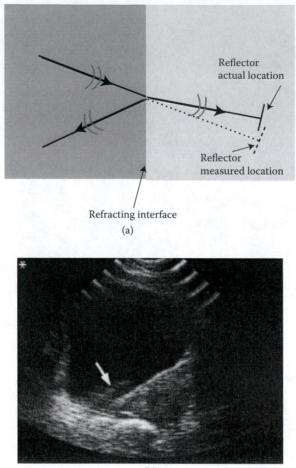

Figure 4.17 (a) Just as for light, the rules of optics hold for sound waves, and reflection and refraction can occur as discussed in Chapter 2. If the ultrasound beam hits an interface at an angle, the refracted beam will produce echoes whose paths are then displaced from those expected in the absence of refraction. A reflector at the actual location indicated (solid lines) will be registered by the scanner at the incorrect apparent location (dashed lines). (b) Refraction can cause artifacts in which images are displaced from their true position. Here, the uterus, shown in cross section at the center of the image, has a region in which its wall appears to have a double layer due to this effect (arrow). (Reproduced with permission, Hylton B. Meire and Pat Farrant, *Basic Ultrasound.* John Wiley & Sons, New York, 1995.)

instrument. These devices are constructed from known materials arranged in a predetermined pattern, so they provide a standard for evaluating the actual ultrasound images obtained from a specific scanner. By making sure the ultrasound device actually can measure the phantom's true structure,

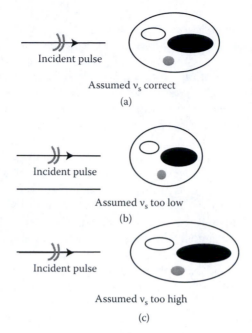

Figure 4.18 Because the value of the speed of sound, v_s, is used to compute distances in computing an image, ultrasound images are distorted if an incorrect value of v_s is assumed by the diagnostic ultrasound instrument. (a) Correct dimensions for a region of the body, measured using the correct value of v_s. (b) Too low a value of v_s results in a compressed image along the direction of the ultrasound beam, while too high a value (c) results in an elongation of the image's dimensions along the pulse direction.

the operator can verify that the scanner is properly calibrated. For example, the correct value of v_s can be determined by making sure known distances between reflectors located in the phantom are correctly determined.

4.11 HOW SAFE IS ULTRASOUND IMAGING?

Since energy is absorbed by the body during an ultrasound scan, it is reasonable to ask if damage results as a consequence. The hazards discovered during the early adoption of x-rays and other forms of radiation in medicine have prompted physicians to study this question carefully. The safety of ultrasound imaging has been determined by two major types of study: (1) laboratory experiments on isolated cells, plants, and animals subjected to ultrasound; and (2) population studies that follow large numbers of persons who have received ultrasound exams to be sure they do not encounter higher incidences of medical problems than does a similar, unexposed control population.

The results of the population studies to be described shortly are reassuring. However, there is no doubt that extremely high intensities of ultrasound can cause damage in laboratory experiments. For example, isolated experiments have found changes in the structure and genetic material of cells exposed to waves of ultrasound, and very high levels can cause lesions due to heating. How can sound present a danger? When very high-intensity ultrasound is absorbed by the body, energy is lost from the sound waves and converted into a new form; the longer the exposure, the greater the amount of energy transferred. This absorbed energy can directly heat tissue, or mechanically disrupt its cells. However, heating can be controlled for by limiting both the intensity and the time of ultrasound exposures to values observed to cause no significant temperature increase.

A phenomenon called **cavitation** is mainly responsible for mechanical cell disruption. You may be familiar with the fact that water boils at a lower temperature at higher altitudes, due to the lower pressures encountered there. Similarly, the rarefactions due to a very intense sound wave can create pressures so low that bubbles of water vapor can form even at body temperature. This situation, known as cavitation, can result in such small bubbles forming and collapsing as a result of high intensity sound waves. The collapsing bubbles act like tiny explosions that can disrupt cell membranes and internal structures. In fact, ultrasound tools for surgery produce damage by this very means. Both of these effects have been carefully studied in the laboratory to establish at what intensity levels significant temperature rises and signs of cavitation occur.

Long exposures to very high-intensity ultrasound can indeed cause damage to cells and entire organisms. These mechanisms for heating and disruption are a factor in therapeutic uses, such as ultrasound lithotripsy or treatments for sports injuries, which use higher intensities aimed at *causing* local tissue disruption in the interest of destroying tissue or stimulating healing. On the other hand, how much danger do the intensity levels and exposure times actually used in clinical imaging present? Significant heating does not occur during conditions typical of clinical exposures, as has been confirmed by direct measurements of temperature increases in tissue. However, experimental evidence (summarized in the references at the end of the chapter by Barnett et al., 1994) suggests that bubble formation can occur even under conditions corresponding to high intensity clinical ultrasound.* These effects are most likely to be of concern in pulsed Doppler measurements, which typically involve the highest intensities. While there is no direct experimental evidence that these effects can cause harm in humans, these results do increase the importance of properly performed population studies of ultrasound use to make sure no damage is observed in practice.

---

* These two results are compatible, because the high intensities present during a pulse can cause cavitation, even though the average intensity remains low enough to prevent significant heating.

How ultrasound can break up kidney stones: extracorporeal shock wave lithotripsy. Very intense ultrasound waves, with intensities of hundreds of watts/cm² or more, can be used to disrupt gallstones and stones in the urinary tract, and high-intensity focused ultrasound is under study as a means for destroying tumors. How can sound waves be focused to a high enough intensity to break apart even hard, mineralized kidney stones? In one method, a special source is used, consisting of two underwater electrodes between which an electric current passes swiftly enough to heat and vaporize water. The resulting rapid expansion and collapse of vapor bubbles creates shock waves of sound with extremely large associated pressures. These sound waves spread out from the source through a water bath and hit the walls of a reflective tank shaped at one end like an ellipse. The reflection of sound waves from the walls of this tank follow the same specular reflection rule as do rays of light. In addition, an ellipse has the special property that all rays emitted from a source located at one of two special points (called the foci) are reflected through the second focus. This special property refocuses the highly intense sound wave by reflection at the second focus of the water bath's ellipse. A different imaging technique (such as fluoroscopy, covered in Chapter 5) is then used to carefully place the region to be treated at this second focus. For example, Figure 4.19 shows how this procedure would look for a person undergoing treatment for a kidney stone. Transducers with built-in focusing elements also can be used to produce highly intense ultrasound for therapy in other parts of the body.

Studies of the safety of ultrasound imaging in humans have focused mostly on the effects of clinical ultrasound performed during pregnancy. Several large human population studies have been performed in which thousands to tens of thousands of women in low-risk pregnancies are assigned randomly to either control groups or routinely exposed groups. The control groups are assigned to receive no routine ultrasound exams, while the routinely exposed groups are examined on a set schedule, regardless of need. Women in either group are given ultrasound exams if a problem arises that makes the exam medically necessary, but no women are moved between groups after their initial assignments. (This ensures that women who develop problems during pregnancy aren't steadily moved from the control to the routinely exposed group. Were this the case, it would not be surprising that the incidence of problems would increase in the routinely exposed group.) All but one of the large studies show no significant physiological effects, even for the large populations studied. (See the RADIUS [for Routine Antenatal Diagnosic Imaging with Ultrasound] study [Bernard G. Ewigman et al., 1993; Saarri-Kemppainen et al., 1990] and references therein.) One study

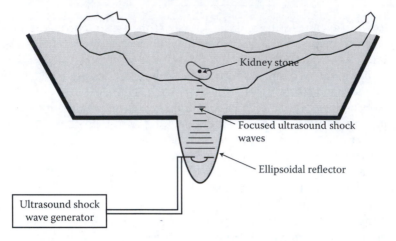

Figure 4.19 Schematic illustration of the extracorporeal shock wave lithotripsy, a method for crushing mineralized deposits in the body with sound waves. The patient shown sits immersed in a water bath. An electrical discharge is used to create a strong sound shock wave, which is reflected from the elliptical sides of the chamber. The reflected sound waves are focused onto the location of the stones to be broken up. The focused sound waves have an extremely high intensity, producing forces within the kidney stones sufficient to break them into smaller fragments.

(Newnham et al., 1993) did see an increase in the percentage of low-birth-weight babies in an intensively examined group vs. a control group receiving a very low average number of exams; apart from this difference, the two groups had identical pregnancy outcomes. However, similarly conducted studies (Bernard G. Ewigman et al., 1993; Saarri-Kemppainen et al., 1990) examined much larger populations, and found no problems. Newnham also notes that there was no difference in the health of the routinely exposed vs. the control babies, and that the average difference in birth weights between the two groups was very small, so that their finding could have been a statistical accident due to the small numbers of cases.

Many physicians have also been inclined to consider diagnostic ultrasound safe enough for routine use in screening each and every pregnant woman to monitor the health of the mother and the fetus. However, some studies do not bear out advantages from routine ultrasound for low-risk pregnancies (Bernard G. Ewigman et al., 1993; Newnham et al., 1993). These studies are always designed to exclude women who already have indications that their pregnancies will present problems, the assumption being that ultrasound exams offer a net benefit for pregnancies with known risk factors. However, some physicians think that these studies underestimate the benefits of routine ultrasound; objections such as these are aired in the correspondence following (Bernard G. Ewigman et al., 1993; Newnham et al., 1993). Improvements in ultrasound imaging technology also could shift this debate in the future.

Most of the population studies listed below only follow women through pregnancy and birth, but some are of long enough term to study children past infancy (Scheidt et al., 1978; Stark et al., 1984). These are again reassuring, although the numbers of children followed is much smaller than in the studies of infants immediately after birth. One study widely reported in the media (Campbell et al., 1993) proposed a correlation between delayed speech in older children and exposure to ultrasound in the womb. However, the relatively small size of the groups studied (only 72 children with delayed speech were included), and several problematic aspects of the study (e.g., the condition can be psychological, rather than physiological, in origin) led even its authors to report that they did not consider their work evidence that ultrasound imaging causes this condition.

In summary, based on many years of large population studies, physicians now believe that ultrasound imaging can safely be performed with no known risks so long as the intensities and exposure times are kept within safe levels. The U.S. FDA, which has authority over medical devices, reviews all diagnostic instruments for premarket approval to ensure that they do not exceed safety standards for peak intensities. To accommodate the unlikely event of a small associated risk, present medical wisdom holds that, ideally, ultrasound imaging should be used only when medically indicated. That is, its benefits are thought to far outweigh any hypothetical risks when there is a specific need for its use. However, studies like RADIUS raise questions about what is the right level to apply this technology. At roughly $200 per procedure in the U.S. in 1994, the RADIUS group estimated that applying routine screening to *all* pregnancies, rather than just those in which it is indicated, would add $1 billion to the nation's healthcare bill. Thus, the economics of healthcare, rather than the scientifically determined safety of diagnostic ultrasound, may provide a practical limit on how widely this technique is applied.

4.12 OBSTETRICAL ULTRASOUND IMAGING

Ultrasound in fact is used widely as a routine part of prenatal care in the U.S., with many women receiving at least one mid-pregnancy ultrasound exam. Diagnostic obstetrical ultrasound is usually performed using a transducer placed against the woman's abdomen, although in some cases a vaginal transducer is required to provide a higher resolution image. The technique offers important information to the parents and obstetrician. For example, it can be used to check the gestational age and overall fetal development by examining various anatomical features during the pregnancy. Ultrasound imaging also can help in the diagnosis of serious conditions early in pregnancy, such as potentially dangerous ectopic pregnancies, in which the egg improperly implants in the fallopian tube rather than the uterus. Other common uses include the detection of multiple fetuses (Figure 4.20a) and determining whether the placenta is placed so as to obstruct the birth

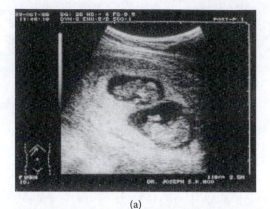

(a)

(b)

Figure 4.20 (a) Ultrasound image of twins at 10 weeks' gestation. (b) Image of a 14-week-old fetus in the womb. The head, seen in profile, is at the right. (Used with permission courtesy of Dr. Joseph Woo.)

canal, a dangerous condition known as **placenta previa**. Obstetricians utilize ultrasound as an important tool in monitoring the fetus' health in high-risk pregnancies such as those where the mother has had a history of difficult gestations, or suffers from a disease such as diabetes.

Obstetrical ultrasound imaging is performed with frequencies of roughly 3.5 to 7 MHz, and pulses roughly 1 microsecond long. These values give spatial resolutions of approximately 1 to 2 mm and adequate penetration of the pulses to permit imaging of the entire fetus within the uterus (Figure 4.20b). Ultrasound images collected at this spatial resolution look much blurrier than a typical x-ray image, and single frames taken from an exam are often more difficult for the patient to interpret than the actual moving image. In addition, ultrasound can be used to detect the fetal heartbeat, which can be measured with a simple hand-held Doppler device without imaging capability.

A normal pregnancy lasts 40 weeks on average; by convention, gestation is divided into three roughly three-month-long periods called **trimesters**. Obstetrical ultrasound imaging can be performed anytime after approximately the fifth week of pregnancy, at which point the gestational sac is visible in the uterus, although more information is gleaned the further along the pregnancy is. Early ultrasound can confirm the pregnancy, and distinguish between normal and abnormal pregnancies (such as a "blighted ovum" in which no fetus can be seen in the amniotic sac). By about seven weeks, the fetal heart motion is visible, and the broad outlines of the developing fetus can be resolved (Figure 4.20b). Later exams can distinguish in great detail many anatomical features of the fetus and placenta.

Knowing the gestational age of the fetus can be difficult. The estimated date of delivery is poorly determined if the woman's menstrual cycle and an external examination are the only factors used for prediction. If the actual date of conception is poorly known, ultrasound measurements of the fetus' development early in pregnancy can be utilized to give an extra clue to the true age. Many measures can be used to predict gestational age, including the dimensions of easily imaged parts of the skeleton, and the circumference of the abdomen. For example, two common measurements used to gauge gestational age early in the pregnancy are the biparietal diameter (BPD), the side-to-side diameter of the skull (Figure 4.21a), and the crown–rump length (CRL) (Figure 4.21b), the length from the top of the fetus' head to the bottom of its rump. Ultrasound can also be used to see if the fetus is developing at a normal rate. This may seem contradictory, since ultrasound is also used to help *determine* gestational age; in fact, ultrasound exams made earlier in the pregnancy more accurately determine gestational age, while scans at a later date can be used to check for normal growth and development.

By examining the ultrasound image at various checkpoints in the pregnancy, the obstetrician can monitor the development of the extremities, the spine, heart, kidneys, bladder, and stomach. Well into the second trimester, both the anatomy and functioning of the larger organs can be assessed. The heart can be seen beating and its four chambers visualized in detail. Congenital heart defects and blood flow within the umbilical cord can be detected with the Doppler techniques to be discussed later in this chapter. The presence of either excessive or inadequate amounts of amniotic fluid can be visualized, and obstructions in the urinary tract or digestive system detected. Movements of the fetus, such as the beating of the heart and "pseudo-breathing" within the womb, can also be readily observed. The structure of the brain can be examined, allowing an assessment of the rate of brain development and a check on any structural abnormalities. The kidneys, liver, and stomach can be checked on and their sizes estimated. The fetus' position within the womb can be monitored if a difficult presentation (such as a breech birth, in which the baby is not born head first) is anticipated.

Such exams make possible the prospect of treating severe problems (such as urinary tract obstructions) surgically before birth, entailing surgery for

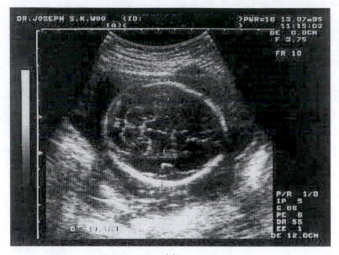

(a)

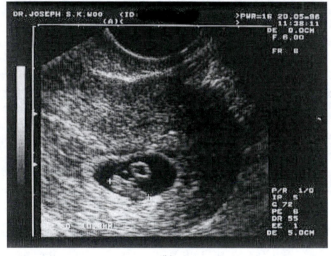

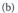

(b)

Figure 4.21 Examples of the ultrasound measurements used to characterize fetal growth early in gestation. (a) Cross-sectional image of the head, showing the bright elliptical outline of the skull, with the brain structure visible within. The dashed line extending across the sides of the head is used to measure the biparietal diameter, to track the growth of the head and skull. (b) Cross-hairs located at the top of the head and rump of the fetus allow the measurement of the Crown Rump Length used to estimate gestational age of the fetus. (Used with permission courtesy of Dr. Joseph Woo.)

the mother as well as the fetus, and possibly an uncertain outcome for the pregnancy even if the surgery is successful. Concerns about the risks involved so far limit such extreme interventions in pregnancy to unusual, severe cases.

One of the most common justifications for ultrasound is its association with other forms of prenatal testing, such as **amniocentesis** and **chorionic villus sampling (CVS)**. In amniocentesis a small amount of the amniotic fluid that surrounds the fetus is suctioned into a long hypodermic needle inserted through the wall of the mother's abdomen. Physicians utilize simultaneous ultrasound imaging to guide the needle so as to avoid the fetus, the placenta, umbilical cord, and uterine arteries. The goal is to recover cells expelled from the developing fetus into the amniotic fluid. These cells are then grown in culture and examined for chromosomal abnormalities indicative of genetic diseases such as Down's syndrome and Tay-Sachs disease; this test also reveals the sex of the fetus. The test results are made available to the parents, who receive the information along with genetic counseling to help them understand their significance. Amniocentesis also makes possible testing for birth defects called neural tube defects, in which the brain or spinal cord fails to develop properly. It also can be used for the detection of lung maturity during the third trimester by testing the amniotic fluid to determine whether the lining of the lungs has developed far enough to allow the fetus to breathe. Without this lining, prematurely born infants develop a dangerous condition called hyaline membrane disease. In a case where an early birth is likely, these levels can be monitored to make sure a delivery is not attempted before lung maturity has been reached. CVS provides a similar ability to detect genetic defects, but cells are sampled from the chorion, a part of the placenta, using a needle inserted either through the vagina or through the abdomen. Again, ultrasound is used to safely guide the needle. For both techniques, the woman remains fully conscious throughout. Amniocentesis is typically performed between 16 and 20 weeks of gestation (in the second trimester), while CVS can be performed earlier, at the end of the first trimester.

Diagnostic ultrasound during pregnancy can offer both reassurance for the parents and unprecedented information about serious complications. Its existence makes possible safe amniocentesis and CVS, leading to increasingly common prenatal genetic testing. For many parents, however, the impact is psychological—ultrasound is remembered by most as providing their first astonishing sight of the child to come.

4.13 ECHOCARDIOGRAPHY: ULTRASOUND IMAGES OF THE HEART

Cardiologists can now utilize ultrasound to directly image cross sections of the beating heart and major blood vessels (Figures 4.1c and 4.14b). They

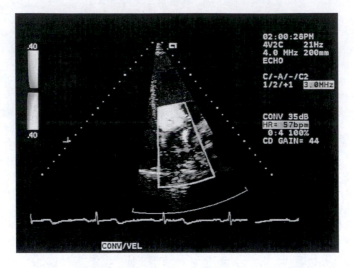

Figure 4.22 (See color figure following page 78.) Cross-sectional image of the four chambers of the heart and map of the flow of blood within the heart obtained by color-flow ultrasound. The schematic drawing shows the heart's structure. The normal flow of blood from the left atrium through the mitral valve into the left ventricle is indicated in blue. The red regions indicate "regurgitating" blood flowing upward through the defectively closed mitral valve. (Reproduced with permission courtesy of Acuson Corporation.)

can use the same ultrasound transducer to measure the flow of blood within the body while displaying this information simultaneously with the moving image (Figure 4.22). This remarkable technique uses the **Doppler effect**: the fact that echoes reflected from moving objects, such as blood cells, will have a frequency different from the original ultrasound pulse. By measuring this shift in frequency, one can determine the blood's flow.

The Doppler effect holds true whenever there is movement of either the source or the receiver of *any* type of sound, not just in the case of ultrasound echoes. Most people have experienced this effect by noticing that the pitch of a passing ambulance's siren changes. When the ambulance is approaching, the siren is shifted to a higher pitch relative to its sound when standing still; the siren of a receding ambulance has a lower pitch. We can begin to understand the origin of this change in frequency by considering situations where either the source or the receiver of sound moves.

4.14 ORIGINS OF THE DOPPLER EFFECT

Before we think about the actual situation encountered in ultrasound imaging, we will consider a simpler example. Figure 4.23 shows a person in a stationary car and a loudspeaker emitting sound waves; regions of

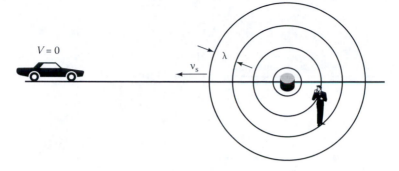

Figure 4.23 Figures 4.23 through 4.25 show how the Doppler effect influences the perceived frequency of sound. In the first case considered, illustrated here, neither the source of sound nor the receivers are moving, and both perceive the same frequency, f_o.

compression in the sound wave are represented as expanding circles one wavelength, λ, apart.

A person standing still near the loudspeaker and a listener in the car both hear the same frequency of sound, f_o. The frequency determines how many sound wavefronts reach either listener in an interval of time. It is proportional to the speed of sound and inversely proportional to wavelength (because the further apart the wavefronts are, the fewer that pass by every second):

$$f_o = \frac{v_s}{\lambda} \tag{4.16}$$

Let us now contrast this with a stationary source of sound, such as a fixed loudspeaker, and a listener in a car moving at a speed, V (Figure 4.24). The person in the car perceives sound waves with a frequency shifted from the unaltered frequency, f_o, heard by the person standing still. This is because the person in the car is *moving toward* the sound, so that the apparent speed of the sound waves is *increased* by the car's speed; that is, the person in the car perceives sound waves approaching with a greater speed, equal to $v_s + V$ (Figure 4.24a). This has the effect of causing the driver to encounter the sound waves more frequently than in the case of the stationary listener. If the car were *receding* from the source, then the apparent speed of the sound waves would be *decreased* by the speed of the car, and they would appear to be traveling at $v_s - V$ (Figure 4.24b). Our reasoning here relies on the fact that the apparent *wavelength* does not change when the reeiver moves (that is, the circles representing compressions remain uniformly spaced one wavelength apart), but the *effective speed of sound* perceived by the receiver does.

The exact relationship between frequency, f', heard by the listener in the car moving at speed V and by the stationary listener on the ground, f_o, can be determined by using these differing speeds of sound in Equation 4.16:

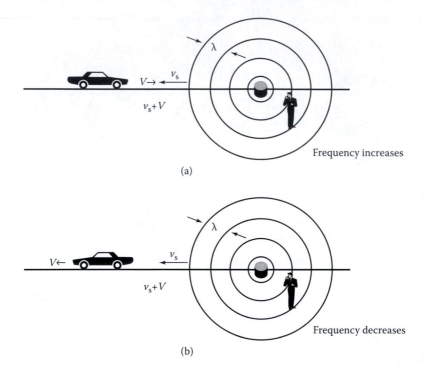

Figure 4.24 When the receiver of sound moves [illustrated here by a person driving a car toward (a) or away from (b) the source at right], it perceives a frequency shifted relative to the frequency heard by a stationary receiver (such as the person standing still at right). The stationary listener still hears the frequency transmitted by the source, but the moving receiver hears a higher (a) or lower (b) frequency, due to the fact that the sound waves are encountered faster (a) or slower (b), due to the relative motion.

$$f' = \frac{v_s + V}{\lambda}$$

$$= \frac{v_s}{\lambda} + \frac{V}{\lambda} = \frac{v_s}{\lambda} + \frac{v_s}{\lambda}\frac{V}{v_s} = \frac{v_s}{\lambda}\left(1 + \frac{V}{v_s}\right)$$

$$= f_o\left(1 + \frac{V}{v_s}\right) \qquad\qquad (4.17a)$$

$$f' = \begin{cases} f_o + f_o\dfrac{V}{v_s} & \text{Advancing case} \\[2ex] f_o - f_o\dfrac{V}{v_s} & \text{Receding case} \end{cases}$$

The final two equations summarize the results for the shifted frequency for a moving receiver either advancing or receding from the listener. The shifted frequency has increased by an amount Δf relative to the f_0. This shift in frequency, Δf, is called the **Doppler shift**, and its value is equal to:

$$\Delta f = f' - f_o = \begin{cases} +f_o \dfrac{V}{v_s} & \text{Advancing} \\[2em] -f_o \dfrac{V}{v_s} & \text{Receding} \end{cases} \qquad \text{Moving receiver} \qquad (4.17b)$$

Again, the plus sign corresponds to the advancing case, the minus sign to the receding case. The change in perceived speed of sound shifts the frequency heard by the moving listener relative to that heard by the stationary one. This Doppler shift is proportional to the receiver's speed, V; it also depends upon the original frequency and speed of sound, v_s. The Doppler shift results in the pitch increasing (becoming shriller) as the car approaches, and lower pitch as it recedes. The greater the speed of the listener, the larger the corresponding Doppler shift.

Consider now the case where the listeners (in this case two people standing on the ground) remain stationary while the *source* of sound moves, as shown in Figure 4.25 for a car moving at speed V while sounding a siren. In this case, the car moves in between each sound wave emitted, so that the expanding waves of sound will be centered at different points. The sound waves bunch up in the direction of travel and spread out behind the car's motion, resulting in a shorter (in the advancing direction) or longer

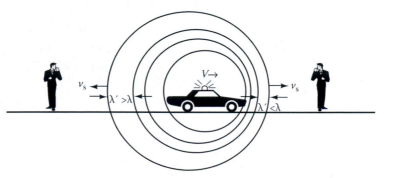

Figure 4.25 When the source of sound—such as a car's siren—moves, the two stationary receivers (the persons at right and left) hear frequencies different from the transmitted frequency. The person at right will hear sound waves that have a wavelength shortened by the source's motion, while the person at the left encounters sound waves with a wavelength lengthened by the motion. Since the sound moves through the air with the same speed in either case, the advancing case (right) results in a higher frequency, while the receding case (left) results in a lower frequency.

(in the receding direction) wavelength, λ', perceived by the listeners. This bunching and spreading also alters the frequency with which the listeners encounter wavefronts, since it alters the *distance* between waves. We can calculate the Doppler shift caused by a moving source of sound by using the change in wavelength (distance between compressions) shown. The change in frequency turns out to be proportional to the speed, V, in this case also. The shorter wavelengths in the advancing direction again result in higher frequencies, the longer ones in the receding direction in lower frequencies. Once more the Doppler shift gives a measurement of the speed of the object that emitted the sound. As before, the frequency at which the sound was emitted and the speed of sound must first be known in order to compute the speed, V, from the Doppler shift. All of these conditions are met in medical ultrasound, so it is in practice possible to measure the motion of moving objects within the body.

Now we will compute exactly the Doppler shift for this case. For the stationary listener, the apparent wavelength, λ', is either decreased (advancing case) or increased (receding case) by the motion of the car in between emitting each wavefront. Since the distance the car moves is given by the product of its speed, V, and the wave's period, T, this given for λ':

$$\lambda' = \lambda - V\,T$$

$$= \lambda - V\frac{1}{f_o} = \lambda - V\frac{\lambda}{v_s} \qquad \text{Moving source} \qquad (4.18a)$$

$$= \lambda \times \left(1 - \frac{V}{v_s}\right)$$

Here, the math has been worked out for the case of an advancing source (shorter wavelength); a similar conclusion results for the receding case, with a "plus" sign replacing all "minus" signs. This change in wavelength, λ', leads to an altered frequency, f', heard by the stationary listeners:

$$f' = \frac{v_s}{\lambda'} = \frac{v_s}{\lambda \times \left(1 - \dfrac{V}{v_s}\right)}$$

$$\cong \frac{v_s}{\lambda} \times \left(1 + \frac{V}{v_s}\right) \qquad \text{Moving source} \qquad (4.18b)$$

$$= f_o \times \left(1 + \frac{V}{v_s}\right) \qquad \text{for } V \ll v_s$$

(The simplified result in the second line is derived using a mathematical approximation to the fraction in the first line, which is true only for speeds

V small compared to the speed of sound, v_s. We will see that this condition holds for medical ultrasound applications of the Doppler effect.) Once again, this derivation applies to the case of an advancing source. This gives a Doppler shift equal to:

$$\Delta f = f' - f_o \cong \begin{cases} + f_o \dfrac{V}{v_s} & \text{Advancing} \\[2em] - f_o \dfrac{V}{v_s} & \text{Receding} \end{cases} \qquad \text{Moving source} \quad (4.18c)$$

We will use this simplified form for the cases encountered in medicine, where the speeds of blood flow are much slower than the speed of sound.

Sample calculation: A fairly large speed for flowing blood would be 75 cm/s, so the ratio between V and v_s is:

$$\frac{V}{v_s} = \frac{75 \text{ cm/s}}{1540 \text{ m/s}} = 0.00049 = 0.049\% \ll 1 \qquad (4.19)$$

which is such a small ratio that the assumption that $V \ll v_s$ is well justified.

4.15 USING THE DOPPLER EFFECT TO MEASURE BLOOD FLOW

In Doppler ultrasound, frequency shifts are generated when the ultrasound beam hits moving red blood cells or other moving objects within the body (Figure 4.26). Because we are interested in the *echo's* Doppler shift, there are *two* frequency shifts to be considered:

1. The moving red blood cells act like a moving receiver hearing an altered frequency, f_1, which is Doppler shifted relative to the original frequency f_o.
2. The red blood cells then act like a moving source when they reflect the ultrasound. Now f_1 plays the role of the source frequency and the echo has a new frequency f_2 which is also Doppler shifted relative to f_1.

The result of these two frequency shifts gives a total shift of the returning echo equal to two times the simple Doppler shift described earlier. We

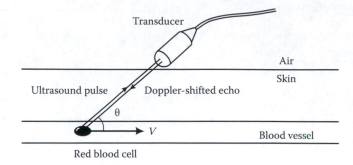

Figure 4.26 Illustration of how the Doppler effect works in ultrasound imaging. Pulses of ultrasound are absorbed by moving receivers of ultrasound (for example, blood cells)—giving one Doppler shift—which then re-emit the ultrasound as moving sources when they generate echoes, leading to a second Doppler shift.

must also take into account the effect of the angle, θ, between the ultrasound transducer and the moving blood because it can change the velocity of blood flow detectable by the transducer. These considerations give us a total Doppler shift equal to:

$$\Delta f = f_2 - f_o = 2f_o \frac{V}{v_s} \cos\theta \qquad (4.20)$$

The maximum Doppler shifts are seen when the transducer's pulses travel directly toward, or exactly opposite to, the flow. For example, if the transducer points directly along the flow, the cosine term gives $\cos 0° = +1$; if the transducer points exactly opposite we have $\cos 180° = -1$. For an angle of 90°, the transducer would be perpendicular to the blood flow and there would be no apparent motion toward or away from the transducer; hence, no Doppler shift would be seen since $\cos 90° = 0$.

We see that measuring this frequency shift allows us to measure the blood flow speed, V, once the Doppler shift has been measured. Because Doppler ultrasound can be performed along with ultrasound imaging, the physician can use the image to orient the transducer's pulses to lie within a small angular range very close to either 0° or 180°. Small errors in orientation do not affect the accuracy of the flow measurements; in fact, variations in angle of 10° or less will result in errors of only a few percent. The imaging information can also be used to estimate the actual angle, in order to obtain a quantitative measurement of blood flow.

Sample calculation: We can compute how large an error in the blood flow measurement will result from mismeasuring the angle between the transducer and the flow. If we assume that the intended angle is 08, where the cosine term equals 1, then we can compute the cosine factor for nearby angles: cos 10° = 0.9848, which gives an error of 1.5%, because:

$$\cos 0° - \cos 10° = 1.000 - 0.9848 = 0.0152 = 1.5\% \qquad (4.21)$$

Similarly, we have cos 20° = 0.940, which gives an error of 6%. So long as the detector is oriented within a few degrees of zero, this will not cause an appreciable error in the measurement of blood flow.

4.16 COLOR FLOW IMAGES

Sometimes Doppler ultrasound is used to monitor only one particular motion. For example, fetal heart monitors utilizing the Doppler effect can measure fetal heart rates from outside the mother's body. Similarly, simple Doppler flow meters can be constructed that use electronics similar to those used in FM radios to detect the frequency shift in a continuous wave of ultrasound reflected from flowing blood. This flow information can be plotted as a function of time to show the changes expected with the pulsatile flow of blood in the circulatory system. Since the frequency shifts due to the Doppler effect are audible frequencies, flow information from a particular region also can be converted into a sound that is played during the exam. By becoming familiar with the audible signatures of various types of flows, the physician can "hear" abnormal flow conditions.

Often, however, the blood flow velocity, V, is measured *simultaneously* with the distance information. These techniques are variously called **echocardiography** and **color flow ultrasound,** and they measure flow rates at many points on the ultrasound image by detecting the Doppler effect for multiple echoes. How can one display all of the information that is collected, since this ultrasound technique can distinguish not only a single velocity, but the velocity of flow at many points on a black-and-white image? If the velocity were plotted as a function of position, the physician would have to digest many plots per image; some simplification is clearly necessary if flows at more than one position are to be monitored.

One useful way of displaying complex flow information involves the use of color overlaying the black-and-white ultrasound image on a computer screen, a technique called **color flow mapping.** The flow velocities are indicated by the colors present on that part of the ultrasound image

(Figure 4.22). For example, bright reds can be used to indicate large approaching flows, while dim reds can represent weak approaching flows. Similarly, blue can be used to represent receding flows. Thus, both the magnitude and direction of the flow are made apparent at a glance. Yellow or green can be used to indicate turbulent flows lacking a well-defined flow direction. This selective coloring in of the black-and-white image wherever there is motion allows the physician to continuously monitor both anatomy and variation in flow.

Color flow mapping can be used, for example, to locate faulty valves in the heart or major blood vessels that may allow blood through when they are supposed to be entirely closed. It can also reveal defects in the septa (or walls) separating the chambers of the heart, through which blood can leak. In the case of large blood vessels such as the aorta or carotid arteries, the variation in flow across a vessel partially blocked by plaque can be visualized.

This use of color flow mapping supplements angiocardiography, which allows the x-ray imaging of the circulatory system using an x-ray-absorbing contrast dye injected into the patient's heart, arteries, or veins. This technique requires exposure to x-rays, and it exposes patients to a small risk of a serious reaction to the injected contrast medium. By comparison, echocardiography can be performed from outside the body (or in some instances through a transducer inserted into the esophagus) using portable imaging equipment that can be wheeled to the bedside, and it does not require the introduction of foreign substances into the circulatory system. In spite of this reduced invasiveness, it allows the cardiologist to see the heart's anatomy in motion, as well as many details of the blood's circulation. Many different imaging techniques are used to study the heart and circulatory system, each with its own advantages and disadvantages, so echocardiography does not entirely displace other imaging methods.

4.17 THREE-DIMENSIONAL ULTRASOUND

While diagnostic ultrasound has become a mature technology, relatively inexpensive and available at virtually every hospital, new advances still continue to offer better images. For example, improvements in the quality of beam focusing can counter the effects of beam absorption to allow the use of higher frequencies and improved spatial resolution. Advances in phased-array development building upon research in radioastronomy have also led to sharper images. Another important advance is the development of safe contrast agents for ultrasound imaging. For example, tiny microbubbles of gas only a few microns in diameter are useful for generating stronger echoes in many imaging applications; these can be safely introduced via the circulatory system and they are completely biodegradable.

Clever new techniques have been developed to beat some of the limitations due to ultrasound absorption and artifact formation. One of the newer is the use of **harmonic imaging**, in which ultrasound of one frequency (the

fundamental) is transmitted, but echoes at frequencies that are multiples of the original (the **harmonics**) are detected. For example, if a contrast agent or an interface within the body generates reflections at twice the original frequency, the ultrasound imaging device can transmit lower frequencies (for improved tissue penetration), while selectively receiving only the higher frequency echoes. The higher frequency echoes are attenuated less, because they need to make only the return trip to the transducer. This technique eliminates many artifacts, which occur only at the fundamental frequency, and has proved especially useful in patients traditionally difficult to image in cardiology because of obesity, a very thick chest wall, or other conditions that can block image formation.

Another major advance is scanners equipped with sophisticated computer graphics that permit the reconstruction of a three-dimensional image of the region being probed. The idea is a simple one: each ultrasound image constitutes a view of only one slice of the body; by taking multiple cross-sectional scans of the patient's body, the physician images many adjacent cross-sectional slices (Figure 4.27a). In most scanners, these cross-sectional images are viewed one at a time. Instead, computer graphics can be used to automatically scan the transducer, and display a total three-dimensional image made up of many stacked slices (Figure 4.27b). These three-dimensional pictures can be displayed on a television screen in a variety of formats. By specifying that the image should be constructed from regions generating a particular echo intensity, a complete picture of the heart or a fetus can be displayed. Special viewing headsets are being developed, which project the reconstructed image onto the plane of vision; in an obstetrical ultrasound scan, this would result in the imaged fetus

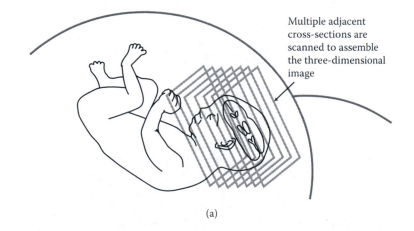

Multiple adjacent cross-sections are scanned to assemble the three-dimensional image

(a)

Figure 4.27 (a) Schematic illustration of how a three-dimensional ultrasound scanner accumulates images by assembling multiple cross-sectional images. (b) Reconstructed three-dimensional ultrasound image of a fetal face at 32 weeks' gestation. (Reproduced with permission courtesy of Horst Steiner, M.D.)

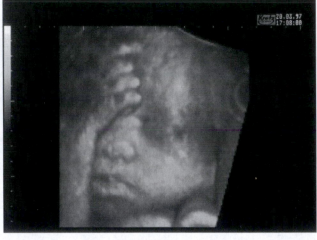

(b)

Figure 4.27 (continued).

appearing to lie inside its mother's abdomen in the proper position and orientation. Similarly, the computer associated with the diagnostic instrument can display only part of a structure, such as the skeleton, and ignore other features that would complicate the image.

It is easy to forget while pondering these advanced technologies that the basis of ultrasound imaging remains the simple idea of seeing with echoes—a complex and useful technology inspired by the ability of bats to navigate in the dark.

4.18 PORTABLE ULTRASOUND—APPROPRIATE TECHNOLOGY FOR THE DEVELOPING WORLD

While portable ultrasound imaging devices have been on the market for some time, recently these units have achieved image qualities comparable to those of standard console-sized units. For example, current units can as small as a laptop computer, weighing only several pounds and requiring only battery power, and consequently can be just as portable. As a result, now ultrasound imaging can be used in a greater variety of locations, including in the field of emergency medicine and veterinary medicine (Figure 4.28a). Another major application is the use of ultrasound as a preferred imaging modality in developing countries where healthcare systems are presently inadequate and strained for resources (Figure 4.28b).

There are multiple reasons that the World Health Organization has identified ultrasound as a preferred technology for imaging in developing nations. First, the units are dramatically less expensive than the alternatives,

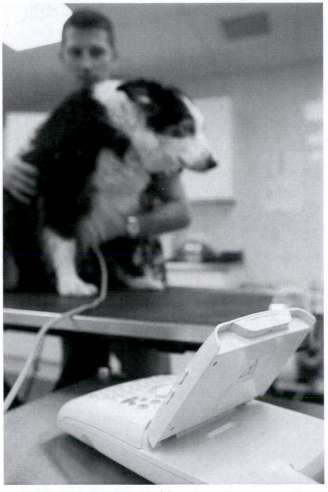

(a)

Figure 4.28 (a) Veterinarians now can make use of portable, battery-powered ultrasound scanners in the clinic and in the field. (b) These light-weight scanners can be applied in settings in the developing world where stable electrical power sources are unreliable and other imaging modalities are too expensive, complex, or unavailable. (Reproduced with permission courtesy of Sonosite, Inc.)

such as magnetic resonance imaging (MRI) or computed tomography (CT), and it is relatively inexpensive to maintain them and purchase necessary supplies. Portability means that units can be deployed in rural locations, as well as without the need for consistent power (although console-units can serve the purpose if supplied with a stable and reliable backup source of elec-tricity). Ultrasound scanners are compact and do not take up much space in small clinics or hospitals. Ultrasound imaging provides three-dimensional

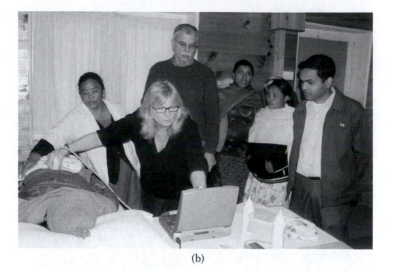

(b)

Figure 4.28 (continued).

information at high resolution, as well as functional Imaging, without the use of ionizing radiation, an advantage over x-ray imaging, and it has unique capabilities for obstetrics, cardiology, and other specialities. Ultrasound examinations can be achieved in minutes for many purposes, making their use practical in large-scale screening applications by mobile clinics providing care to rural areas lacking in healthcare options. Because images are inherently digital, local physicians can consult with remote doctors using the internet to transfer images and supporting information. One limitation now being addressed is the severe shortage of physicians and sonographers qualified to perform ultrasound exams in these settings. Programs such as the Jefferson Ultrasound Research and Education Institute (JUREI) and www.Sonoworld.com offer training and resources for training physicians and technicians worldwide, through programs in the U.S., in the countries of interest, and through distance learning. Through a feature called Teaching the Teachers, physicians from emerging countries are trained both in ultrasound imaging methods and in how to pass on their training to others. Thousands of physicians have been educated through these programs, returning to their communities skills in a genuinely appropriate and much-needed technology.

SUGGESTED READING

E. Carr Everbach, "Medical diagnostic ultrasound," *Phys. Today*, pp. 44–48, March 2007.
Frederick Kremkau, "Seeing is believing? Sonographic artifacts," *Phys. Today*, pp. 84–85, March 2007.

Textbooks for learning more about the details of ultrasound imaging

Frederick W. Kremkau, *Diagnostic Ultrasound: Principles, Instruments, and Exercises*. W.B. Saunders, Philadelphia, 2006.

Hylton B. Meire and Pat Farrant. *Basic Ultrasound*, John Wiley & Sons, New York, 1995.

T. Szabo, *Diagnostic Ultrasound Imaging: Inside Out*. Elsevier Academic Press, Burlington, MA, 2004.

References on obstetrical diagnostic ultrasound and studies of ultrasound safety

S.B. Barnett, G.R. ter Haar, M.C. Ziskin, W.L. Nyborg, K. Maeda, and J. Bang, "Current status of research on biophysical effects of ultrasound," *Ultrasound Med. Biol.*, Vol. 20 (1994), pp. 205–218.

Bioeffects and Safety of Diagnostic Ultrasound, American Institute of Ultrasound in Medicine, Rockville, MD, 1993.

J.D. Campbell, R.W. Elford, and R.F. Brant, "Case-control study of prenatal ultrasonography exposure in children with delayed speech," *Can. Med. Assoc. J.*, Vol. 149 (Nov. 15, 1993), pp. 1435–1440; see also related correspondence in the same journal, Vol. 150 (March 1, 1994), pp. 647–649.

B.G. Ewigman, J.P. Crane, and F.D. Frigoletto, "Effect of prenatal ultrasound screening on perinatal outcome," *New Engl. J. Med.*, Vol. 329 (1993), pp. 821–827.

E.A. Lyons, C. Dyke, and M. Toms, "In utero exposure to diagnostic ultrasound: a six year followup," *Radiology*, Vol. 166 (1988), pp. 687–690.

John P. Newnham, Sharon F. Evans, Con A. Michael, Fiona J. Stanley, and Louis I. Landau, "Effects of frequent ultrasound during pregnancy: a randomised controlled trial," *Lancet*, Vol. 342 (Oct. 9, 1993), pp. 887–891; see also related correspondence in the same journal, Nov. 27, 1993, pp. 1359–1361; and Jan. 15, 1994, p. 178.

A. Saarri-Kemppainen, O. Karjalainen, P. Ylostalo, and O.P. Heinonen, "Ultrasound screening and perinatal mortality: controlled trial of systematic one-stage screening in pregnancy. The Helsinki Ultrasound Trial," *Lancet*, Vol. 336 (1990), pp. 387–391.

P.C. Scheidt, F. Stanley, and D.A. Bryla, "One-year follow-up of infants exposed to ultrasound in utero," *Am. J. Obstet. Gynecol.*, Vol. 131 (1978), pp. 743–748.

C.R. Stark, M. Orleans, and A.D. Havercamp, "Short- and long-term risks after exposure to diagnostic ultrasound in utero," *Obstet Gynecol.*, Vol. 63 (1984), pp. 194–200.

Electronic resources

Dr. Joseph Woo's website on obstetrical ultrasound imaging: http://www.ob-ultrasound.net/.

Mark Deutchman, ed., with John Hobbins, *Obstetrical Ultrasound: Principles and Techniques* CD-ROM, SilverPlatter, Norwood, MA. (Peer reviewed by the American Medical Association.)

A review of three-dimensional ultrasound imaging techniques

Horst Steiner, Alf Staudach, Dietmar Spitzer, and Heinz Schaffer, "Three-dimensional ultrasound in obstetrics and gynaecology: technique, possibilities and limitations," *Hum. Reprod.*, Vol. 9 (Sept. 1994), pp. 1773–1778.

Ultrasound surgery

J.E. Kennedy, G.R. ter Haar, and D. Cranston, "High intensity focused ultrasound: surgery of the future?" *Br. J. Radiol.*, vol. 76 (2003), pp. 590–599.

History of ultrasound

Edward Yoxen, "Seeing with sound: A study of the development of medical images," in *The Social Construction of Technological Systems: New Directions in the Sociology and History of Technology*. Bijker W., Hughes T., Pinch T. (eds). The MIT Press, Cambridge, MA. 1987: 281–303.

QUESTIONS

Q4.1.   Sketch the sequence of events during an ultrasound scan, showing the path of the ultrasound pulse and indicating how the final picture is constructed. Describe in words anything you cannot draw.

Q4.2.   Using the ideas set forth in this chapter, can you explain why bats have evolved to use ultrasound for hunting and navigating, rather than audible sound, which many animals use to communicate?

Q4.3.   We think of old-fashioned fog horns as having a deep, pleasing bass tone. However, fog horns were invented to fulfill a practical need: the desire to warn ships of obstacles in heavy fogs. Why would low frequency sound be a good choice in this situation?

Q4.4.   If using a higher frequency gives you higher spatial resolution in ultrasound imaging, explain why one can't simply increase the frequency indefinitely, permitting ultrasound imaging of cells or even smaller structures.

Q4.5.   Name three effects that can cause distortions of the ultrasound image. How can each of these be corrected for or avoided?

Q4.6.   If a cardiologist sees no color in a region on a color Doppler map of the heart, does that mean that there is no blood flow in that region? Explain why or why not, using a drawing if necessary.

Q4.7   Describe the ideal ultrasound contrast agent. Give the ideal properties of its acoustic impedance, speed of sound and half-intensity-length, compared, for example, to those for soft tissue, blood, etc.

PROBLEMS

Basic physics of sound waves

P4.1. (a) A diagnostic ultrasound imaging instrument uses a frequency of 6.0 MHz. What is the corresponding wavelength in soft tissues in the body? (b) What would the wavelength associated with this frequency be in air?

P4.2. (a) It is desired to have an ultrasound wavelength of 0.50 mm for imaging soft tissues in the body. What frequency should be used to achieve this value? (b) In some unknown material, the wavelength associated with an ultrasound frequency of 2.0 MHz is equal to 1.75 mm. What is the speed of sound in that material?

Echo ranging and echo intensity

P4.3. (a) An ultrasound transducer detects an ultrasound echo 20 milliseconds after sending a pulse. How far away is the interface that generated this echo? (You may assume the speed of sound corresponds to 1540 m/s, although distances in this problem will not necessarily correspond to values possible within the human body.) (b) Two interfaces are 5.0 cm apart. How much time elapses between the echoes received by the transducer from each interface?

P4.4. (a) Use Table 4.2 to determine values for the acoustic impedances of bone, various types of soft tissue, and air, and compute the intensity of reflected sound for normal incidence between each of the following interfaces: (i) fat and muscle, (ii) bone and soft tissue, and (iii) air and soft tissue. (Use ratios or percentages to compare numbers.) (b) Use your results to explain why this presents difficulties for ultrasound imaging of the brain. (c) Use these results to explain why sonographers use a gel between the ultrasound transducer and the patient's skin.

P4.5. A fundamental limitation on how fast ultrasound scanners can work is the transit time for sound to cross the body and return to the transducer as an echo. In this problem, you will make some rough estimates of the times necessary to perform abdominal ultrasound scans. Throughout this problem you may assume a beamwidth several times the wavelength of sound used; similarly, you should make reasonable estimates for all unknown distances and parameters.

    a. Estimate how long it would take for an ultrasound pulse to travel entirely across your abdomen and return, to get an upper bound on this transit time. To do so, use a ruler or meter stick to make measurements on yourself in order to get a representative value for this distance. Use a typical number for the speed of sound in soft tissue.

    b. After you have computed the transit time for one pulse to cross the abdomen and return, next estimate how long an entire ultrasound scan of your abdomen would take. Use values for typical beam widths and your results from part (a). Make a drawing to show approximately how many pulses would be necessary to complete an entire scan. (You may wish to consult Figure 4.9.) Explain your reasoning.

c. What motions of the body might interfere with the completion of an entire scan? That is, which ones are fast enough to occur over times shorter than the typical duration of an entire scan?

P4.6. Scans of the fetal brain can reveal structure within the skull. For example, this could be used to measure the location of the midline between the two hemispheres of the brain. (See Figure P4.6.) During such a brain scan, the echoes from the right side of the skull, the midline of the brain, and the left side of the skull are observed after times of 0.10×10^{-4}, 1.26×10^{-4}, and 2.40×10^{-4} s, respectively. The speed of sound can be assumed to be 1540 m/s everywhere along the path (ignoring variations in the speed of sound due to the skull). (Adapted from *General Physics*, Morton M. Sternheim and Joseph W. Kane, John Wiley & Sons, New York, 1991, p. 576.)

a. Where is the midline of the brain compared to its normal location halfway between the sides of the skull?

b. Which one of the hemispheres of the brain is larger?

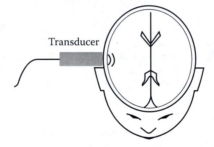

P4.7. (a) Assume that the speed of sound is roughly the same (1540 m/s) in all of the soft tissues in the schematic drawing shown in Figure P4.7, and that their acoustic impedances have the values shown. Explain which interfaces will be easiest/hardest to see, by computing the reflected intensities from each interface along the pathway indicated. (b) Make a *rough* sketch of the echo intensity as a function of time, indicating which echoes come from which interfaces. (For simplicity, assume the original beam is not focused. You do not have to account quantitatively for absorption or geometry, but show how these effects would qualitatively affect your results.)

Material	Acoustic impedance (kg/m²-sec)
Blood	1,660,000
Fat	1,300,000
Muscle	1,650,000
Cartilage	2,200,000

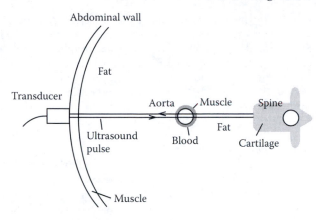

Absorption of ultrasound

P4.8. An ultrasound pulse of frequency 3.0 MHz and wavelength 0.50 mm can penetrate as deeply as 10 cm into a person's abdomen before being almost entirely (97%) absorbed. This represents a possible ultrasound frequency used for abdominal imaging. Given this information, what wavelength and frequency would you suggest using to probe the structure of the human eye to high resolution? To solve this problem, first assume that for soft tissues, the following relationship holds between the absorption of sound and its frequency:

$$L = \frac{C}{f}$$

where f = frequency, L = the depth at which 97% of the intensity has been absorbed, and C is some constant with a value to be determined in this exercise.

First, use Figure 3.28(a) and some reasonable estimates of the relevant dimensions of the eye to decide to what distance you think the beam should be able to penetrate into the eye. Explain your answer. Then use the numbers given above to find a value for C. Now, assuming that roughly the same value of C will apply for both the abdomen and the eye, use this value of C to estimate what the new frequency, f_{eye}, of ultrasound for optical exams should be. What wavelength of sound waves, λ, does this correspond to? Compare this result to actual features of the eye, estimating their sizes with a ruler on the figure. Which features will you be able to resolve with this frequency?

Sources of distortion

P4.9. Assume that a diagnostic ultrasound scanner has been miscalibrated, so that in performing its imaging calculations, it incorrectly assumes the speed of sound in a soft tissue path is 1400 m/s, when the true value is 1540 m/s. As a result, the scanner will display distorted images of structures in the body. Sketch the distortions that will result from this miscalibration, compute their magnitude, and explain your reasoning.

P4.10. In soft tissue, two interfaces that generate ultrasound reflections are separated by d = 1.0 mm along the direction of the beam. The criterion for resolution is that the two interfaces be at least half the pulse length apart, and that pulses must be at least one wavelength long. What is the minimum frequency that will resolve these interfaces?

P4.11. Recall that we can use the results for geometrical optics described in Chapter 2 for light waves to describe sound waves as well. Consider Figure P4.3, in which a uniform region of tissue with one speed of sound has embedded in it a lens-shaped organ with a different speed of sound. Sound waves refract when they hit the interface between the two media, changing their direction of travel as shown. What can you say qualitatively about the relative values of the speeds of sound in the two tissues? (Hint: No calculations are required to answer this question.)

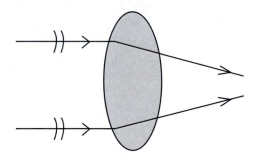

Doppler ultrasound

P4.12. Reproduced in Figure P4.12 is a color-flow image of a cross-sectional ultrasound scan of the human heart. Draw arrows to indicate the blood flow velocities and their directions for the color Doppler map of the heart using the following key:

> Blue = receding flows
> Red = advancing flows
> Yellows, greens = mixing, turbulence
> (Brighter colors indicate higher flow rates.)

Use the direction of the arrows to indicate flow direction, and the lengths of the arrows to indicate flow speed. Explain why the flows have the orientations you have indicated.

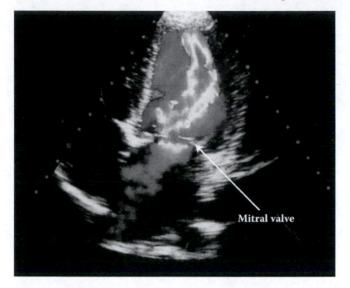

Figure P4.12 (See color figure following page 78.)

P4.13. Compute the frequency shift due to a blood flow velocity of 30 cm/s for a 3.0 MHz beam incident upon the blood vessel at 30° to the flow. Make a drawing of the geometry for measurement that you have assumed. What percentage shift in frequency is this? What is the shift in Hz?

P4.14. A cardiologist uses an ultrasound scanner with an operating frequency of 3.5 MHz that can detect Doppler frequency shifts as small as 0.1 kHz. What is the smallest flow velocity detectable with this device?

ANOTHER USEFUL SOURCE OF PROBLEMS ON ULTRASOUND IMAGING

Frederick W. Kremkau, *Diagnostic Ultrasound: Principles, Instruments, and Exercises*. W.B. Saunders, Philadelphia, 1993.

5   X-ray vision

Diagnostic X-rays and CT scans

5.1 INTRODUCTION

The 1995 centennial of the discovery of x-rays also marked one hundred years during which x-ray imaging reigned as the preeminent imaging technique of modern medicine. X-ray imaging is so widely used that virtually every reader of this book has had at least one diagnostic x-ray, while every year about seven out of every ten U.S. citizens receive at least one x-ray. As these numbers indicate, x-rays remain a workhorse of medical imaging, providing low-cost glimpses inside the body where ultrasound cannot penetrate and fiber optic scopes cannot go. **Radiography** (the science of medical x-ray images) was revolutionized in the 1970s by the widespread introduction of **computed tomography (CT)**, a computerized mathematical technique that permits the reconstruction of three-dimensional images from x-rays. With the invention of the CT scanner, x-ray imaging has become an even more sophisticated and sensitive probe of anatomy and function. Using a combination of CT and MRI (Chapter 8), physicians can noninvasively analyze the anatomy of any part of the body, including the brain. The wide utility of CT has led to an explosive growth in its use, with an estimated 62 million or more CT scans per year estimated to occur in the U.S. alone. Increasingly, CT is being combined with other methods of imaging, such as PET, to provide complementary imaging of body anatomy and function or pathology.

The basic idea behind taking diagnostic x-rays is quite simple. **Radiographs**—images colloquially called "x-rays"—are shadows created when all or part of a beam of x-rays are absorbed by a part of the body (such as the skeleton) (Figure 5.1a). Those x-rays that do not get absorbed by the body travel on to be sensed by a detector. The resulting image is a **projection** of all of the **radiopaque** (x-ray-absorbing) objects in the x-ray's path. Since there is no way to detect if one object was in front of or behind another, the two overlap on the image. This means that diagnostic x-rays inherently lose depth information, and provide only a flattened planar image of the body (Figure 5.1b). CT scans can distinguish between the many structures that overlap on a diagnostic x-ray, presenting instead a cross-sectional view

Image receptor

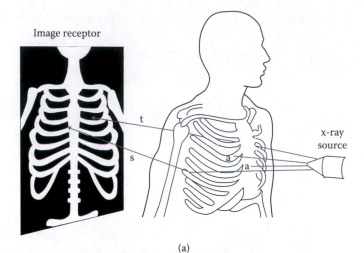

(a)

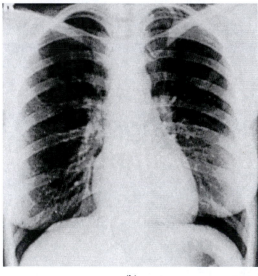

(b)

Figure 5.1 (a) Schematic drawing showing how radiographs are formed as x-ray projections. The x-ray image is formed when a beam of x-rays are shone through the body (in this case, the chest) toward a detector or image receptor, such as x-ray film. The image is formed by the variations in x-ray absorption between different parts of the body. For example, bones are much more effective at blocking x-rays than are muscles, organs, the lungs, etc., hence the film is exposed less behind the skeleton than behind the soft tissues of the chest. (b) Example of an actual chest x-ray taken with x-ray film. The ribs and other parts of the skeleton are seen clearly, and the outline of the heart is apparent at the center of the image. (Reproduced with permission courtesy of John H. Juhl and Andrew B. Crummy, eds., *Paul and Juhl's Essentials of Radiological Imaging*, J.B. Lippincott, Philadelphia, 1993.)

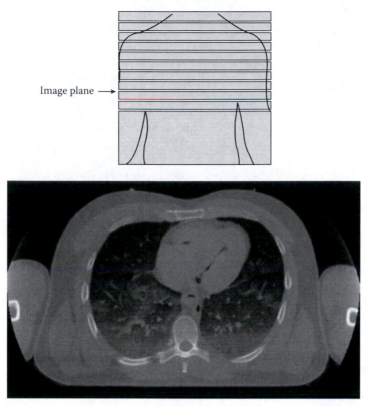

(c)

Figure 5.1 (continued) (c) Cross-sectional CT scan of the chest, taken in a horizontal (axial) plane through the level of the heart (inset). The spine is at the bottom of the image, and the heart at the top center. (Used with permission courtesy of the National Library of Medicine's Visible Human Project, at http://www.nlm.nih.gov.)

of body anatomy (Figure 5.1c) or a computer-generated, three-dimensional reconstruction.

Note how this procedure differs from the operation of a camera, even though film was traditionally used to capture the x-ray image. A camera uses lenses to collect the light from an object and focus its image onto film, while the projected x-ray image is merely an unfocused shadow. This is because no materials exist that can be used to make practical x-ray lenses for medical imaging. Using the language of Chapter 2, the index of refraction is virtually the same for almost all materials, so refraction essentially does not occur. Diagnostic x-rays are formed in a method similar to the contact prints made when children lay objects directly atop photographic paper, then use sunlight to expose only the uncovered parts of the film.

In spite of their many advantages, diagnostic x-rays make use of ionizing radiation, and thus inherit its associated risks. In Chapter 7, we will examine the issue of how the effects of exposure to low levels of radiation are evaluated and weighed against medical benefits, in the context of the use of x-rays in therapy.

In this chapter, we first examine what actually is measured in a diagnostic x-ray: that is, how x-rays interact with the tissues within the body, and how this impacts the imaging of different parts of the body. We next discuss how organs ordinarily not visible on an x-ray can be made visible using x-ray contrast media. We then describe how x-rays are generated, and what types of detectors are used to sense their presence. The important application of mammography to the screening of women for breast cancer is considered in depth as a special case. Finally, the powerful new technologies of digital x-ray imaging and CT are explained. The chapter ends with a description of how these techniques can be used in screening for osteoporosis.

5.2 DIAGNOSTIC X-RAYS: THE BODY'S X-RAY SHADOW

X-rays and **gamma rays** are very energetic photons, with wavelengths shorter than 10 nm and with many times the energy of a photon of visible light. Table 3.1 shows how x-rays fit into the larger scheme of the electromagnetic spectrum. In medical physics, the term *x-ray* is generally used to characterize such photons when they are generated in a continuous spectrum of energies from, for example, an x-ray tube source, while photons of specific energies emitted during radioactive decays are called *gamma rays* (Chapter 6). (The definitions of gamma and x-rays used in medical physics actually differ from the way other physicists use these terms. Physics texts generally define gamma rays as having more energy than x-rays, with the exact energy ranges being left somewhat unclear.) We measure these photon energies using the electron-Volt (eV), a unit roughly comparable to the average chemical bond energy in the body. The energies used in radiographic imaging range from 17 to 150 **kiloelectron-Volts** (**keV**, where kilo means one thousand). The photons used in radioisotope imaging (Chapter 6) and cancer therapy (Chapter 7) have more energy than those used in diagnostic x-rays. Because of their much greater energy, x-ray photons are absorbed by processes that differ from those discussed in Chapter 3 for visible light. Several different interaction mechanisms can come into play, and which are important is determined by the energy of the photon and the characteristics of the absorbing material.

Let us now consider how diagnostic x-ray images are produced in more detail. The basic geometry is shown in Figure 5.1(a), with Figure 5.2 showing the process in more detail in cross section. The source of x-rays is generally a device called an **x-ray tube**, which emits x-rays at many different angles. The person being examined lies between the x-ray source and the detector (or **image receptor**). The geometry for formation of images is now apparent: a particular point on the detector corresponds to one pathway x-rays can take

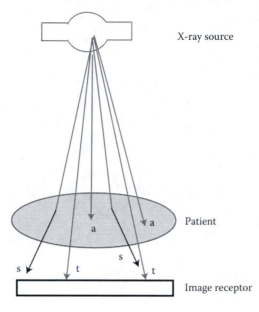

Figure 5.2 Cross-sectional view of the basic geometry for forming a radiograph, or diagnostic x-ray image. X-rays are generated by a source, usually an x-ray tube, which emits radiation at many different angles. X-rays travel through the body before encountering an image receptor. The actual image is formed by those x-rays that are not absorbed by the body, but which actually are either transmitted or scattered so as to reach the image receptor. Absorbed x-rays are indicated by a, transmitted x-rays hitting the detector by t, and scattered x-rays by s.

through the body. We can describe the possible outcomes of an encounter between x-ray photons and matter using the same three processes discussed for visible radiation in Chapter 3: transmission, absorption, and scattering. The image receptor measures the total number of x-rays transmitted through the part of the body in a line of sight between the source and that part of the detector, plus any scattered x-rays. In images such as Figure 5.1(b), the whiter regions correspond to where *fewer* x-rays hit the image receptor (radiopaque regions), and the darker regions indicate where *more* x-rays hit the image receptor (x-ray transparent or **radiolucent** regions).

Since variations in x-ray absorption along different pathways are the essential quantity influencing image formation, to understand x-ray image formation, we first address ways to understand how body tissues differ in their abilities to absorb x-rays.

5.3 TYPES OF X-RAY INTERACTIONS WITH MATTER

We will now explore the processes by which absorption and scattering occur for the x-rays used in diagnostic procedures. Which of these fates

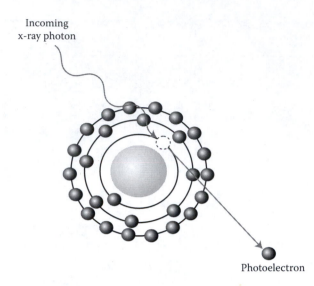

Incoming
x-ray photon

Photoelectron

Figure 5.3 The photoelectric effect. An x-ray photon interacts with an atom within the body, resulting in the excitation of an inner-orbital electron. The resulting photoelectron is free to travel, while the x-ray photon is entirely absorbed.

befalls an x-ray photon depends upon its energy, and the properties of the body tissues through which it travels.

We begin with the **photoelectric effect,** which dominates the absorption of x-rays with energies below approximately 25 keV. In this phenomenon, an incoming photon interacts with a tightly bound electron inhabiting an innermost orbital of an atom (Figure 5.3). For example, the atom might be carbon, oxygen, hydrogen, or nitrogen in the soft tissues, or calcium in the bones. There is a chance that this interaction results in the complete absorption of the x-ray photon, giving the electron enough energy to escape its orbital and hence become free altogether of the atom. Such a freed electron is called a **photoelectron.** Any energy left over from promoting it from its orbital appears as kinetic energy of the electron. In the photoelectric effect, *all* of the photon's energy is transferred to the photoelectron and the original photon no longer exists. The photoelectrons are free to travel throughout the body, but in general they only travel very short ranges before their energy is reabsorbed. Meanwhile, the vacant electron orbital is quickly refilled by the capture of an electron. The energy released when this occurs usually shows up as a photon called a **characteristic x-ray,** which can contribute to scattering if it escapes the body.

All interactions between x-rays and matter are probabilistic: that is, for each encounter there is only a likelihood of either complete transmission or absorption of the photon. The odds that an x-ray photon is absorbed by the photoelectric effect depend on the chemical elements in the absorbing material. The important quantity is the number of protons—and hence electrons—in the nucleus of an atom of that element, a quantity called the **atomic number, Z**. The likelihood of the photoelectric effect *increases* as the cube of the atomic number, Z^3. The photoelectric effect is more likely to occur in materials that have many atoms with relatively large values of Z because of this relationship. For example, heavy metals such as lead (Z = 82) are good absorbers of x-rays, so they can be used in, e.g., lead aprons for shielding parts of the body during diagnostic x-rays. Soft tissues of the body consist primarily of low Z atoms such as carbon (Z = 6), nitrogen (Z = 7), oxygen (Z = 8), and hydrogen (Z = 1). The probability of absorption by the photoelectric effect in a material depends upon its average value of Z, so soft tissues' low average $Z_{soft\ tissue}$ = 7.4 means they have a low probability of absorbing x-rays by the photoelectric effect. For example, water has an effective Z of 7.42, while muscle is closer to 7.46—different by only slightly over half a percent—and fat has an effective Z of about 5.92. By contrast, bone is 10% calcium (Z = 20) by weight, which boosts its effective atomic number to approximately Z_{bone} = 12.7. Reasoning from the dependence on Z^3, one would estimate that the average atom in bone is about $(Z_{bone}/Z_{soft\ tissue})^3 = (12.7/7.4)^3 \approx 5$ times as likely to absorb x-ray photons as one in soft tissue. The density of the material also influences how many atoms the x-ray encounters when it passes through a given thickness of material, so denser materials are generally better absorbers of x-rays than less dense ones. This dependence also makes the relatively denser bone and much denser lead better at absorbing x-rays than soft tissues.

As a general rule, the probability of the photoelectric effect drops rapidly as the x-ray energy increases (Figure 5.4). However, whenever the x-ray energy coincides with the exact amount of energy required to promote an electron to a higher energy orbital, the likelihood of absorption is considerably enhanced and we call that energy an **absorption edge** (Figure 5.5). The energy at which absorption edges occur is determined by the chemical element, and hence the Z, of the atoms in material. Later in the chapter, we will see how radiologists take advantage of this effect by choosing x-ray energies to coincide with important absorption edges in a contrast medium or an x-ray detector.

As the x-ray photon energy increases, a different process called the **Compton effect** becomes more important in soft tissue above approximately 25 keV. In this process, an x-ray photon can be thought of as colliding with a loosely held outer orbital electron, transferring enough energy to it to free it from its host atom (Figure 5.6). Exciting such an electron requires less energy than for the photoelectric effect. Indeed, the x-ray energy is so large compared to the energy binding the electron to the atom that the x-ray interacts with the electron as though it were not bound. This situation results in significant differences in the photon–electron interaction in comparison with the photoelectric effect. In fact, the Compton effect is analogous to having a pool ball (the x-ray photon) hit another pool ball (the electron, acting as though it's free of its associated atom), setting the second ball in

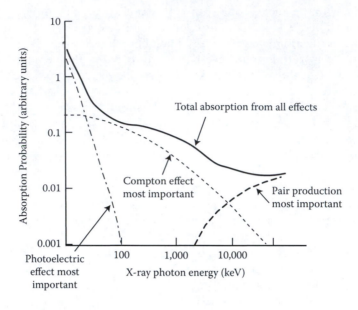

Figure 5.4 Absorption of x-rays in water as a function of energy, indicating the separate contributions due to the photoelectric effect and the Compton effect. The third absorption mechanism that dominates at high energies, called pair production, is described in Chapter 6.

motion while itself recoiling. Like a pool ball striking multiple other balls, a single x-ray photon can undergo multiple Compton effect encounters, gradually losing energy each time. (By contrast, recall that in the photoelectric effect, the photon is instead entirely absorbed.) We say that the resulting photon has been **Compton scattered** as it travels in a direction different from the original x-ray photon; scattered photons can corrupt the eventual x-ray image because of this loss of directional information.

Since in the Compton effect, x-ray photons interact with electrons as though they were not bound to an atom, only the *total number* of electrons in a block of material matters. Thus, only the thickness of an absorber and its density are important for x-ray absorption at higher energies by this mechanism. There also is no enhancement of the Compton effect near absorption edge energies. Thus, the Compton effect distinguishes between materials with different chemical compositions only because their densities can be different. Because most soft tissues have very similar densities, the Compton effect is relatively insensitive to variations in anatomy compared to the photoelectric effect (Table 5.1).

Figure 5.4 summarizes how each process enters into determining the *total* attenuation of x-rays in water; here attenuation refers to any mechanism by which photons are lost, including absorption and scattering. We summarize the interaction of x-rays with body tissue by specifying a quantity called the **attenuation coefficient**, μ (the Greek letter *mu*), measured

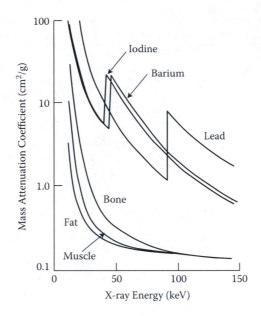

Figure 5.5 The variation of mass attenuation coefficient (μ/ρ) with x-ray energy for bone, muscle, and fat, as well as lead (used for shielding x-rays for safety purposes), and the contrast agents iodine and barium. The jumps due to absorption edges for iodine, barium, and lead are shown. To get the attenuation coefficient, the mass attenuation coefficient is multiplied by density, so the differences in attenuation between higher density bone, iodine, or lead, and less dense soft tissues, such as muscle and fat, are even more pronounced in practice. (Adapted in part from John R. Cameron and James G. Skofronick, *Medical Physics*, John Wiley & Sons, 1978.)

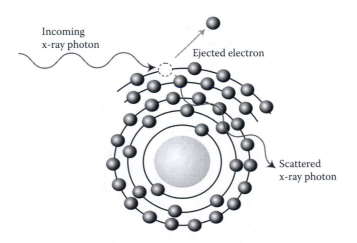

Figure 5.6 The Compton effect. An incident x-ray photon scatters from an outer shell electron, leading to the ejection of the electron and a scattered x-ray photon.

Table 5.1 Attenuation coefficient at 60 keV and density for
some materials important to medical x-ray imaging

Absorbing material	Attenuation coefficient at 60 keV, $\mu(cm^{-1})$	Density $\rho(g/cm^3)$
Fat	0.1788	0.91
Soft tissue other than fat (muscle, body fluids)	0.2045	1.00
Water	0.2055	1.00
Brain	0.2061	1.00
Air	~3 ×10⁻⁴	0.00129
Bone	0.466 to 0.548	1.65 to 2.0

in units of cm^{-1} (1/cm). This quantity determines the average intensity of x-rays of a particular energy transmitted by a particular material. The higher its attenuation coefficient, the more readily a material attenuates x-rays of that energy. The reciprocal of the attenuation coefficient $(1/\mu)$ is equal to the **range** of travel of the x-rays in the material, explaining the peculiar units of one over distance. After passing through a thickness equal to the range $(1/\mu)$, only 37% of the original x-rays remain. Each chemical element has its own specific attenuation coefficient, and a material, such as a body tissue, has an attenuation coefficient that depends upon the average for all of the chemicals constituting it.

The number of x-rays absorbed or scattered depends upon how many electrons are encountered along the x-ray's path through the body. This increases when the thickness or density of electrons within the absorbing material increases. The absorber's chemical composition is important because different atoms absorb x-rays with varying efficiencies depending on Z and how near the x-ray energy is to any absorption edges. These two effects can usefully be separated by breaking the attenuation coefficient into multiplicative factors: density, ρ (measured in units of g/cm^3) and **mass attenuation coefficient**, μ/ρ, the attenuation coefficient *per unit density* (measured in units of cm^2/g). The last quantity depends solely upon chemical composition and photon energy, and it is determined by the probability of x-ray attenuation. These numbers are multiplied to get the total attenuation coefficient:

$$\mu\left(cm^{-1}\right)=\rho\left(g/cm^3\right)\times\mu_m\left(cm^2/g\right) \tag{5.1}$$

The exact mathematical expression for the intensity, I_{trans}, of **monoenergetic** (single energy) x-rays transmitted by a material of thickness x and attenuation coefficient μ, is given by:

$$I_{trans}=I_o e^{-\mu x} \tag{5.2a}$$

where I_o is the intensity of x-rays incident upon the absorber. In addition, we can compute the intensity transmitted through two or more consecutive regions with thicknesses x_1, x_2, x_3, x_4, etc. and attenuation coefficients μ_1, μ_2, μ_3, μ_4, etc., respectively. Since each diminishes the transmitted intensity by a factor given by Equation 5.2(a), we repeatedly multiply the initial intensity by the correct factor for each region:

$$
\begin{aligned}
I_{trans} &= I_o e^{-\mu_1 x_1} e^{-\mu_2 x_2} e^{-\mu_3 x_3} e^{-\mu_4 x_4} \times \dots \\
&= I_o e^{-(\mu_1 x_1 + \mu_2 x_2 + \mu_3 x_3 + \mu_4 x_4 + \dots)}
\end{aligned}
\tag{5.2b}
$$

The exponents simply add, yielding a relatively simple expression for the absorption due to multiple layers. In addition, the intensity of x-rays *attenuated* is equal to:

$$
I_{atten} = I_o - I_{trans}
\tag{5.3}
$$

These expressions will prove useful in our later discussion of contrast formation.

Sample calculation: Let us compute some typical numbers for the x-ray transmissions encountered in a chest x-ray. First, how many x-rays are transmitted through a region of soft tissue approximately 20 cm thick? We can use this to model the tranmission through the upper chest for a small person. For 20 keV x-rays, the linear attenuation coefficient, $\mu = 0.77$ cm^{-1} for soft tissue.

$$
\frac{I_{trans}}{I_o} = e^{-\mu x} = e^{-0.77 \text{cm}^{-1} \times 20 \text{cm}} = 2.1 \times 10^{-7}
\tag{5.4}
$$

This means an extremely small fraction of the x-rays are transmitted at 20 keV, making this choice of photon energy a poor one for chest x-rays: virtually all x-rays are absorbed rather than being transmitted to form an image. For 60 keV x-rays, the linear attenuation coefficient is very different, $m = 0.21$ cm^{-1}, so we have instead:

$$
\frac{I_{trans}}{I_o} = e^{-\mu x} = e^{-0.21 \text{cm}^{-1} \times 20 \text{cm}} = 1.5 \times 10^{-2} = .015 = 1.5\%
\tag{5.5}
$$

This is still a small percentage of the original x-ray intensity: only 1.5% of the incident x-rays are transmitted, but it's dramatically higher than for 20 keV. Consequently, higher energy photons are used to image thicker body sections, as in chest x-rays, because of this dramatic difference in transmission.

So far, our discussion of absorption has assumed that the radiation has a single energy. However, x-ray generators for radiography actually emit photons with many different energies, each with a different attenuation coefficient. This means the attenuation of medical x-rays is even more complicated than the preceding discussion indicates. To characterize the actual situation, a quantity called the **half-value layer** (HVL) is used. The HVL defines a distance in which 50% of x-rays are absorbed in a tissue or other material (Figure 5.7a). Upon first entering the body, medical x-rays have half-value layers of roughly 4 to 8 cm for most soft tissues. However, the x-rays remaining after this first half-value layer are the less readily absorbed, hence more energetic, photons. This selective absorption of low energy and transmission of higher energy x-rays results in an enriching of the remaining beam with a higher content of higher energy photons, a phenomenon called **beam hardening** (Figure 5.7b). The next 4 to 8 cm of travel consequently result in fewer than 50% of those higher energy photons being absorbed. (In other words, the half-value layer becomes successively *larger* for the remaining increasingly higher energy x-rays.) The resulting complex dependence of x-ray absorption on energy must be taken into account in shielding for safety and in choosing x-ray source characteristics. Computers can be used to carry out the mathematical modeling necessary to determine the exact falloff of x-ray intensity with distance for actual x-ray sources.

5.4 BASIC ISSUES IN X-RAY IMAGE FORMATION

Three criteria determine the quality of an x-ray image: contrast, spatial resolution, and noise. In addition, absorption and scattering both contribute to the x-ray dose—a measure of the amount of energy transferred from the x-rays to the body, and the important quantity for determining the procedure's level of risk. The formation of good x-ray images requires a balancing act between low radiation dose and sufficient x-ray transmission to form a useful diagnostic image. Balancing these many concerns generally entails compromises peculiar to the procedure of interest.

For x-ray imaging we can define contrast, C, as the percent difference in the detected x-ray signal due to x-ray transmission between two x-ray paths in the body (Figure 5.8).

$$C = \frac{I_1 - I_2}{I_1} \tag{5.6}$$

where I_1 and I_2 are the x-ray intensities transmitted through paths 1 and 2 in the figure. Thus, to achieve adequate contrast on an image, the x-ray transmission of the object of interest must be sufficiently different from its surroundings to distinguish it. In many essential problems in medical imaging, such as mammography, achieving adequate contrast and spatial

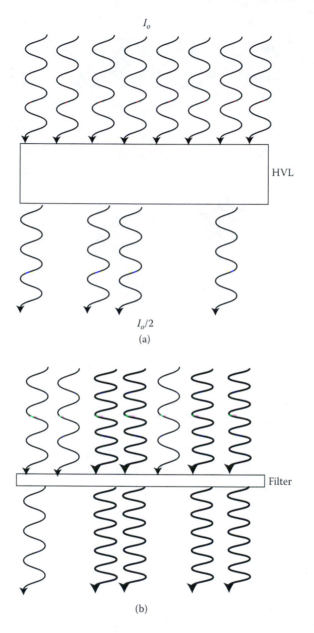

I_o

HVL

$I_o/2$

(a)

Filter

(b)

Figure 5.7 (a) Definition of the HVL (half-value layer). (b) Illustration of beam hardening. Since the range of lower energy photons is generally shorter than that of higher energy photons, passage through an absorber results in the selective absorption of lower energies first.

resolution is a difficult goal. The contrast within an x-ray image is determined by the energy of the x-ray beam, characteristics of the source and image receptor, scattered x-rays, sources of noise, and the x-ray absorption

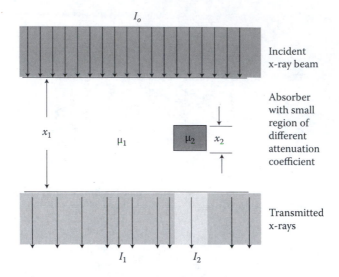

Figure 5.8 Illustration of the definition of contrast for radiography, considering the difference in x-ray transmission along two pathways, one of which contains the absorber to be imaged.

characteristics of the object being imaged. We first consider qualitatively the effect of differing x-ray absorption properties on contrast formation; this aspect of image formation is due to a combination of the chemical properties (effective atomic number) and density of the x-ray absorbing material itself, the thickness of the absorbers, and the energy spectrum of the x-rays used.

Using Equations 5.2(a) and 5.6, we can re-express the contrast in terms of the quantities that determine its value:

$$C = \frac{I_1 - I_2}{I_1}$$

$$= \frac{I_0 e^{-\mu_1 x_1} - I_0 e^{-\left(\mu_1\left(x_1 - x_2\right) + \mu_2 x_2\right)}}{I_0 e^{-\mu_1 x_1}}$$

$$= \frac{I_0 e^{-\mu_1 x_1}\left(1 - e^{-\left(-\mu_1 x_2 + \mu_2 x_2\right)}\right)}{I_0 e^{-\mu_1 x_1}}$$

$$= 1 - e^{-\left(\mu_2 - \mu_1\right)x_2}$$

(5.7)

If two tissues have very different x-ray absorption properties for a particular x-ray energy, they give good contrast and show up as distinct structures (Figure 5.9a). This could be due to differences in density, mass

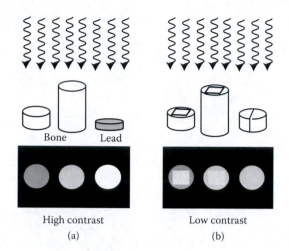

Bone   Lead

High contrast   Low contrast
(a)   (b)

Figure 5.9 Examples of situations in which (a) high contrast and (b) low contrast
occur in an x-ray image. (a) Absorbers with very different x-ray absorption properties result in good contrast, with a clear difference in the
number of x-rays transmitted. This can be caused either by large differences in the mass attenuation coefficient, density, and/or thickness.
(b) Small differences in x-ray absorption result in very low contrast.
This can be due either to very similar mass attenuation coefficients and
densities (rightmost figure), or a very thin absorber embedded in a much
thicker absorbing region (leftmost figures).

attenuation coefficient, or thickness, since Equation 5.7 depends upon all
three through the values of μ and x_2. (We will see shortly how the thickness of the surrounding tissue enters into determining the level of scattering, which can degrade contrast.) For example, it is easy to distinguish the
ribs from the surrounding soft tissues on a chest x-ray, because they satisfy
all three criteria (Figure 5.1b). However, if two adjacent tissues have very
similar x-ray absorption properties, then they are not distinguishable on
a radiograph, because the contrast is very small. This is true for virtually
all soft tissues (Figure 5.9b); for example, little detail is seen within the
heart in Figure 5.1(b). If a small region of high absorption is embedded in a
thicker region of low absorption, then it may not provide enough contrast
to make its presence noticeable (Figure 5.9b). This is the case for the mineral deposits called microcalcifications, that can indicate the presence of a
breast tumor, as well as for small masses in the lung called nodules that can
be either cancerous or benign. While x-ray absorption is one major issue
in contrast formation, scattering, the image receptor's sensitivity, and the
exact geometry for forming x-ray images also play important roles.

Attenuation coefficient values for different parts of the body for 60 keV
x-rays are given in Table 5.1. Consider that the values of attenuation coefficient for *all* soft tissues, including fat, muscle, water, and brain tissue,
differ by only a few percent, due mostly to small variations in chemical

composition and density. As a result, radiographers must work with limitations imposed by inherently low contrast between different types of soft tissues. The attenuation coefficient of bone is over twice that for soft tissues, due to both its higher density and higher effective atomic number, Z: as a consequence, the skeleton is generally distinguishable from soft tissues on radiographs. The air-filled lungs are also easy to distinguish, since their lower density results in little attenuation in comparison with the rest of the body. These effects are clearly apparent in radiographs such as the chest x-ray in Figure 5.1(a).

As the previous discussion shows, the choice of x-ray energy has important implications for the creation of effective medical x-ray images. However, there is no one obvious correct value to use, and different procedures represent different trade-offs. For example, the number of x-rays absorbed is greater for thicker body sections than for thin ones. We can see from Figure 5.7(b) that since higher energy photons are less strongly attenuated, they are transmitted more readily. This means that imaging of thicker parts of the body (as in, for example, chest x-rays) should be performed with higher energy photons so enough x-rays are transmitted to expose the image receptor adequately at safe patient doses. (Conversely, very low energy x-rays would be primarily absorbed or scattered before reaching the detector, and hence contribute only to the radiation dose.) However, this choice results in x-ray attenuation taking place mostly through Compton scattering, resulting in decreased contrast. For thinner body parts—for example, the breasts in mammography—lower energy x-rays can be used because there is less thickness to absorb them. Then the greater contrast due to the lower energy photons can be used effectively without delivering undesirably high radiation doses.

As Figure 5.2 makes clear, scattered x-rays also expose the x-ray image receptor. Still worse, scattered radiation is more readily detected because it tends to be lower in energy and travels at more oblique angles than the transmitted x-rays (also called the **primary beam**). In general, scattered photons emerge from the body traveling in a new direction, and some fraction of these hit the image receptor. Since scattering destroys information about the actual pathways the x-ray took through the body, these x-rays hit the image receptor uniformly, causing an overall fogging, which reduces image contrast. This fogging due to scattering can be an appreciable effect—up to 50% to 90% of the total x-rays hit the image receptor for some types of exams.

This effect is illustrated in Figure 5.10(a), which models the effect of scattering on the contrast, C, due to a small absorber. The extra intensity due to scattering is denoted as RI_1 (because the entire volume contributes to the scattering, so the scattering does not depend greatly upon the smaller region), and it is assumed to uniformly expose the image receptor. The effect is to leave the difference in intensities due to the absorber unchanged, while increasing the overall level of exposure. This reduces the contrast, C_s, with scattering by a factor of $(1 + R)$:

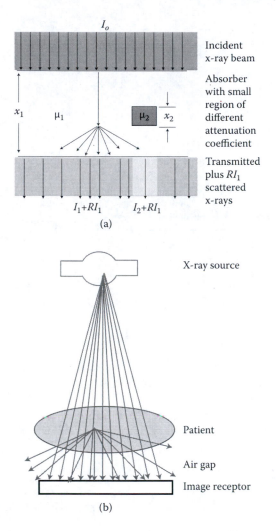

Figure 5.10 (a) Scattering uniformly exposes the image receptor, resulting in an overall reduction of contrast. (Compare to Figure 5.8.) Illustration of how (b) air gap and (c) grids can be used to reduce the amount of scattered x-rays hitting the image receptor.

$$C_s = \frac{\left(I_1 + RI_1\right) - \left(I_2 + RI_1\right)}{\left(I_1 + RI_1\right)}$$

$$= \frac{I_1 - I_2}{I_1\left(1 + R\right)} \qquad\qquad (5.8a)$$

$$= \frac{C}{1 + R}$$

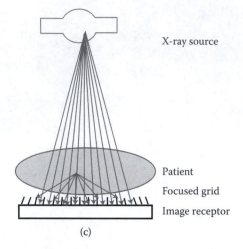

X-ray source

Patient

Focused grid

Image receptor

(c)

Figure 5.10 (continued).

Sample calculation: The ratio of the scattered intensity to the total intensity of x-rays hitting the image receptor is called the scatter fraction, F. If $F = 50\%$ for a particular exam, then half the intensity forming the image is due to scattering. By what factor is the contrast degraded?

The total intensity hitting the image receptor is equal to the sum of the transmitted (I_1) and scattered radiation (RI_1), so the scatter fraction is:

$$F = \frac{RI_1}{I_1 + RI_1}$$

$$= \frac{R}{R+1}$$

(5.8b)

If $F = 50\%$, then $R/(R + 1) = 50\% = 1/2 = 1/(1 + 1)$ and $R = 1$. We can then use Equation 5.8a to show that $C_s = C/(1 + R) = C/(1 + 1) = (1/2)C$; for this case, the contrast is reduced to half its value in the absence of scattering.

One of the goals of effective x-ray image formation is discovering how to reduce or remove scattering. Several techniques can be used to prevent scattered x-rays from hitting the image receptor. Since the entire irradiated volume creates scattering, restricting the x-ray beam to hit only the regions of interest reduces scattering. If an air gap is left between the patient and the image receptor, then fewer scattered x-rays will be intercepted (Figure 5.10b). This is because the scattered x-rays emerge from the body with a greater range of angles than do the transmitted photons. Thus, moving the image receptor away from the patient allows more of the scattered x-rays to miss the image receptor. To reduce scattering, a device called a **bucky** (a grid of extremely thin lead strips separated by radiolucent spacers, resembling a Venetian blind) can be placed between the body and image receptor to absorb scattered x-rays (Figure 5.10c). The thin channels between the lead strips absorb all x-rays except those traveling with a narrow range of angles, a process referred to as **collimating** the transmitted x-rays. Again, this idea takes advantage of the greater divergence of the scattered x-rays by providing a channel that favors passage of the primary beam's x-rays. Because the primary beam's x-rays travel along paths that radiate from the source, **focused grids** can be constructed to select for only this beam geometry. In applications where the shadow created by the slits is a problem, the grid can be oscillated from side to side so as to exposure the image receptor uniformly. Scattering is not only a problem for image quality; since x-rays are scattered throughout the room, scattering contributes to radiation exposure to distant parts of the patient's body, as well as any nearby medical personnel. In general, shielding is used to block as many of these scattered photons as possible.

In radiography, the major source of noise is generally due to statistical fluctuations in the number of photons hitting the detector, an effect called **quantum noise**. For high levels of noise, the resulting mottled grainy texture that noise imparts to radiographs can degrade contrast and spatial resolution. (You may be familiar with this effect if you have ever taken a photograph at too low a light level.) Figure 5.11 illustrates this effect for two different levels of exposure. The grid of squares in the low noise (left) and higher noise (right) cases represent the number of transmitted x-rays hitting small areas of the image receptor. The average number hitting the low noise image is 10,000 per square, while the higher noise case has only 100 per square. However, each square registers an actual exposure, which includes fluctuations about the average. A statistical measure called the standard deviation can be used to describe the typical magnitude of these fluctuations; for this situation, the standard deviation is equal to the square root of the number of x-rays detected, as indicated. Although the standard deviation is higher for the low noise case (100 vs. 10) it is lower *as a percentage of the average* (1% vs. 10%), which is what determines the extent to which the noise corrupts contrast and spatial resolution. Quantum noise can be minimized by using maximally efficient detectors, by lengthening the exposure time, and/or by increasing the incident x-ray intensity. However, the last two solutions also increase the patient dose, leading to instances in which safety concerns limit the optimal image quality.

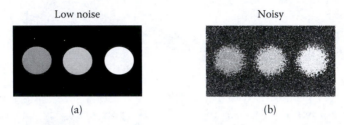

9,995	10,114	9,865
10,086	10,007	9,932
10,002	9,980	10,019

101	104	89
91	95	116
104	94	106

Average 10,000 x-rays per square
$10,000 \pm \sqrt{10,000}$
$10,000 \pm 100$
$100/10,000 = 1\%$ noise

Average 100 x-rays per square
$100 \pm \sqrt{100}$
100 ± 10
$10/100 = 10\%$ noise

Low noise

Noisy

(a)   (b)

Figure 5.11 Example showing the effect of two different average x-ray exposures on the amount of quantum noise in an image. The images at the bottom illustrate the effects of the two noise levels in contrast.

As usual, the spatial resolution (also called **blur** or **unsharpness** in radiography) of the image limits the size of the smallest detail discernible on the image and can degrade contrast (Figure 5.11b). The properties of the x-ray source and image receptor and the geometry used for imaging all determine the spatial resolution. Movement during an exposure also can cause blurring. Spatial resolution can be specified by giving the smallest spacing between two thin lines that can be resolved using the imaging technique. Another criterion used is determining the size of the image of a tiny object approximating a true mathematical point. Under optimal conditions, spatial resolutions as small as 0.1 mm are achievable in radiography, while CT scans have typical resolutions of 1 mm.

5.5 CONTRAST MEDIA MAKE SOFT TISSUES VISIBLE ON AN X-RAY

One way of getting around the similarities in x-ray absorption of many tissues is to utilize **contrast media**—radiopaque materials introduced into the soft tissues of the body. This is necessary, for example, in imaging the heart and the digestive tract, where the very similar densities and effective Z values of water, blood, and muscle make distinguishing any differences in x-ray absorption particularly difficult. Barium (Z = 56) and iodine

(Z = 53) are the two elements most commonly incorporated into contrast media. The high Z of these elements makes them absorb x-rays much more strongly by the photoelectric effect than soft body tissues (Figure 5.5); in addition, the compounds into which these elements are incorporated for imaging are denser than water. Barium and iodine in particular are chosen because their main x-ray absorption edges (called the **K-edge**) fall at 37.4 and 33.2 keV, respectively, in a range corresponding to typical diagnostic x-ray energies. As Figure 5.5 illustrates, the mass attenuation coefficient of iodine and barium rises abruptly just above their K-edge energies, resulting in significantly enhanced x-ray absorption by the contrast medium if x-rays with this energy range are used. The contrast agent's greater radiopaqueness creates large contrasts in absorption with surrounding soft tissues, making their presence easily discernible on a radiograph. This means that if the contrast agent is introduced into a specific region of the body, then the anatomy of that region can be easily visualized in turn. Contrast media are designed to be nontoxic compounds used in liquid form which are retained in the body long enough for image formation, then excreted naturally. While they signal their presence on radiographs as bright white regions, contrast agents merely absorb x-rays—they themselves do not emit x-rays, nor are they radioactive. Their apparently glowing appearance is due only to the convention that radiographs represent strongly *absorbing* regions as bright white.

To see why contrast media are necessary, consider Figure 5.12(a), which shows an ordinary radiograph of the abdomen. While the skeleton clearly shows up, few details of the abdominal organs are visible. A similar view is shown in Figure 5.12(b), but with the important distinction that the person imaged has been given a barium enema before the exam. As a result, a barium contrast agent fills the lower part of the gastrointestinal tract, making it appear as radiopaque as the skeleton, and revealing any abnormalities. Barium or iodine contrast media can be administered as drinks or enemas, depending on whether the lower or upper gastrointestinal tract is to be studied. A combination of barium contrast and air can also be used to delineate these regions by creating regions of, respectively, high and low x-ray absorption. Since the barium contrast medium moves gradually, it is also possible to watch its progress to get dynamic information about function.

Similarly, iodine compounds are used to make the anatomy of the urinary tract visible in studies such as **pyelograms** (diagnostic x-rays of the kidneys) and **urograms** (x-rays of the urinary tract). These studies can be performed to watch the functioning of the urinary tract by following the excretion of a contrast agent introduced by injection. The contrast media are organic iodine compounds of two types. The traditional choice, called ionic agents, are associated with a small risk of severe reactions—even death—in less than 1 in 40,000 cases. Nonionic media are more expensive, but offer a lower overall complication rate. It is significant to note that in either case, the risks due to reactions from contrast agents greatly exceed the small risk due to the radiation itself.

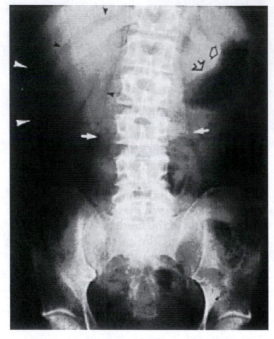

(a)

Figure 5.12 (a) The radiography of a normal abdomen shows little detail apart
from the skeleton. A dark region corresponding to air in the gut is
indicated by open arrows. (b) With the addition of barium contrast
medium, the structure of the gastrointestinal tract becomes quite clear.
(Reproduced with permission courtesy of John H. Juhl and Andrew B.
Crummy, eds., *Paul and Juhl's Essentials of Radiologic Imaging*, J.B.
Lippincott, Philadelphia, 1993.) (c) Angiography apparatus. (Reproduced with permission courtesy of Siemens Medical Systems.)

X-ray angiography, x-ray imaging of the circulatory system with contrast
media, also makes use of organic iodine compounds. Although the outline
of the heart itself is visible in even an ordinary chest x-ray (Figure 5.1a), an
injection of contrast media is necessary to see details of the blood vessels
(Figure 5.12c). This is usually performed by means of a catheter threaded
through a large vein into the blood vessel or heart chamber of interest;
the injection can then be made locally, using only a small amount of contrast dye. X-ray angiography remains the "gold standard" for imaging the
heart and circulatory system at high spatial resolution. Its use significantly
expands the ability of diagnostic x-rays to study and treat cardiovascular
disease, by far the leading cause of death in the U.S. For example, coronary
angiography can be used to detect the narrowing of major blood vessels,
which indicates the presence of coronary artery disease. This technique
is important, in large part because angiography makes possible cardiac
catheterization procedures, which now replace many types of open surgery

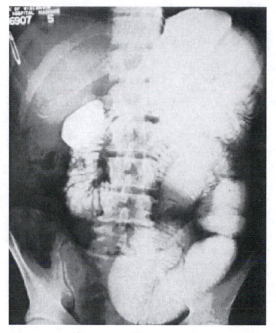

(b)

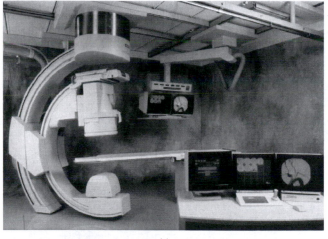

(c)

Figure 5.12 (continued).

on the heart and large blood vessels. These less invasive and risky procedures can be used for numerous operations—from the insertion of cardiac
pacemakers to balloon angioplasty techniques for opening up blood vessels
occluded by plaque.

5.6 HOW X-RAYS ARE GENERATED

The way x-rays are generated plays a major role in determining the quality and characteristics of the resulting images. The x-rays used in diagnostic imaging are produced using a source called an x-ray tube (Figure 5.13). In this device, an evacuated container houses several components used to generate x-rays by the conversion of energy from electrical power to x-radiation, and—as an unavoidable by-product—heat. The first step in this process involves producing free electrons. Within the chamber, a fine spiral **filament** of tungsten (much like those found in incandescent lightbulbs) is heated by passing an electrical current through it. At sufficiently high temperatures, some of the electrons in the filament have enough thermal energy to escape their attraction to the filament's metal atoms and to boil off to form a cloud. Surrounding the filament is a cup-shaped metal assembly called a **cathode**. At some distance from the cathode and filament is the metal **anode** (or **target**). In a fixed target x-ray tube, the target remains stationary, while in **rotating anodes**, it is a bevelled disk that rotates at high speeds. A very high electrical voltage is applied between the cathode and anode, with the polarity of this voltage chosen to render the anode positive and the cathode negative. The positive electrical charge on the anode strongly attracts the freed electrons, and this electrical force accelerates them toward the anode. The cathode is shaped so as to focus by electrical forces the beam of accelerated electrons so they strike only a thin line on the anode. After traversing the gap, each electron has an energy in keV equal to the accelerating voltage in kiloVolts (kV). This actually motivates the definition of the unit electron-Volt (eV): 1 eV is the kinetic energy an electron has after accelerating across a gap with 1 volt of electrical potential difference between the two sides.

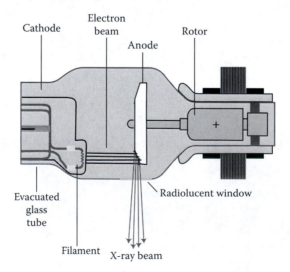

Figure 5.13 The construction of a rotating anode x-ray tube.

That is, if the cathode-anode voltage, called the peak kiloVoltage (**kVp**), is 150 kV, then the electrons will have a kinetic energy equal to 150 keV just before they hit the anode. (In practice, this voltage varies in time in a complex way not covered here.)

Upon colliding with the anode, the electron's kinetic energy is released in interactions with atoms within the metal anode. Less than 1% of the electrons' energy actually goes toward x-ray production, and the remaining energy going toward heating the anode. This heat serves no purpose in x-ray production, and it must in fact be removed to prevent it from damaging the x-ray tube. Indeed, the advantage of rotating anode sources over fixed target x-ray tubes is that they allow the point at which electrons strike the anode to be constantly moved as the anode rotates rapidly. This spreads the heat to be dissipated over a greater area, enabling more electrons to strike the anode, and hence produce more x-rays, without melting the target.

Two mechanisms produce x-rays as the fast electrons hitting the target slow down. The first, called **bremsstrahlung** (German for *braking radiation*), corresponds to the case where the electrons interact via electrical forces with atomic nuclei, gradually slowing down and changing direction. Whenever a charged particle like an electron changes its velocity, it emits radiation (Figure 5.14a). The energy of an x-ray photon produced by this mechanism depends upon how much energy the electron loses in a particular collision with a nucleus. Glancing collisions will produce low energy x-rays, while the maximum x-ray energy possible corresponds to a collision in which all of the electron's original energy is converted into

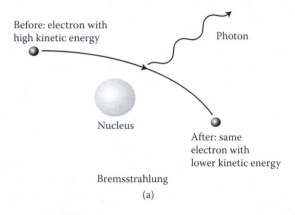

Figure 5.14 (a) Bremsstrahlung, the emission of x-rays by electrons when they accelerate due to electrical interactions between the negatively charged electrons and the positively charged atomic nuclei. The energy carried by the emitted photon is equal to the kinetic energy lost by the electron. (b) A high energy electron can knock out another electron bound to an atom in the anode, leaving a vacancy (open circle). (c) Characteristic radiation results when the vacancy is filled.

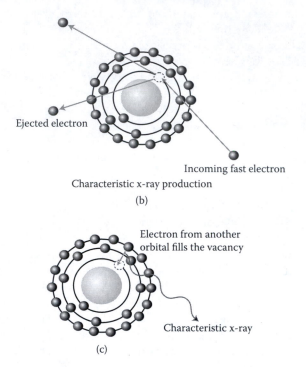

Characteristic x-ray production

(b)

(c)

Figure 5.14 (continued).

a photon. Tube voltages commonly used in diagnostic applications range from 25 kV to 150 kV, with corresponding maximum x-ray energies of 25 keV to 150 keV. (The lowest energy x-rays emitted from the tube are typically about 15 keV, since lower energy photons are absorbed by materials in the x-ray tube.) A radiolucent window allows the x-rays emitted to emerge from the x-ray source as a beam useful for imaging.

The emission spectrum of an x-ray source is a plot of the number of x-rays produced at different energies. Figure 5.15 shows emission spectra for two popular anode metals used in imaging, (a) tungsten, and (b) molybdenum. In both spectra, the radiation from bremsstrahlung produces x-rays at many energies, rather like the broad spectrum of a lightbulb. Because the x-ray sources are also operated at different voltages, the maximum x-ray energy emitted differs: in (a), the kVp of 100 volts results in x-rays with an energy range extending approximately to 100 keV, higher than in (b), where the kVp is only 30 volts. The overall number of x-rays produced by bremsstrahlung is influenced by the atomic number of the anode metal as well. The higher atomic number of tungsten (74) relative to molybdenum (42) means its nuclei are more effective at accelerating the electron beam, and hence produce more x-rays for the same operating conditions. Tungsten and molybdenum also have the advantage of having a high melting temperature and good thermal properties for heat dissipation.

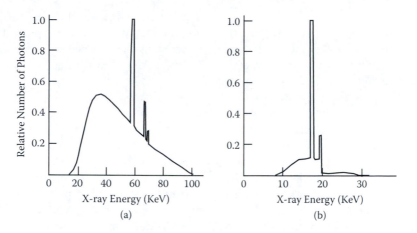

Figure 5.15 Emission spectra of two x-ray sources showing the number of x-ray photons emitted at various energies. (a) Tungsten anode at a voltage of 100 kVp, with a 2.5 mm aluminum filter, settings typical for imaging thick body sections, as for chest x-rays. (b) Molybdenum anode at a voltage of 30 kVp, and a 0.03 mm molybdenum filter, typical settings for mammography. Note especially that the range of energies in (b) is much lower than in (a). (Adapted from Steve Webb, *Physics of Medical Imaging*, Institute of Physics Publishing, Bristol, U.K., 1988.)

Another reason different metals are used in anode construction is that x-ray tubes also emit **characteristic x-rays** at specific energies characteristic of the anode metal. For example, careful inspection of Figure 5.15(a) and (b) shows that tungsten and molybdenum anodes also produce sharp x-ray peaks in their emission spectra; these peaks are located at different energies for the two anode materials. The peaks result when an energetic electron from the incident beam collides with an inner electron bound to an atom of the anode metal. If the energy of the incident electron is at least as great as the orbital energy of the bound electron, this collision can result in the transfer of enough energy to the bound electron to free it altogether from its orbital (Figure 5.14b). After this collision has taken place, a vacancy remains in the orbital; in time, the empty orbital is filled by an electron from a higher energy orbital. As it moves from a higher to a lower energy orbital, this electron can release its excess energy as a characteristic x-ray photon (Figure 5.14c). Because the emitted photon's energy is exactly equal to the difference in electron orbital energies, the emitted x-rays have a spectrum peculiar to the anode metal's electronic structure. Because there are often several orbitals that can easily supply electrons to fill the vacancy, a variety of characteristic x-ray energies can appear in the emission spectrum. The tube voltage does not affect the energy at which characteristic radiation occurs, apart from setting an upper limit to the highest energy photon that can be produced. Characteristic radiation is a significant factor in x-ray production, and the total emission spectrum must be taken into account in selecting an appropriate anode metal.

X-rays radiate from the focal line where the electrons hit the anode. Because this line is presented edge-on to the image receptor, it appears as a focal *spot* (see Figure 5.16a), with dimensions determined by the width of the line and the angle at which the line is oriented. Longer lines and greater angles give larger focal spots. The choice of focal spot size is a trade-off between greater spatial resolution at smaller spot sizes vs. better heat dissipation at higher spot sizes. We can see why by using Figure 5.16(b) to derive the relationship between focal spot size and spatial resolution. There, a point-sized hole in a perfect x-ray absorber is placed between an x-ray source with width a, creating an image with width b; this situation is meant to present a simplified model for how well small objects can be imaged. Note that even though the transmitting hole is represented as a true mathematical point, its x-ray image has a significant width, B. The relation between B and focal spot width a is determined by the distances between the source and object (d_1), and the object and the image receptor (d_2). Figure 5.16(b) shows the geometry that allows us to use similar angles to solve for B:

$$B/d_2 = a/d_1$$
$$B = a \; d_2/d_1$$

(5.9)

Thus, the smaller the focal spot, a, the smaller the image of the point absorber, and hence the higher the spatial resolution. Greater values of a result in blurring, as is apparent at the edges of a wide block of strongly absorbing material (see Figure 5.16c). The contribution of the focal spot size to the blurring of x-ray images is also related to the distance between the patient and image receptor, d_2. If the tissue to be imaged is very close to the image receptor, a small d_2 value reduces the resulting blur. However, there is another trade-off resulting from the competition between image magnification and blurring. We can see from Figure 5.16(c) that when the strongly absorbing block from Figure 5.15(b) is imaged (here the focal spot a is very small for simplicity) that its image size (I) is larger than its original size O; we describe this using a magnification factor, $M = I/O$. Again, using similar angles we can show that:

$$\frac{I}{d_1+d_2} = \frac{O}{d_1} \quad \text{or}$$
$$M = \frac{I}{O} = \frac{d_1+d_2}{d_1}$$

(5.10)

Thus, the magnification is increased by increasing d_2, at the cost of greater blur and reduced spatial resolution. (This effect can be readily

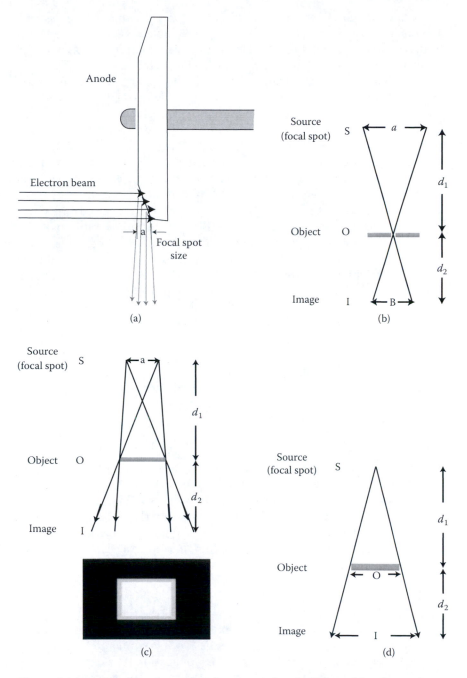

Figure 5.16 (a) Focal spot geometry for x-ray tube. (b) Effect of focal spot size on spatial resolution. Illustration of how blur (c) and magnification (d) are caused by imaging geometry and focal spot size.

observed with light. Use either a flashlight or a lamp with a clear glass bulb to make hand shadows on the wall, using varying distances between your hand, the lamp, and the wall. You can easily visualize the trade-off between the degree of blurring at the edges of the shadows and magnification.)

Heat dissipation is important because the power of the electron beam hitting the target amounts to many kilowatts. If this high power level is deposited into too small an area on the anode, it will melt the metal target. Thus, a larger focal spot allows a higher rate of x-ray production, because it can accommodate the higher heat production necessary. Longer exposure times must be used at lower powers with the smaller spot sizes to avoid melting the target. However, longer exposure times increase the chance of motion that can also blur the image. X-ray tubes can have filament sizes ranging from a large focal spot (typically a few mm in size) used when high resolution is not essential, to a very small focal spot (≥ 0.1 mm), used for specialized exams requiring exceedingly high resolution images.

The number of electrons striking the anode determines the number of x-rays produced for all energies. (Graphically, this quantity is proportional to the area under the emission spectrum curves in Figure 5.15 because this process corresponds to summing all x-rays produced at all energies.) This is set by the electron current, or **milliamperage** (*mA*), a direct measure of the number of electrons flowing per second between the cathode and anode, which is controlled by adjusting the filament temperature. The total number of x-rays produced during an exposure is then set by the **milliampere-second** (*mAs*), the product of exposure time in seconds, t, and electron current, mA:

$$mAs = mA \times t \qquad (5.11)$$

Longer exposure times t naturally result in more x-rays contributing to the production of a radiograph, and, for fixed kVp, the total number of x-rays produced per second is proportional to the mA. This determines not only how many x-rays strike the image receptor, but the overall patient dose as well. The milliamperage and exposure time must be chosen carefully to optimize the conditions for image formation, taking into account time constraints such as relevant body motions (which could blur the image if too long an exposure were used).

To summarize, the exact x-ray spectrum emitted is determined by the anode metal, tube voltage, electron current, and the filtration used. Since x-ray absorption depends strongly on photon energy, these variables allow considerable flexibility in selecting the emission spectrum and x-ray fluence most appropriate for a particular imaging application. For example, tungsten anodes operated at higher tube voltages produce both bremsstrahlung and characteristic x-rays at the higher energies useful for imaging thicker body sections in exams such as chest x-rays (Figure 5.15a). This is because the penetrating properties of higher energy x-rays are better suited for transmission through thicker body parts. Aluminum or copper filters can be used to absorb the less penetrating lower energy x-rays, which would otherwise be absorbed entirely within the body, contributing to the radiation dose without enhancing image contrast. Conversely, for thinner body sections, such as the hand and forearm, molybdenum anodes operated at lower tube voltages are often more appropriate (Figure 5.15b). More soft x-rays are transmitted through the thinner tissues and can contribute to image formation. This choice allows these applications to take advantage of the higher subject contrast available at lower energies. Molybdenum filters can be used to reduce the amount of high energy x-radiation above 20 keV (the K-edge for molybdenum); this is important because this "harder" radiation is almost entirely transmitted by the thin body sections, and hence reduces contrast. These practical physical constraints on source selection will be explored further in the context of a specific application in the section on mammography.

5.7 X-RAY DETECTORS

The image receptor used in forming a radiograph also plays an essential role in determining the contrast, spatial resolution, and noise level of the image, as well the patient's radiation dose. X-ray film remains in use for many applications, including imaging the chest and lungs, the skeleton, and the gastrointestinal tract (with barium contrast), as well as in dentistry. Increasingly, however, electronic detectors can now offer advantages over conventional film techniques. In addition, fluoroscopy is useful for imaging motion in real-time. We will now survey the essential characteristics of these basic types of image receptors to understand what features and limitations each can offer.

Film was the standard choice for recording x-ray images for decades after the early days of radiography. Even now, film has numerous advantages, including extremely good spatial resolution, good sensitivity, low price, wide availability, and permanency for record keeping. The film used in radiography consists of a film base (a transparent polyester or acetate sheet) that supports one or two coatings of the **emulsion**, which actually captures the image. The emulsion is a suspension of tiny silver bromide grains in gelatin. When the film is exposed, photons interact with the grains, sensitizing them to form a **latent image**. The sensitized grains are retained and blackened during the process of development, rendering those regions opaque, while unsensitized grains are removed, leaving only the transparent base. The radiographic image is formed by the resulting pattern of transparent and opaque regions of film, corresponding, respectively, to radiopaque and radiolucent regions of the body.

While this basic process can indeed be used to create a radiograph, by itself photographic film is not especially sensitive to x-rays. However, the sensitivity can easily be increased by placing the film in proximity to one or two thin **intensifying screens** of fluorescent material, forming what

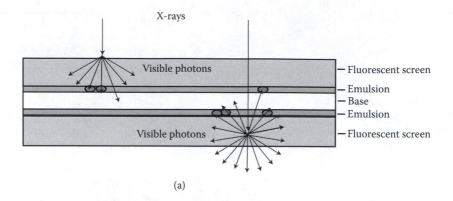

(a)

Figure 5.17 (a) Construction of a screen-film combination image receptor. Sandwiching film between fluorescent screens improves the efficiency of capturing x-rays, but creates blur due to the spread of visible light photons within the image receptor. (b) X-ray film characteristic curves for good contrast, but low latitude, film (top), and lower contrast, wider latitude film (bottom).

is called a **film-screen combination**. In such a system, an x-ray photon hits an intensifying screen, which then emits visible photons; these visible photons finally hit and expose the film emulsion. Phosphors in the screens efficiently absorb x-rays and re-emit their energy as visible light (Figure 5.17a). For example, one 50-keV x-ray photon can be converted into roughly 2000 photons of visible light in this way. Because photographic film is much more sensitive to visible light than it is to x-rays, this means that the combined detection system registers a much higher fraction of the x-rays hitting it than would film alone. To improve the detection efficiency yet further, the x-ray film can be made with an emulsion on both sides. The entire system finally is encased in a light-tight cassette for handling.

Improving the efficiency of x-ray detection with fluorescent screens permits the same quality x-ray image to be obtained at a much lower radiation dose to the patient. Research has resulted in a variety of newer phosphors made from rare earth compounds much more efficient at converting x-rays to light than the traditional calcium tungstate phosphor. However, an undesirable effect of phosphor screens is the reduction of the spatial resolution of the image produced. When an x-ray photon is directly absorbed by the film, it exposes the film at the precise location of impact with a spatial resolution of about 0.020 mm. When an x-ray produces visible photons in the fluorescent screen instead, these visible photons fan out and expose a larger area of film (Figure 5.17a), blurring the image. Good values for this type of image receptor are consequently limited to roughly 0.1 to 0.2 mm. These effects can be minimized by using only one screen, and by keeping the film

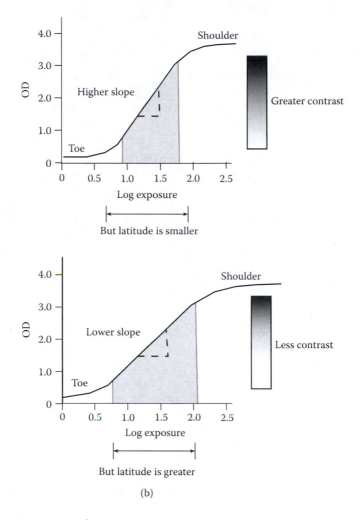

Figure 5.17 (continued).

and screen(s) in close proximity. Some phosphors, such as cesium iodide, can be grown so as to form oriented arrays of tightly packed, needle-like crystals; each crystal then acts like an optical fiber (Chapter 2), confining the re-emitted visible photons and avoiding blurring.

While x-ray film can be magnified, very few other manipulations can be performed to enhance the quality of images. Another problem with film is its limited ability to distinguish between subtle variations in absorption of x-rays, restricting its ability to image contrast. Typically, films are viewed by a radiologist in transmission, illuminated from behind with a lightbox. The perceived extent of film transparency and opaqueness can be made quantitative by using the **optical density** (or **OD**), defined as

$$OD = \log \frac{I_o}{I} \hspace{4cm} (5.12)$$

where I_o and I are the visible light intensity before and after the film, respectively. A plot of the variation in OD as a function of exposure is called the film's **characteristic curve** (Figure 5.17b). As Figure 5.17(b) illustrates, a high (low) OD corresponds to more (less) blackening because of greater (lesser) exposure to x-rays. (Be sure to note that the OD is not a density per se, but a measure of film opaqueness.) Very high exposures saturate the film (corresponding to the curve's shoulder), and very low ones do not expose it beyond an unavoidable level of fogging (as in the curve's toe). In between these limits lies the useful region of the curve, where OD varies strongly with exposure (shaded region of Figure 5.17b). The difference in contrast for an exposure difference due to a given difference in x-ray absorption is greater for larger slopes. The upper curve thus can generate images with greater contrast than can the lower. However, the useful range of variation in exposure (called the **latitude** of film and **dynamic range** more generally) is smaller for greater slopes. Since the latitude of x-ray film extends over a factor of less than 100, this is a crucial limitation in practice. While lower slopes lead to lower contrast, they increase the latitude. Thus, there is an inherent trade-off between the desirable features of high contrast and wide latitude. In practice, this limitation means that the film can register variations either in highly absorbing structures, or in weakly absorbing ones, but not both at the same time.

Understanding logarithms: When we need to plot or describe a quantity that varies over a tremendous range, perhaps over many orders of magnitude, the logarithm function is extremely useful. For example, the photon energies and mass attenuation coefficients in Figure 5.4 are plotted as logarithms to capture their dependencies over the range of interest. A logarithm is essentially an exponent (power) that describes the number of interest. A fixed number—10 in our case—is chosen as the base for constructing the logarithm. Then, the exponent required to represent a given number is computed. For example:

$$1 = 10^0 \quad \text{so } \log 1 = 0$$

$$10 = 10^1 \quad \text{so } \log 10 = 1 \hspace{3cm} (5.13)$$

$$100 = 10^2 \quad \text{so } \log 100 = 2$$

and so on.

(continued on next page)

Since exponents add, when two numbers, A and B, are multiplied, their logarithms are added. That is, if:

$\log A = a \quad$ then $10^a = A$

$\log B = b \quad$ then $10^b = B$

$A \times B = 10^a \times 10^b = 10^{a+b}$ $\qquad\qquad$ (5.14)

$\log(A \times B) = a + b$

This means, for example, that whenever you add 1.0 to a logarithm of a number, it has the same effect as multiplying the number itself by a factor of 10. For example, in Figure 5.4, the separation between 0.01, 1, 10, 100, etc. on the axes are all the same. In Figure 5.17(b), the lowest achievable *OD* is 0, corresponding to 1, or 100% transmission. The lowest achievable *OD* for low exposures in Figure 5.17(b) is called the baseline fog, and it has a value of roughly 0.2. From Equation 5.12, we see that this means that the most transparent x-ray film with this characteristic curve only transmits $1/10^{0.2} \approx 1/1.6 \cong$ 63% of the light incident upon it.

Radiography that makes use of image receptors based on electronic detectors to record and storage the image is called **digital radiography**; increasingly film-based radiography is being replaced by digital techniques, as discussed in a later section. Electronic detectors are divided into two types: indirect detectors employ phosphors to capture x-ray photons and re-emit visible light that is then detected, while direct detectors sense the x-rays themselves without first converting their energy into visible light. Since direct detectors avoid the blurring inherent in the intensifying screen, they can achieve higher spatial resolution. Another distinction is between digital radiography detectors that produce a usable image immediately after the x-ray exposure, and those that require further processing; the latter, called **computed radiography (CR)** systems, often use storage phosphors that can replace screen-film cassettes in existing x-ray systems. Exposing the CR storage phosphor to x-rays results in a stored image that can be read out later in a separate step, including to a digital format. X-ray images can be measured using solid state detectors, usually made of silicon-based electronic integrated circuits such as CCDs (first mentioned in Chapter 2) and CMOS electronic detectors found in digital cameras. These can be used to capture radiographs if intensifying phosphor layers are used first to convert the x-ray image to visible light, an indirect approach. X-ray images collected in either way can easily be stored in electronic format on a computer, for use with the digital image methods discussed later in the chapter. Direct electronic detectors made from thin film transistors made of amorphous (noncrystalline) selenium (a material adapted from xerography) are another alternative technology for solid-state image receptors for mammography and other applications.

In addition, some x-ray imaging apparatuses, such as CT scanners, use electronic **point detectors**, which only measure x-ray transmission through a line. The x-ray intensity is measured at many points to build up an entire image, so these detectors are either used in arrays or are scanned to measure x-ray intensities at different positions. Two popular point detectors are **scintillators** and **gas ionization detectors**. Both these detectors provide an electronic signal proportional to the x-ray intensity; the result is stored in a computer, which then assembles the total image from a series of measurements. While these point detectors might seem needlessly complex compared to film, they have appreciably greater dynamic range; that is, they are able to measure many orders of magnitude wider ranges of variation in transmitted x-ray intensity than can film. This ability contributes to an improved ability to distinguish, for example, the low contrast between soft tissues.

Scintillator detectors use a crystal that absorbs x-rays and reemits their energy as visible light photons (Figure 5.18). These visible photons next enter a device called a **photomultiplier tube**. Inside the photomultiplier tube, they hit a photocathode, a device that converts light to photoelectrons via the photoelectric effect. However, these photoelectrons are too few in number to produce an appreciable electrical signal. To overcome this problem, the photoelectrons are accelerated by a large voltage toward a positive electrode called a **dynode**. The collision between the energetic incoming electrons and the dynode metal frees many more electrons. These in turn are accelerated to the next dynode, further multiplying the signal when they in turn collide and release more electrons. After many such multiplications, a very large electrical signal has been produced from each original x-ray.

A gas ionization detector consists of a box fitted with an x-ray transparent window and filled with highly pressurized xenon gas. The element xenon is chosen because its high atomic number Z makes it a good x-ray

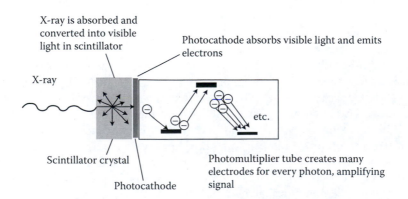

Figure 5.18 Scintillator detector. See text for description.

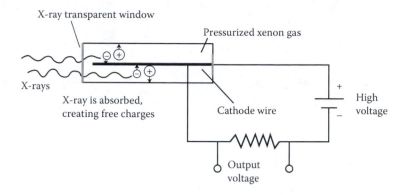

Figure 5.19 Gas ionization detector. See text for description.

absorber (Figure 5.19). A wire runs down the length of the box, and a very large voltage is applied between the inside walls of the box and this wire. When x-rays enter the detector, they interact with xenon atoms and ionize them by one of the absorption processes. The free electrons thus created are accelerated by electrical forces toward the central wire. The resulting electrical current is measured, and its magnitude is proportional to the original x-ray's energy.

Fluoroscopy is a form of real-time x-ray imaging used for imaging motions within the body, and for many interventional procedures done under x-ray guidance (Figure 5.20a). For example, fluoroscopy must be used to follow the catheter's progress through the body in the cardiac catheterization techniques discussed earlier (Figure 5.12c). This dynamic imaging technique

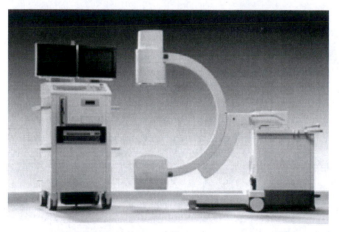

(a)

Figure 5.20 (a) Fluoroscopy apparatus. (Reproduced with permission courtesy of Siemens Medical Systems.) Schematic illustrations of the operation of (b) a fluoroscopy apparatus and (c) an image intensifier.

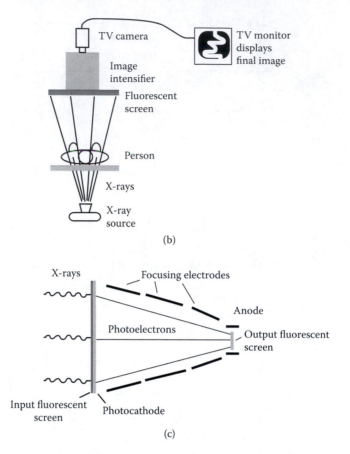

Figure 5.20 (continued).

typically uses fluorescent materials to convert x-rays into visible light on a phosphor screen (Figure 5.20b). However, the dim resulting image is difficult to see when safe radiation exposures are used. Traditional fluoroscopy units employ a device called an **image intensifier** to increase the brightness of the original dim image (Figure 5.20c); a video camera is used to record the visible light image. In an image intensifier, the fluorescent screen is placed against a photocathode, like that used in a scintillation detector. In the photocathode, the visible photons are converted into photoelectrons. These photoelectrons are accelerated and focused by electrical forces onto a second, smaller phosphor screen, where they form a tiny version of the original x-ray image. The brightness of the original image is increased by two processes: both the concentration due to focusing and the energy added to the photoelectrons produce more light on the output screen. Increases of a factor of 1000 to 5000 in brightness can be achieved this way. The resulting brighter image can be viewed directly, but it is more common to view it with a video camera and display it on a monitor. The resulting images can also be converted into an electronic format for further analysis by computer. However, fluoroscopy can now take advantage of detectors like those used for digital radiography, such as flat panel electronic arrays.

Since relatively higher and continuous irradiation must be used throughout the procedure, fluoroscopy results in higher radiation doses than imaging by film. Individual images are in general of much lower quality than can be achieved with image receptors in terms of spatial resolution, noise, and contrast. Consequently, fluoroscopy is used only in applications where its unique ability to see motion is needed, such as x-ray studies used to guide interventional procedures, or to follow a process involving flow within the body.

5.8 MAMMOGRAPHY: X-RAY SCREENING FOR BREAST CANCER

Throughout the world, breast cancer is a common—and often fatal—form of cancer in women. Within the U.S., it is the second most deadly cancer for women, after lung cancer, estimated to have caused approximately 40,000 deaths in 2007. Since 1990, there has been a 2.2% per year decrease in the death rates for this disease, due at least in part to advances in cancer treatments and diagnosis. Breast cancer appears to be one form of cancer in which early detection and treatment pay off. Mammography has been proven effective at detecting many breast tumors at early stages of formation, when they are most responsive to treatment. The success of surgery, radiation therapy, chemotherapy, and hormonal therapies is significant enough to warrant hope that screening programs for early detection will enable more women to survive this disease, and to take greater advantage of effective, less-disfiguring therapies.

Public health screening for breast cancer encompasses several major components, including regular physical examinations by a physician and mammograms during the years of highest risk. Mammograms can detect tumors when they are too small to be felt upon examination; the National Cancer Institute estimates that mammograms detect at least 80% of all breast cancers, with even better detection rates for older women.

Exams are performed on a dedicated mammographic x-ray system (Figure 5.21) specially designed for breast exams. Figure 5.22(a) shows the geometry used, and Figure 5.22(b) shows an actual exam in process. The woman being examined typically stands before the mammography unit, and a technician positions her breast between two plates. The breast is then compressed between the plates to thin out the breast tissue to a D-shape several centimeters thick. X-rays are then transmitted through the breast toward an image receptor (either an electronic detector or a film-screen cassette) on the bottom plate. The entire unit can rotate about a horizontal axis, permitting images to be taken at more than one angle to allow overlapping structures to be distinguished. Another view of the breast is taken after rotating the assembly 90°; four films (two views of each breast) are

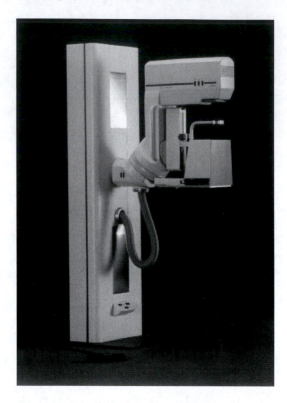

Figure 5.21 X-ray system for mammography. (Reproduced with permission courtesy of Siemens Medical Systems.)

typical. Collimation of the x-rays, shielding of the equipment, and having
the woman wear a lead apron can all be employed to reduce the radiation
dose to the rest of the body.

After the exam, a radiologist carefully examines each image, searching for
signs that may indicate a tumor's presence (Figure 5.22c). Mammography is
only a *screening* technique, that is, it cannot definitely identify those women
who suffer from breast cancer, but rather, offers some indication of which
women are most likely to have breast cancer upon further examination. All
a mammogram can detect is a region of increased radiopaqueness—there is
no definitive x-ray signature of a malignant tumor; only a biopsy can prove
that a mass actually is cancerous. The majority of mammograms appear
normal, but in a few percentages of all cases, a suspicious finding warrants
more investigation. The woman examined is informed about the results of
her mammogram and given advice on any necessary follow-up exams. The
next step after a positive (suspicious) mammogram may be a second mammogram performed with magnification and at higher spatial resolution.
Another common follow-up exam is the use of high resolution ultrasound
to distinguish between cysts and solid tumors (Chapter 4). Benign, fluid-
filled cysts can also be diagnosed by aspiration with a needle to remove

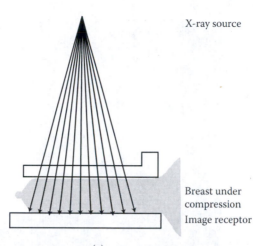

X-ray source

Breast under
compression
Image receptor

(a)

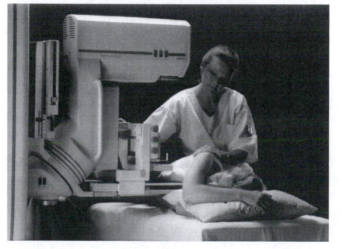

(b)

Figure 5.22 (a) Schematic illustration of the imaging geometry for a mammogram.
(b) Actual exam in progress. (Reproduced with permission courtesy
of Siemens Medical Systems.) (c) Mammogram showing a radiopaque
tumor (white mass at upper right). (Reproduced with permission courtesy of Dr. Steven E. Harms.)

fluid. If a solid mass indicative of a tumor is found, even this does not mean
cancer since many tumors are benign. A biopsy must be performed to distinguish between benign and malignant tumors.

Since in mammography asymptomatic women are screened by the millions, mammograms have been designed to keep the x-ray doses administered at low levels. As discussed further in Chapter 7, such extremely low
doses are used that even the most conservative estimates give negligible

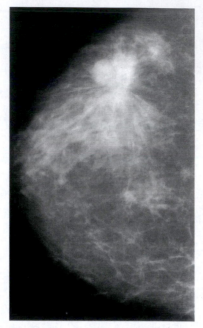

(c)

Figure 5.22 (continued).

risk of cancer from this cause. However, the two competing constraints of low dose and best quality image make designing mammographic systems a challenging application of medical physics. Careful selections of x-ray source characteristics, x-ray detectors, and imaging geometries all contribute to optimizing image contrast while minimizing the x-ray dose. We will return to a more careful consideration of mammography risk vs. benefit in Chapter 7.

Recall that higher energy x-rays are more penetrating, but lower energy x-rays give better contrast between different tissues. Thus, although using lower energy x-rays increases the dose, it improves contrast. This is especially important in mammography, where the radiologists seek inherently low contrast structures. In part this is because the x-ray absorptions of different types of soft tissue are all very similar. Breast tumors do not absorb x-rays appreciably differently from breast gland tissue, so their subject contrast is inherently poor; better contrast occurs when the tumor is surrounded by fat, which is somewhat less absorbing than glandular tissue at low energies. This is one reason mammograms are usually only prescribed for older women; younger women have denser breasts, with more gland tissue and less fat, but with advancing age the balance shifts toward a higher fraction of fat. This means that tumors are more effectively imaged in older women. (Breast cancer also occurs less frequently in younger women, making screening tests less effective because of the lower incidence.)

As a result of the difficulty in directly imaging tumors, in mammography the tumor itself often is detected indirectly by observing **microcalcifications**: tiny calcium deposits resembling minute grains of salt that can be associated with a tumor. These microcalcifications resemble bone in their high x-ray linear attenuation coefficient, but they are so small—deposits 0.1 mm and under must be imaged—that they offer little contrast; hence their detection requires both excellent contrast and extremely high spatial resolution.

> **Why must the breast be compressed during a mammogram?** Breast compression can be quite uncomfortable (but not dangerous) for the woman being examined, but it is necessary. The answer to the question lies in the physics of x-ray image formation. Compression spreads out the breast tissue, enabling exams to be performed at lower x-ray doses, because the breast itself has been rendered thinner and better able to transmit x-rays. As a result, lower-energy x-rays then can be used to examine the thinned breast, resulting in higher contrast images. It also improves spatial resolution, because there is less blurring due to motion, and less separation between the breast and detector. In addition, compression results in less overlap of different tissues and in the production of fewer scattered x-rays, so the images are easier to interpret.

Specialized x-ray tubes incorporating molybdenum anodes operating at relatively low voltages are used for mammography; these are used in conjunction with molybdenum filters to absorb x-ray energies above 20 keV, which would uniformly penetrate the breast without providing appreciable contrast (Figure 5.15b). Specialized electronic detectors and film-screen combinations also have been developed to detect the images. These can incorporate phosphors such as cesium iodide with absorption edges carefully matched to the molybdenum anode emission spectrum and thicknesses chosen to optimize detecting x-rays at this energy range. Research into efficient new phosphors optimized for absorbing low energy x-ray photons and emitting light absorbed well by x-ray film or electronic detectors have resulted in large dose reductions in the past several decades. However, the inherent blurring due to the image receptor limits the spatial resolution to about 0.1 mm for an ordinary screening mammogram. Because the smallest microcalcifications can be difficult to resolve with these constraints, follow-up mammograms employ different imaging geometries to provide magnification of the breast in order to better resolve any possible tumor masses and microcalcifications. Because the use of magnification would involve increasing the blur for fixed focal spot size, a very small focal spot size is required to provide the high spatial resolution necessary for such exams.

Dramatic improvements in image quality were one reason mammograms became more widely prescribed during the 1980s. Equally important are the skills of radiologists experienced in painstakingly interpreting large numbers of mammograms routinely, searching for subtle indications of disease. New digital imaging technologies being developed with the hope of helping radiologists catch **false negatives** (cancers missed by the examiner) will be discussed in the next section. **Scintimammography** (Chapter 6) and **breast magnetic resonance** imaging (**breast MR**) (Chapter 8) are being investigated as follow-up exams that could help reduce the number of **false positives,** the 65 to 85% of suspicious mammograms in which no cancer is found in follow-up biopsies. Medical researchers hope that someday these methods may help to reduce the number of biopsies required, as well as locate an even higher number of cancers than can mammography by itself.

How effective are mammograms? This question has been addressed through two main methodologies: epidemiological population studies and statistical analyses of databases containing information about breast cancer screening, treatment, incidence, and mortality. Both approaches reinforce the argument that mammography is an effective screening tool for breast cancer that saves lives. Many major population studies of women regularly screened using mammograms have been performed.* Earlier detection tends to artificially increase the time between diagnosis and death even in the absence of effective treatments, so to be effective, screening must reduce mortality from a disease over the long term, where mortality is defined in terms of death rate (for example, the number of deaths due to breast cancer each year per 100,000 women) to control for changes in population size. Reduction of mortality rates of 20% to over 39% in women over 50 has been consistently seen in the major population studies of mammography, although so far the record on benefits from screening before age 50 is mixed. The measure for whether reductions in a death rate are believable is **statistical significance;** a finding meets this standard only if it is extremely unlikely to have resulted from chance alone. (See Chapter 7.) The results of several studies of women over 50 meet this rigorous criterion. A 2007 review of the literature on population studies for women between age 40 and 49 also saw evidence for a decrease of 7 to 23% in breast cancer mortality, although few randomized, controlled clinical trials have been performed for this age group.†

Because of the long time over which populations must be studied in order to see any beneficial effects, the mammograms performed in most studies were done many years, even decades, ago. Mammography quality has improved considerably in the meantime, while radiation doses have gone down, so the net benefit is expected to be higher in the future.

---

* L.L. Humphrey, M. Helfand, B.K. Chan, S.H. Woolf, "Breast cancer screening: a summary of the evidence for the U.S. Preventive Services Task Force," *Annals of Internal Medicine,* volume 137, pp. 347–360 (2002).

† K. Armstrong, E. Moye, S. Williams, J.A. Berlin, E.E. Reynolds, "Screening mammography in women 40 to 49 years of age: a systematic review for the American College of Physicians," *Annals of Internal Medicine,* volume 146(7), pp. 516–526 (2007).

However, many population studies have been criticized on the basis of not meeting standards for randomized, controlled clinical trials.* As a result, in 2005, the NIH National Cancer Institute released results from a major study of databases containing information on breast cancer mortality, treatment and screening in the U.S. for the period 1990 to 2000, a period over which breast cancer mortality declined by 24%.† This study used seven different statistical approaches to determine to what extent improvements in treatment and mammography screening influenced this decline. The researchers concluded that between 28% to 65% of the decrease was due to mammography, with the rest primarily due to improved treatment.

Based on these findings, the NIH National Cancer Institute now recommends regular mammographic screening for all women every one or two years after age 40; women with risk factors, such as a family history of breast cancer, are advised to consult with a physicians about the wisdom of starting such exams earlier. Meanwhile, improvements in treatments, and in mammographic techniques discussed in the next section, all promise hope that the decrease in mortality due to this disease will continue.

5.9 DIGITAL RADIOGRAPHY

Traditionally, anatomical information can lie buried in an x-ray film, indicated only by subtle contrasts in x-ray absorption, invisible to the eye even with optimum lighting and magnification. This is due to a combination of factors: the inherent limitations in the range of intensities that x-ray film can capture (its latitude or dynamic range), as well as the fixed format for viewing x-ray film. The use of digital detectors and computerized display systems have lifted both constraints, leading to the present era where digital radiography is becoming the method of choice for many procedures.

For example, digital detectors have a large dynamic range, so they record even tiny differences in x-ray transmission, while computer monitors can display thousands of different shades of gray, allowing the differentiation of tissues with subtly different contrast. Computerized image processing also can be used to enhance the x-ray image by selecting gray-scale levels to emphasize differences in contrast, smoothing out image mottling due to noise and otherwise making the most out of the data available in challenging imaging scenarios.

---

* O. Olsen, P. Gøtzsche, "Cochrane review on screening for breast cancer with mammography." *Lancet*, volume 358 (9290) pp. 1340–2 (2001).

† Donald A. Berry, Kathleen A. Cronin, Sylvia K. Plevritis, Dennis G. Fryback, Lauren Clarke, Marvin Zelen, Jeanne S. Mandelblatt, Andrei Y. Yakovlev, J. Dik F. Habbema, Eric J. Feuer, "Effect of screening and adjuvant therapy on mortality from breast cancer," *New England Journal of Medicine*, volume 353(17), pp. 1784–1792 (2005).

As one dramatic example, in **digital subtraction radiography**, a radiograph taken after injection with a contrast agent will show enhanced absorption due to the dye, but there will also be a large background of absorption due to the surrounding tissue (Figure 5.23a). If the blood vessels containing the contrast agent are small, the resulting contrast will be quite low. However, if a **mask** x-ray image is taken before the injection, then only the background absorption is imaged (Figure 5.23b). The *difference* between the two images (with and without contrast) is due only to the blood vessels containing the contrast medium. If these two images are subtracted mathematically, point by point, the difference image shows

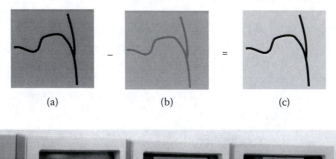

(a)   (b)   (c)

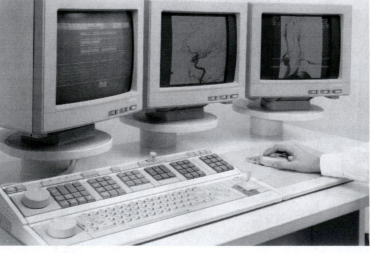

(d)

Figure 5.23 Illustration of the concept behind digital subtraction radiography. (a) A radiograph may show only small contrast between an interesting structure, such as a contrast-enhanced blood vessel, and the surrounding tissue. (b) A mask image without contrast media also is obtained. (c) The difference image formed by subtracting images (a) and (b) shows absorption due only to the contrast agent, greatly enhancing contrast at the expense of increasing the noise level. Such manipulations can be done simply and routinely when x-ray images are captured by computer. (d) Actual DSA images. (Reproduced with permission courtesy of Siemens Medical Systems.)

only the blood vessels containing the contrast (Figure 5.23c). In **digital subtraction angiography (DSA)** and arteriography, this technique is valuable since many blood vessels are too small to offer appreciable contrast without image enhancement (Figure 5.23d). Subtraction not only improves the contrast; it also removes the distracting images of bones and other strong x-ray absorbers that can hide information. X-ray film itself can be manipulated to give such difference images. More usefully, digital radiography allows these and other manipulations to be performed flexibly and quickly by computer, to minimize the effects of noise, enhance contrast, and otherwise improve image quality after the fact. In **digital fluoroscopy**, subtraction techniques can allow good image acquisition using lower concentrations and smaller volumes of contrast medium, both measures that reduce the risk to the patient. Digital fluoroscopy benefits from all the same advantages as digital radiography, with the additional benefit that the real-time computerized measurement process allows the radiation dose to be reduced in several ways. For example, the x-ray tube operating parameters can be continuously adjusted to provide the optimal image quality at lowest dose, the cumulative radiation dose can be displayed on the monitor and watched to avoid radiation burns (Chapter 7), and the x-ray tube can be pulsed so it only emits x-rays during image acquisition.

For digital radiography, the image must first be recorded in a form compatible with modern computers. The computer file that stores the information about an x-ray image actually contains a matrix of transmitted x-ray intensity values, as shown in Figure 5.24(a). The smallest element that makes up such an image is called a **pixel** (short for *picture element*); television and computer screens also build up pictures from many pixels. Each intensity measurement is assigned an integer value and identified by its location in the matrix by a row and column assignment. In real life, the transmitted x-ray intensity can have any value starting at zero and ranging to 100% transmission. The location of features within an image is also defined by continuously varying distances; such smoothly varying values are called **analog** numbers. For example, the optical density of an x-ray film image is an analog quantity. However, in a digital image, the x-ray absorption is assigned to one of a fixed number of steps in absorption between the maximum and minimum measurable absorption (Figure 5.24b). This resembles the pricing of items in a currency: we arbitrarily say that an item can cost $1.50 or $1.51, but do not allow finer differences in price. When we describe a quantity using numbers that can only change by discrete steps, we say we are using **digital** numbers. This conversion of continuous information about intensity and location into discrete numerical values is what we mean by digital imaging.

Why does forcing the x-ray absorption into a digital number not lose important information about differences in structure? Consider that the actual transmitted intensity is measured in terms of the transmission of discrete numbers of x-ray photons, and thus is rendered uncertain by noise from fluctuations in the number detected. For example, if one wants to

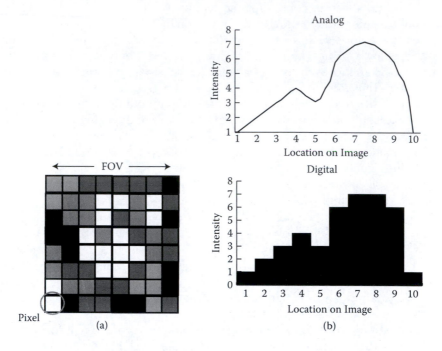

Figure 5.24 (a) Illustration of the matrix of gray-scale values which make up a digital image. (b) Comparison of the digital and analog approach to representing numbers.

image differences of 1% in x-ray absorption, then using 200 evenly spaced possible values between zero and the maximum absorption of interest will be perfectly adequate, since each step would then be equal to 1/200 = 0.5% of the total absorption range. Digital computers are used to store and manipulate the measured intensities using the computer standard **binary** format. We can best understand how this number system works by recalling how one interprets the more commonly used decimal numbers (Figure 5.25). Each digit in a decimal number is a number from 0 to 9 that multiplies a power of 10. The rightmost number is interpreted as the 1's place (1 = 10^0), the next the 10's (10 = 10^1), 100's (100 = 10^2), etc. Binary notation is similar, except digits (called **bits**) multiply powers of 2 instead of 10, and each digit can only take on the values 0 or 1. (The ease of storing strings of only two easily distinguishable values is one of the features making this notation attractive for computers.) The smallest difference between two binary numbers is also one bit, which plays the role of one cent ($0.01) in the pricing example. The number of bits used ranges from 8 to 12 bits. As Figure 5.25 shows, the maximum number of different intensities describable by an N-bit binary number (the highest attainable **contrast resolution**) is 2^N. This gives between 256 (= 2^8) possible values of intensity per pixel for an 8-bit binary number. To return to our earlier example, an 8-bit number would be more than adequate to store 1% differences in contrast since

$$235 = 2 \times 100 + 3 \times 10 + 5 \times 1$$

$$= 2 \times 10^2 + 3 \times 10^1 + 5 \times 10^0$$

Decimal

1101 in binary is "13" in decimal:

$$13 = 1 \times 8 + 1 \times 4 + 0 \times 2 + 1 \times 1$$

$$= 1 \times 2^3 + 1 \times 2^2 + 0 \times 2^1 + 1 \times 10^0$$

Binary

An N-bit binary number can represent 2^N different values:

Example: a 3-bit number can take on $2^3 = 8$ different values:

000	100
001	101
010	110
011	111

(a)

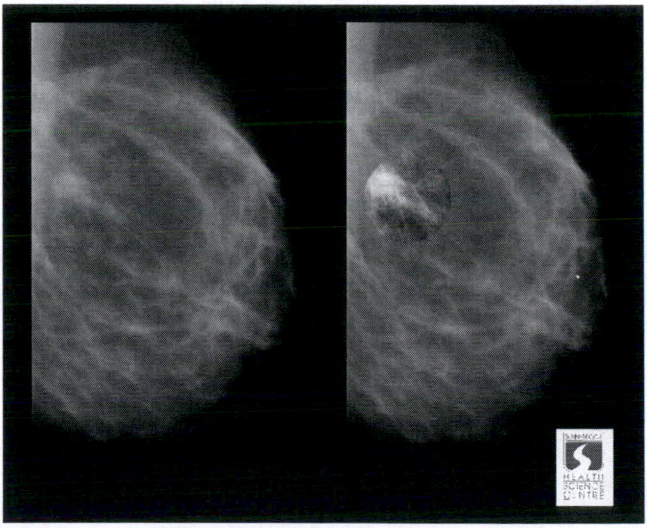

(b)

Figure 5.25 (a) Illustration of the decimal and binary number systems. (b) Digital mammography image illustrating how computer magnification and image processing can enhance tumor detection. Left: unenhanced image. Right: the computer-enhanced digital image provides clearer indications that the region might be malignant. (Image reproduced courtesy Dr. Martin Yaffe, Imaging Research Program, Sunnybrook & Women's College Health Sciences Centre, Toronto, Canada.)

1/256 ≈ 0.4%, while techniques such as mammography, which require higher contrast resolution, would necessitate using more bits. For example, current digital radiography systems featuring 12 or 14 bits to define x-ray transmissions would be able to distinguish among 4096 (= 2^{12}) and 16,384 (= 2^{14}) different values, respectively.

The dimensions of a pixel are determined by the total number of pixels in each row and column forming the image, and the **field of view (FOV)** (spatial extent of the image) by the formula:

$$\text{Pixel size} = \frac{\text{FOV}}{\text{\# pixels in row or column}} \tag{5.15}$$

The pixel size cannot be smaller than the smallest detector element, although it is also determined by the way the image is stored electronically. Present digital radiography systems can feature pixel sizes on the order of 100 to less than 50 microns. By itself, the pixel size puts a lower limit on the spatial resolution of an imaging technique, so small detector elements and large matrices are necessary. Matrices with thousands of pixels along an edge are typical of modern digital imaging systems. (By comparison, the computer this book was written on has a screen with 1280 × 800 pixels.)

Of course, the body itself is not divided up into tiny squares or cubes of tissue; this artificial division of the image results from the use of point detectors and the requirements of computer storage. However, if the pixels are small enough, our eyes cannot distinguish the true grainy nature of the image, which appears as smooth as an actual object (Figure 5.23d). Television screens, computer monitors, and pictures in magazines and newspapers also consist of tiny dots, but we are only aware of this upon close examination. We also experience this same effect in the post-impressionist paintings by Georges Seurat, which can look realistic at a distance, but dissolve into meaningless dots of paint at close range.

Digital radiography is one reason among many why medicine is becoming increasingly reliant on information technologies; all the imaging technologies discussed in this book similarly produce vast amounts of information that place new demands on hospitals for its storage, distribution, and display. Equally important is establishing standards so images can be shared among a wide variety of different computer programs for treatment and surgery planning, comparison with other imaging methods, etc. **Picture Archiving and Storage Systems (PACS)** serve this function. PACS define formats for computer files (such as **DICOM**, for **Digital Imaging and Communications in Medicine**) that include standards for image information as well as patient records; they help control the sheer size and cost associated with storing such large quantities of information and they interface with other healthcare management software so physicians associated with a patient's case can easily access all relevant scans, for example, even if they are not in the facility that performed the exam. Also, as with other forms of telemedicine, sharing of images via teleradiology means that radiologists can consult with remote colleagues to get expert advice on interpreting challenging cases.

Images stored on film can be converted into a digital format using special purpose scanners. However, detectors that measure the transmitted x-ray intensity and store it electronically are more useful for digital imaging than film. Once stored in digital format, an image can be displayed flexibly in numerous ways on a computer screen. One possibility involves mapping a brightness to each pixel corresponding to the transmitted x-ray intensity detected at that point on the image. If the most transmitted x-rays correspond to the darkest pixels, and the fewest to the brightest, this mapping would generate an image similar to an x-ray film. This idea of using degrees of brightness to construct an image on a black-and-white screen is the same gray-scale display first encountered for ultrasound in Chapter 4. However, the information in a radiograph also can be directly converted into x-ray attenuation coefficients, rather than the transmitted intensities themselves. The average attenuation coefficient for each pixel can be extracted mathematically by taking the logarithm of the transmitted intensities; gray-scale values on the computed image then indicate variations in x-ray absorption directly. Numerous other digital imaging computational techniques have been developed to enhance images or even automatically search for important features. For example, the noise in an image can be reduced by averaging over the intensity values of neighboring pixels, at the expense of blurring the image. Similarly, the noise in a fluoroscopy image can be greatly reduced by averaging over successive video frames. We will discuss another important technique, called **windowing**, in the next section.

Digital subtraction radiography, as discussed earlier, is one technique that takes advantage of the ease of manipulating images stored on a computer to enhance contrast. The same idea can be used even without contrast agents, by subtracting images taken at different x-ray energies. Such **dual energy radiography** can also enhance the contrast between tissues, since the x-ray absorption of many tissues depends upon x-ray energy. For many tissues the absorption coefficients are very similar at high energies, but differ significantly at lower energies. (See, for example, Figure 5.5.) Then the difference between a high energy image (125 kVp) and a low energy image (85 kVp) will result in a new image that emphasizes the differences in absorption between the two energies. All of these capabilities are put to use dramatically in computed tomography.

Digital mammography differs from traditional film-based methods only in its use of electronic detectors and subsequent computerized display technologies; however, the implications of these changes are significant. Digital detectors can now be made with a combination of efficiency at detecting x-ray photons, good spatial resolution and excellent dynamic range that results in improved contrast compared to film. Since film isn't used, the limits it imposes on x-ray energy and exposure are not relevant, so x-ray sources and filtering can be optimized in energy for each woman's individual breast composition and thickness. As with digital camera images, digital mammograms can be made brighter or dimmer, higher or lower contrast on the computer without taking a second image, which can minimize the number of procedures repeated to improve image quality. For all these reasons, digital mammography can result in slightly lower radiation doses per procedure.

After images are recorded, doctors can magnify images, zoom in on suspicious regions, and use mathematical image processing to find and enhance the greatest change in transmission, which might otherwise appear featureless or unclear (Figure 5.25b). Computers programs also can be used to analyze a database of x-ray images and known diagnoses, and the results used to produce a **Computer Aided Diagnosis (CAD)** algorithm that predicts the diagnosis associated with new x-ray images Although it has so far not been shown to improve diagnosis, CAD has been widely implemented; so far a major NIH-sponsored study released in 2007 showed no improvement in mammography results when CAD was used.

To see if digital mammography is more effective than film for detecting breast cancer and reducing mortality, the NIH is performing a large clinical trial, the Digital Mammography Imaging Screening Trial, featuring 49,500 women. Participants received a digital and film mammogram at the same visit in 2001, then were followed up over several years. Early reports from this study revealed that certain subsets of women benefited from digital mammography, which proved significantly better in screening the 65% of the women enrolled who were under age 50, who had very dense breasts, or who were pre- or perimenopausal (defined in terms of having had a recent menstrual period). However, no benefit was seen for women who did not fit into these categories. In spite of these advantages, only 32% of U.S. breast imaging centers feature digital mammography units at the time of writing; other complications include the need for radiologists to retrain before using digital systems, and the fact that digital systems remain several times the cost of film-based units. Advances in digital mammography on the horizon include **breast tomosynthesis** (the use of mammograms taken at multiple angles to reconstruct a 3D view of the breast, using techniques described in the next section) and the development of contrast agents to heighten the appearance of tumors.

5.10 COMPUTED TOMOGRAPHY (CT)

CT scanners effectively "open up" the body by turning ordinary flat x-rays into cross-sectional images that offer information about the body's anatomy and function in three dimensions. An x-ray projection can be confusing if overlapping structures obscure the anatomy of interest (Figure 5.26). In addition, radiographs can only be obtained easily for a few projections.

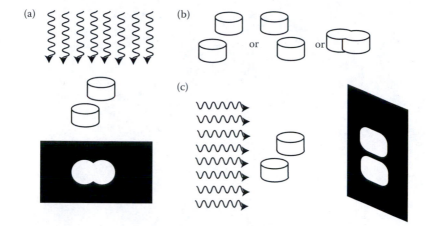

Figure 5.26 (a) Illustration of how a projection cannot distinguish the structure of overlapping objects. It is not clear, for example, which of the three options shown actually corresponds to the absorbers' spatial orientation. (b) Simple demonstration of how adding a second projection to the information available from (a) can clarify the three-dimensional arrangement of the two absorbers. It is now clear that either option 1 or 2 from part (a) is possible, but not option 3. A third projection could be used to distinguish between the two remaining possibilities.

For example, imaging the chest in a horizontal plane such as that shown in Figure 5.1(c) is impossible. With CT, the physician can examine a crisp, detailed image revealing only one plane of the body at a time. Overlaps are eliminated, so different organs can be clearly distinguished and their internal structure analyzed. Because CT has greatly enhanced sensitivity to contrast, the skeleton's x-ray absorption does not overwhelm details from the rest of the body. As a result, CT provides excellent visualization of soft tissues that would be difficult or impossible to see via ordinary radiography. These advantages enable CT images to contribute to better planning for surgery, allowing surgeons to visualize the region to be operated on without incisions. Since CT directly measures the way different parts of the body absorb x-rays, it is an essential part of planning radiation therapy. Furthermore, CT scans can be used to measure the density of body tissues—a useful feature that facilitates the study of diseases such as osteoporosis, as discussed in the next section.

From the outside, a CT scanner resembles a huge doughnut, with a cylindrical hole roughly 70 cm in diameter (Figure 5.27). The person to be scanned lies on a table that can be moved into this opening. Since only one region of the body is examined at a time, the scanner surrounds only that section rather than entire body, so the person being scanned is not uncomfortably confined. This geometry opens up the possibility of interventional surgical medical procedures being performed with CT scanning as a guide.

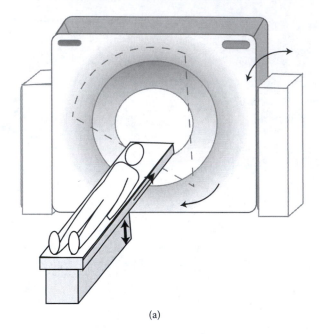

(a)

Figure 5.27 (a) Illustration and (b) photograph of a CT scanner. The patient being examined lies on a table that is progressively fed through the circular opening in the scanner. (Reproduced with permission courtesy of Siemens Medical Systems.)

During the CT scan, a series of x-ray projections are collected for different regions of the body. A computer stores these projections, and then mathematically manipulates them to compute a cross section of the body at that plane. Three-dimensional information can then be discerned by either comparing cross sections taken at different points along the body or by having a computer create a three-dimensional image by "stacking up" these cross sections. Since a CT scan really is no more than an elaborate type of x-ray, it is painless.

Inside the CT scanner lies an elaborate array of equipment, including an x-ray source and many x-ray detectors. While several scanner designs are possible, the easiest to understand is shown in Figure 5.28. There an arc-shaped array of detectors faces an x-ray source that emits a fan-shaped x-ray beam through the person's body. The photon energies used lie in the high end of the diagnostic x-ray range. The relation between the detectors and x-ray tube is fixed, but they rotate together around the patient (Figure 5.28a). A typical design might employ 900 individual electronic or gas ionization detectors in an array. Just as in a normal x-ray, the source emits x-rays that travel in straight lines toward the many individual detectors, each of which measures the x-ray attenuation along one line through the body. In this geometry, collimators can be placed before each detector to greatly reduce the scattered x-rays detected. Unlike a radiograph, the

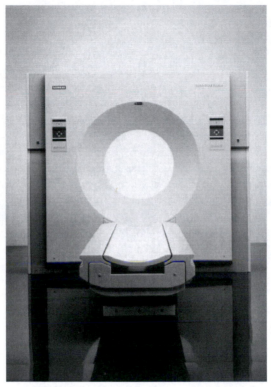

(b)

Figure 5.27 (continued).

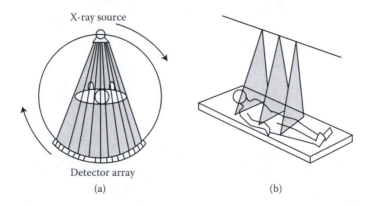

X-ray source

Detector array

(a)   (b)

Figure 5.28 One possible geometry for CT scanner source and detectors. (a) Both the source and arc-shaped detector array rotate in tandem, recording projections through a single plane within the body for many different angles. (b) After enough orientations have been recorded, the patient's body is translated farther into the scanner, and the whole process repeated for a new plane.

detectors only measure the projection of a thin "slice" of the body. However, one projection is recorded for many different orientations of the detector-source array as it rotates around the body.

After completing one circuit around the body section, the entire array moves to a new plane in the body, and the whole procedure repeats (Figure 5.28b). Because of the scanner geometry, the cross-sectional images obtained (**axial projections**) correspond to horizontal planes when a person is standing (Figure 5.28b). The entire CT scanner assembly can tilt to adjust the exact angle of the section (Figure 5.27a).

While the way a CT scanner turns these projections into an image is quite complex, the basic idea resembles the way our eyes use stereoscopic vision to sense depth. By viewing objects from two orientations—one for each eye—one can discern their relations in three dimensions. A variety of mathematical techniques exist for converting these x-ray projections into cross-sectional images, but we will only consider one commonly employed method called **filtered back projection**.

The basic idea behind filtered back projection is illustrated in Figure 5.29. (For simplicity, the x-ray source is shown emitting many parallel x-rays, but the same methods work for the fan-shaped beam.) During a scan, the detectors record what is called a **forward projection**. Each detector in the array measures the x-ray intensity transmitted through the body section. The x-ray intensity without a body present is also known. From this

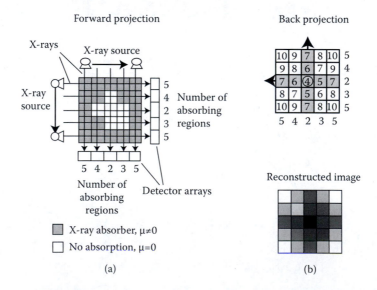

Figure 5.29 Filtered back projection in the production of CT images. The tissue being scanned is represented by a gray scale indicating its absorption coefficient. (a) Creation of forward projections for two source and detector orientations. (b) Reconstruction of the original absorber's cross section, using back projection.

information, one can compute the sum of all x-ray absorptions along one line corresponding to that particular x-ray beam. In Figure 5.29(a), the x-ray absorption measured by each detector is indicated by a number and a shaded box above each detector. After forward projections have been measured for different angles (only two are shown in the figure), we can employ a process called **back projection** to reconstruct the original tissue's pattern of x-ray absorption (Figure 5.29b). Graphically, back projection corresponds to tracing backward along the x-ray's path from each detector; each region of overlap between such back projections is assigned an absorption value based on the sum of each detector's absorptions. The resulting matrix of local x-ray absorptions is then displayed using a gray scale image. By itself, back projection does not give an accurate map of the original absorbers; for example, it can introduce into the resulting image regions that do not correspond to actual x-ray absorbers and assign jagged edges to images of smooth structures. However, if one first subjects the measured forward projections to a mathematical process called **filtering**, this reduces these artifacts in the image reconstructed with back projection.

Reconstructing an image from a CT scan is straightforward mathematically, but involves enormous numbers of repetitive calculations. One reason this technique became feasible only in the early 1970s is that only then did fast, inexpensive computers become readily available. CT images are inherently digital; the pixels that make up each cross-sectional image represent a small volume of tissue called a **voxel** (for *volume element*) (Figure 5.30a). Each voxel is a tiny box having dimensions as small as a third of millimeter or less per side. The voxel thickness is determined by the width of the section examined by the scanning x-ray beam, or defined by collimators on the detector array. The spatial resolution of a CT scan is determined in part by the voxel size, as well as by the same geometrical factors discussed earlier for radiography. In practice, the smallest spatial resolutions achieved are under 1 mm. For a tomographic axial image typically consisting of a matrix of 512×512 or 1024×1024 voxels, this means that over 260,000 or 1 million, respectively, gray-scale values must be stored for each cross-sectional image. Since each 3D image consists of many such cross sections, computers must be used to store and manipulate the enormous amounts of data generated by such imaging techniques.

In theory, increasingly finer spatial resolutions can be achieved with CT when a combination of higher x-ray intensities and longer exposure times are employed. Special micro-CT scanners used for research can see details on the scale of microns (10^{-6} m). However, decreasing the voxel size necessarily involves increasing the total x-ray dose. This is because the major source of noise in CT images is fluctuations in the number of transmitted x-rays detected. When the image is divided into even more voxels to give higher resolution, then the number of transmitted x-rays also is divided up more finely. This means there are even fewer x-rays detected per voxel, and the images become unacceptably noisy unless a more intense x-ray source is

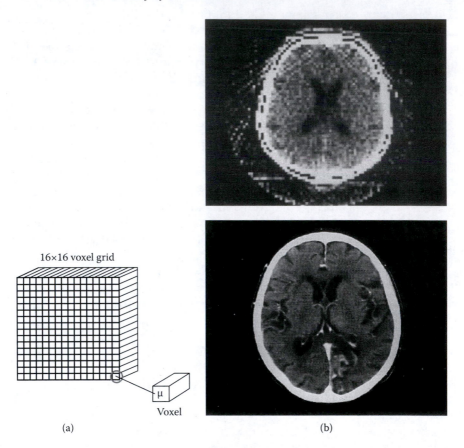

16×16 voxel grid

Voxel

(a)   (b)

Figure 5.30 Constructing an image from voxels. (a) How voxels are represented by
an image matrix. A CT scan measures an average value of x-ray attenuation coefficient, μ, for the voxel corresponding to a small region in
the body. (b) Low (top) and high (bottom) resolution cross-sectional
images of the brain. Individual pixels are evident on the older, low
resolution image, but less apparent in the more modern, higher resolution image. (Reproduced with permission courtesy of Siemens Medical
Systems.)

used or the patient is irradiated for a longer time. Either way involves more
x-rays being absorbed within the body. Thus, the voxel sizes given above
represent the practical limits of this technique. While quite adequate for
many medical diagnostic applications, this resolution is too coarse to allow,
for example, tiny blood vessels, structures within the eye, fine structure of
bones, or individual cells, to be imaged.

CT scanners represent x-ray absorptions using a quantity called the **CT
number**. Measured in **Hounsfield units**, the CT number is equal to the percent difference between the x-ray attenuation coefficient of a voxel and that
of water, multiplied by 1000:

$$\text{CT number} = \frac{\mu_{tissue} - \mu_{water}}{\mu_{water}} \times 1000 \qquad\qquad (5.16)$$

Water is defined to have zero CT number, while fatty tissues have CT numbers less than zero, and most other tissues values greater than zero. The largest CT numbers correspond to the bones, and the lowest to air in the lungs or bowel. The number of bits used to represent CT numbers determines how small a difference in absorption can be stored, as explained in the previous section. The detectors used to measure the x-ray intensities can also discriminate between minute variations, enabling CT scanners to have excellent discrimination between similar values of x-ray absorption coefficient. Tiny variations in x-ray absorption between different types of soft tissues can be easily measured and displayed. CT images can be used to clearly distinguish organs, blood vessels, and other soft tissue anatomy, often eliminating the need for contrast media. When contrast is still needed, principally to study blood flow, smaller amounts of the contrast dyes used in radiography can be used. For example, the inert gas xenon (with $Z = 54$) can be used in CT for imaging blood flow in the brain by having the person to be scanned inhale a mixture of xenon and oxygen. As the xenon is absorbed into the blood, the relatively radiopaque xenon reveals the blood flow pattern without the need for iodine contrast and its associated risks.

All of the flexibility in displaying digital images is available in CT, leading to greatly improved contrast sensitivity relative to ordinary radiography. For example, if a single image encompasses an enormous range of variation in x-ray absorption, a special method of displaying images called **windowing** can be used to make sense of the resulting image. For example, in Figure 5.31, the body section imaged includes both radiopaque bones (the ribs and spine) as well as the highly radiolucent lungs. If the full range of CT numbers were directly mapped onto gray-scale values, the bones would show up as featureless white regions, and the lungs equally featureless black regions. With windowing, the full range of image gray-scale values is restricted to correspond to only a subset of measured CT numbers; for example, the gray scale would correspond to only a small range of CT number variation corresponding to soft tissues. In Figure 5.31(a), such a window is defined that emphasizes only the lungs; CT values close to those corresponding to the lungs are resolvable on this image. Because the lungs have very low CT numbers, all other tissues are effectively "overexposed" and hence show up as all white on the gray scale. Figure 5.31(b) shows the same cross-sectional image, processed with two different windows: one that allows lung structures to be seen, the other that correctly "exposes" the soft tissues.

Since CT images are formed and stored as axial cross sections, one way to obtain a three-dimensional image involves measuring many separate cross-sectional images that overlap by part of a section width, then having a

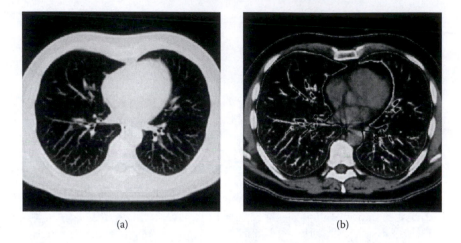

(a)   (b)

Figure 5.31 (a) Cross-sectional image through the chest, using a window that allows
details within the lungs to be resolved. All other more radiopaque tissues show up uniformly white. (b) The same image can be processed
to show variations within both the lungs and soft tissues, using two
different windows. (Reproduced with permission courtesy of Siemens
Medical Systems.)

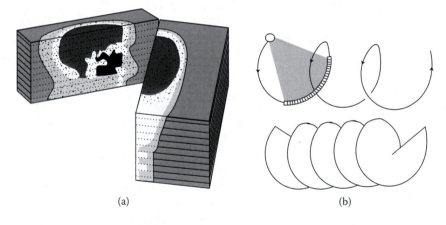

(a)   (b)

Figure 5.32 (a) Stacks of axial sections can be used to compile a three-dimensional
image. Here, a cutaway view shows how stacked horizontal sections
can be used to generate a three-dimensional image. (b) Illustration
of the coupled motion of the x-ray source and detector arrays during a spiral CT scan (top) and the resulting helical section recorded
(bottom).

computer form an image by mathematically "stacking up" the cross sections
(Figure 5.32a). This method of taking a series of axial images while step-
ping the patient through the x-ray beam is called "step-and-shoot." In fact,

modern multislice CT scanners use a combination of a cone-shaped beam (rather than a fan-shaped beam) to irradiate simultaneously many detector rings containing as many as hundreds of individual detectors; such systems can perform multiple axial scans at the same time in under half a minute. **Spiral or helical CT** techniques build on this technology to perform even more rapid scans of yet larger body volumes. Rather than "slicing up" the body into many separate planes, spiral CT involves taking a series of cross-sectional images corresponding to one continuous spiral. (This is rather like the difference between slicing an apple into separate cross-sectional slices vs. slicing it into one continuous spiral ribbon.) This can be accomplished in practice by rotating the detector-source array continuously while simultaneously translating the body through the scanner (Figure 5.32b). Since each cross-sectional slice can be set to overlap with adjacent slices, this means that the spatial resolution can be finer than for "step-and-shoot" cross sections, where the beam width sets the thickness of the slice. As a result, voxels now can have the same dimension in all directions, achieving spatial resolutions smaller than 0.3 mm. Entire spiral CT scans can be completed in seconds or less, depending on the volume imaged. This allows imaging of fast body processes in the beating heart and patients who have difficulty holding still for long times without sedation (such as small children.)

Now that 60% of U.S. hospitals own a spiral CT scanner, the applications of CT imaging have dramatically expanded as fast, large-volume scans are routinely available. One use of spiral CT being studied is imaging of the lungs to detect cancer. In spite of the fact that lung cancer is the most common cause of cancer-related death in the U.S., evidence for benefits from lung cancer screening by chest x-ray or spiral CT is very mixed at the moment. There is a lack of evidence to date that early screening of even high-risk groups, such as smokers, saves lives. Of the 170,000 diagnosed with lung cancer each year in the U.S., 90% die within two years; however, as is true for other cancers, earlier detection can lead to more effective treatment and reduced mortality. While the potential benefit is large, with 90 million current or former smokers at risk in the U.S. alone, the cost of screening is also high, at $300 to $1000 per scan. In addition, there is presently no evidence that spiral CT scans can catch fast-growing lung cancers at an earlier, more treatable stage, rather than just identifying larger, slower-growing tumors, with little improvement in outcomes. Another issue is whether the technique just leads to false positives: detection of suspicious but benign nodules, leading to unnecessary, dangerous biopsies and surgeries. The U.S. National Institutes of Health are presently sponsoring several large scale population studies aimed at clarifying this urgent public health question. The National Lung Screening Trial, begun in 2002, is designed to compare screening by spiral CT and chest x-rays using a large prospective randomized clinical trial capable of determining whether there is a 20% or greater decrease in lung cancer mortality. A group of 50,000 former or current smokers have been randomly assigned to receive a series of either spiral CT or standard chest x-rays to screen for lung cancer, with the follow-up designed to last at least 8 years. The Prostate, Lung, Colorectal and Ovarian (PLCO) Cancer Screening Trial will compare lung cancer mortality in a large group receiving chest x-rays with a control group that does not; preliminary results available from 2006 only show that the chest x-rays indeed detected many early lung cancers, but at the expense of many false positives. The NIH-sponsored Lung Imaging Database Consortium, by contrast, is designed to help understand how to best use spiral CT as a resource for finding lung cancer by creating a database of shared images for use in research, training, and clinical practice; for example, the database can be used to help develop computer algorithms that assist radiologists in identifying likely tumors based on their appearance in spiral CT scans.

Although less commonly used, **Electron Beam Computed Tomography** also improves on these scan times. Rather than having a rotating x-ray source and detectors, these scanners have a ring of fixed detectors and a separate ring of tungsten x-ray targets. An electron beam is then rapidly steered around the tungsten ring, creating beams of x-rays wherever it hits. Because only the x-ray source's electron beam is moved, the scan can take place much more quickly. This can reduce complete spiral scan times to a twentieth of a second. Ultrafast spiral CT scanners have particular utility for imaging the beating heart, imaging the lungs, and studying cardiovascular diseases.

The ability to perform spiral CT scans readily also enables "virtual endoscopy" applications such as **virtual colonoscopy,** in which computer-reconstructed views of the inside of the colon are generated from CT scans, and displayed as a three-dimensional image (Figure 5.33) or video. Early results from clinical studies have shown that virtual colonoscopy can be as accurate as traditional colonoscopy at finding polyps, growths that might indicate colon or rectal cancer. Although the spiral CT approach is noninvasive, less expensive, and appealing for patients who cannot or will not tolerate colonoscopy, it cannot remove or biopsy the tumors or polyps, unlike colonoscopic procedures, it exposures the patient to a radiation dose, and it still requires unpleasant procedures to clear the bowel of all stool.

There are essentially no restrictions on who can be examined by CT, in contrast to the restrictions for MRI discussed in Chapter 8. CT scanners also acquire scans more quickly in general, at a lower acquisition and operating cost than MRI. Although CT has many advantages, it retains some of the inherent limitations of x-ray imaging. Because it relies on x-ray transmission, CT essentially yields only a map of attenuation coefficient or density. This is not a sensitive enough measure of anatomy in some cases, and it is not a measure of body function. We will discuss in Chapters 6 and 8 how hybrid scanners that combine CT with SPECT, PET, or MRI can provide both anatomical and functional imaging. This, along with its widespread and growing applicability, ensures that CT will continue to play a major role in modern medical imaging.

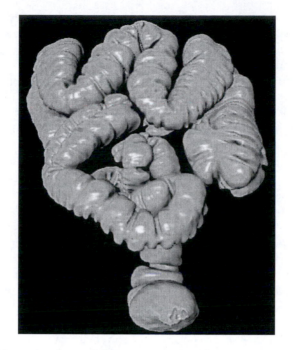

Figure 5.33 (See color figure following page 78.) Three-dimensional reconstruction of the outside and inside of the colon, made using spiral CT for the purposes of virtual colonoscopy. The sequence of images re-creates a "flight" through the colon similar to what is usually seen during an actual endoscopic exam. (Reproduced with permission courtesy of David J. Vining, "Virtual colonoscopy," *Gastrointestinal Endoscopy Clinics of North America*, Vol. 7(2) (April 1997), pp. 285–291.)

5.11 APPLICATION: SPOTTING BRITTLE BONES—BONE MINERAL SCANS FOR OSTEOPOROSIS

A broken bone ordinarily heals readily in a child or young adult, but for an elderly person a broken hip can precipitate a total loss of independence, depression, or even death. Many elderly women and men suffer from a bone-weakening condition, **osteoporosis**, making them extremely vulnerable to fractures. In the U.S., osteoporosis causes an estimated 1.3 million fractures per year, and its financial toll is estimated at billions of dollars each year. Prevention is acknowledged to be the most important tool in the fight against this epidemic, and x-ray measurements play an important role in identifying those most at risk.

Both men and women have a significant chance of developing this condition after age 70, but many women encounter osteoporosis earlier because of reduced hormonal levels after menopause. Preventative measures include increasing calcium intake during childhood and early adulthood, ensuring adequate vitamin D intake, performing weight-bearing exercise regularly, and ceasing smoking and alcohol abuse; drug therapies are now available as well for those diagnosed with the condition or its precursor. While the entire population is advised to follow these dietary and lifestyle changes, there is also an immediate need for determining how to diagnose this condition so as to target those persons most at risk. In order to determine how effective these therapies and preventative measures are, it is also necessary to be able to measure whether bones have become compromised.

The average person is inclined to think of bone as a dead, rocklike substance. In reality, the skeleton is a dynamic organ of the body, its composition in constant flux. The structural framework of the skeleton is built from a mesh of organic molecules, primarily the protein collagen, on which are deposited calcium- and phosphate-rich bone minerals. Bones naturally lose and deposit their bone minerals, changing their shapes in response to the environment, and altering their balance of different types of bone tissue even in adulthood. The bone mass of the body peaks at roughly age 35, and bone minerals are gradually lost thereafter at a rate that increases with age. As the bone mineral density decreases, a person eventually develops an increasing risk of fracture. In osteoporosis, this natural loss of bone minerals with age is accelerated.

The prospect of removing bone samples for regular biopsies to diagnose and track the course of osteoporosis is unappealing, and radiographs can only measure very large ($\geq 35\%$) changes in bone density. Instead, different specialized forms of x-ray measurements can be used for monitoring bone health. To be effective, such a bone mineral density test must accurately measure small bone losses using an apparatus that allows comparisons with earlier measurements and with other individuals. Because they are at highest risk for fracture, the bones most commonly tested include those in the spine and hip; peripheral regions, such as the wrist, heel, and finger, are also tested because they are easy to access. Bone mass testing devices can help evaluate the fracture risk for different parts of the body, and help determine, for example, if drug therapy is indicated.

The basic idea behind most bone mineral density tests involves measuring x-ray transmission along a series of paths through the body (Figure 5.34). These measurements of transmission also determine x-ray absorption, which depends upon the density and mass attenuation coefficient of the body tissues encountered. Since the body's mass attenuations coefficients are known already, this allows density to be determined. However, since any path through the body will include both bone and soft tissues, special x-ray techniques have been developed to single out the effects of bone alone. (Note that these techniques are different from what is colloquially called "bone scans" in medicine; this term is used to refer to radionuclide imaging procedures described in Chapter 6.)

Dual energy x-ray absorptiometry (DEXA or DXA) is the present "gold standard" for osteoporosis screening. DEXA uses collimated x-rays from an x-ray tube source and a scintillation detector positioned so it intercepts x-rays transmitted through the body section of interest, such as the hip,

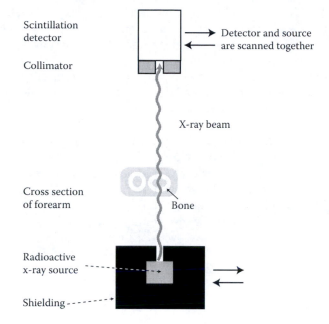

Figure 5.34 Schematic illustration of the operation of a device to measure x-ray absorption through a pathway in the body.

spine or wrist. At each position, a reading yields the sum of transmitted x-ray intensity (and hence x-ray absorption) along one line through the body. This includes the effect of x-ray absorption from both bone and the surrounding soft tissues; however, the absorption due to soft tissue can be compensated for by comparing different beam paths that do (path A) and do not (path B) include bone.

The DEXA tube is operated at two different tube voltages, for example 70 kV and 140 kV; the two different ranges of x-ray energies are used to make two sets of transmission measurements for the same set of paths through the body. In addition, the x-ray mass attenuation coefficients for both soft tissue and bone minerals are known in advance for both energies, as well as the unattenuated beam intensities for both energies. Given this information, the two sets of x-ray absorption measurements can be used to calculate the bone mineral density directly. DEXA scans are short out-patient procedures costing a few hundred dollars in 2007. They deliver a low radiation dose approximately 1/10 that of a chest x-ray and cost less than CT. DEXA does have the drawback that it provides no information about changes in bone structure, rather than density, and it is unable to distinguish between different types of bone.

Quantitative computed tomography (QCT) takes advantage of the ability of standard CT scanners to actually measure the average attenuation coefficient in each tiny voxel of tissue. Since x-ray absorption is related to density, and the mass attenuation coefficient is known in advance

(Figure 5.10), CT also yields the bone mineral density at each voxel, as well as anatomical information. Thus, it can reveal both any changes in the shape of the spine or the hip, and the distribution of bone loss in different types of bone tissue. Since bones can "remodel"—change their shape in response to bone density loss—to recover some strength, this is important information lost in DEXA. QCT presently is used less frequently than DEXA, primarily for measurements on the vertebra.

The applications described in this chapter make clear that applications of x-rays play a major role in the medical effort to control widespread and important diseases such as breast cancer and osteoporosis, with future applications possibly including lung and colon cancer screening. In Chapter 7, we will also see how the combination of CT technology and three-dimensional computer imaging is playing an increasingly important role in the planning of cancer therapy. In these areas and many others, over one hundred years after their discovery, x-rays continue to offer new and exciting opportunities for the diagnosis and treatment of disease.

SUGGESTED READING

Internet and multimedia

There are numerous rapidly changing web resources available through the radiology departments of almost all major medical schools. Many of these feature radiology teaching files that display sample images for a variety of procedures.

Additional sources of problems on x-ray imaging

Bruce Hasegawa, *The Physics of Medical X-ray Imaging*. Medical Physics Publishing, Madison, WI, 1991.

Russell K. Hobbie, *Intermediate Physics for Medicine and Biology*. John Wiley & Sons, New York, 1988.

More advanced discussions of the medical physics of radiological imaging

Thomas S. Curry III, James E. Dowdey, and Robert C. Murry, Jr., *Christensen's Introduction to the Physics of Diagnostic Radiology*. Lea & Febiger, Philadelphia, 1984.

Bruce Hasegawa, *The Physics of Medical X-ray Imaging*. Medical Physics Publishing, Madison, WI, 1991.

Russell K. Hobbie, *Intermediate Physics for Medicine and Biology*. John Wiley & Sons, New York, 1988.

Perry Sprawls, Jr., *Physical Principles of Medical Imaging*. Medical Physics Publishing, Madison, WI, 1995.

Steve Webb, ed., *Physics of Medical Imaging*. Institute of Physics Publishing, Bristol, U.K., 1992.

Breast Imaging

National Council on Radiation Protection and Measurements, *A Guide to Mammography and Other Breast Imaging Procedures: NCRP Report No. 149.* Bethesda, MD, 2004.

QUESTIONS

Q5.1. Describe the different ways x-rays can interact with matter, and explain what characteristics of an absorbing material are important in determining the absorption due to each mechanism.

Q5.2. (a) Explain when the exponential attenuation of x-rays holds true, and when the decrease in intensity is more complicated. Describe the last case qualitatively. (b) A beam of x-rays is emitted by an x-ray tube. A thickness of 2.5 mm of aluminum is required to reduce the intensity of the beam to one-half its original value. Explain why an additional 3.5 mm is required to reduce the intensity by a further factor of 2. (Hint: Consider how much aluminum would be required if the beam were composed of photons having a single energy.)

Q5.3. Air was formerly used as a contrast medium in imaging the brain in a technique called pneumoencephalography in which air was injected into the cerebral ventricles to enable the imaging of tumors or other abnormalities. Explain why this would work. (This painful and potentially dangerous procedure has been rendered unnecessary by improvements in imaging by CT and MRI.)

Q5.4. What is the function of the phosphor in a film-screen cassette for detecting x-rays?

Q5.5. What are the various types of detectors used in detecting medical x-rays? Explain the operation of one in detail, using drawings where necessary.

Q5.6. Examine the following listing of K absorption edges for various types of phosphors used in film-screen receptors for detecting x-rays. Explain why the traditional phosphor calcium tungstate is appropriate for chest x-rays, while the rare earth compounds gadolinium oxysulfide, lanthanum oxybromide, and yttrium oxysulfide are better for mammography. Which of the latter materials would you guess to be most effective, based on this information alone?

Phosphor material	K absorption edge (keV)
Calcium tungstate	69.5
Gadolinium oxysulfide	50.2
Lanthanum oxybromide	38.9
Yttrium oxysulfide	17.1

Q5.7.   Scientists also use x-ray generators to produce x-rays used to study the structure of proteins and other biological molecules. Two types of anode materials are commonly used in this sort of experiment, and only the characteristic x-rays emitted ordinarily are used. For copper anodes, the characteristic radiation most frequently used is 8.0 keV, and for molybdenum anodes 17.4 keV is used. Aluminum (Z = 13) works well for shielding when the copper anode is used, but scientists must be careful to switch to steel or brass shielding when molybdenum anodes are used. Explain why, using information from the following table.

Shielding metal	Z values	Density (g/cm³)
Aluminum	13	2.8
Steel	Largely iron with Z = 25	8
Brass	Alloy of copper (Z = 29) and zinc (Z = 30)	8.5

Q5.8.   Explain the operation of a CT scanner, using drawings to describe how a CT scan is generated.

Q5.9.   CT scanners can resolve contrast differences of less than 0.5% in the x-ray attenuation coefficient, μ, while traditional radiography can only resolve differences of about 2%. Explain how this fact affects how physicians can utilize images obtained from the two techniques. What other relevant differences exist between the two techniques, and how do they affect the effectiveness of these two imaging modalities?

Q5.10. Explain why a single measurement of the x-ray transmission through, for example, one specific line through the wrist, is insufficient to determine bone density. Explain why a technique such as DEXA is adequate. (Hint: Think of the expression for x-ray attenuation and transmitted intensity, and assume you know the mass attenuation coefficient of soft tissue and bone, as well as the density of soft tissue, in advance, but not the density of bone or the thickness of bone or soft tissue.)

Q5.11. Explain why x-rays with energies in the high range of those used in diagnostic imaging are used in CT imaging. Explain why beam hardening is a significant issue for CT as well.

Q5.12. Assuming that one can manufacture x-ray image receptors with increasingly small detector size, explain why this does not mean you can keep decreasing the spatial resolution indefinitely as well without compromising contrast resolution. (Hint: Consider quantum noise.)

Q5.13. In combination with new digital detectors for mammography, physicians are considering whether different x-ray sources might offer desirable features, especially for challenging imaging applications such as dense or larger breasts. Explain why using tungsten anodes with filters made of rhodium (with a K-edge of 23.22 keV) or silver (with a K-edge of 25.5 keV) might offer advantages for this application over standard molybdenum anodes using molybdenum filters. (Hint: Think about the features of the x-ray emission spectrum produced for each source and how it relates to transmission; consider that the contrast resolution for digital detectors is appreciably greater than for film-screen combinations.)

PROBLEMS

Interaction of x-rays with matter

P5.1. Heavy metals such as lead (Z = 82) are excellent x-ray absorbers compared to water (composed of low Z oxygen (Z = 8) and hydrogen (Z = 1)). An average value of Z = 7.42 describes water-rich soft tissues in the body. For safety purposes it is often important to completely absorb x-rays in a protective layer, a process called *shielding*. Lead is often used to construct shields and protective garments, such as aprons, which prevent x-rays from hitting the entire body during localized procedures. Taking into account only differences in absorption due to differing values of Z, calculate how much more strongly an atom of lead absorbs x-rays by the photoelectric effect in comparison with a typical atom in soft tissue. (Here you are ignoring density. Since lead is denser than most materials in the body, this will lead to an even stronger relative absorption.)

P5.2. (a) In many medical imaging procedures, aprons made of a thin layer of lead sandwiched between fabric are used to shield other parts of the body from unnecessary exposure to x-rays. Consider a lead apron that contains a 0.5-mm-thick layer of lead. Using the following information, compute what fraction of 140 keV x-rays incident upon the apron will be transmitted:

The mass absorption coefficient of lead for 140 keV x-rays is: $\mu/\rho = 2.0$ cm^2 g^{-1}.

The density of lead is: $\rho = 11.3$ g/cm^{-3}.
(b) How thick would the lead shielding in a wall of an x-ray experimental laboratory have to be to reduce the intensity of 8.0 keV x-rays to 1% of its original value? The mass absorption coefficient of lead for 8.0 keV x-rays is: $\mu/\rho = 232$ cm^2 g^{-1}.

Contrast, contrast media, and x-ray absorption

The following problems make use of the information in the following table for approximate linear attenuation coefficients for air, water, fat, and bone at two energies.

X-ray energy (keV)	μ_{air} (cm^{-1})	μ_{water} (cm^{-1})	μ_{fat} (cm^{-1})	μ_{bone} (cm^{-1})
20	6.4×10^{-4}	0.76	0.5	4.8
60	3.7×10^{-5}	0.20	0.17	0.47 to 0.55

P5.3. (a) What percentage of the incident x-rays are transmitted by a 1-cm-thick rib embedded in 20 cm of soft tissue for 20 and 60 keV x-rays? Compare to the text's results for 20 cm of soft tissue alone. (b) What percentage of the incident x-rays are transmitted by a 4-cm region of breast tissue for 20 and 60 keV x-rays? (Approximate the soft tissues in both parts as having the same linear attenuation coefficient as water.)

P5.4. What is the contrast for a 1-cm region of (a) bone and (b) air embedded in soft tissue (approximated as having the same linear attenuation coefficient as water)?

P5.5. Compute the contrast between normal fatty breast tissue and a 0.1-mm microcalcification for (a) 20 keV and (b) 60 keV x-rays. We can approximate the breast tissue as having roughly the same linear attenuation coefficient as fat, while the microcalcification is modeled as having the same linear attenuation coefficient as mineralized bone. Do the same calculation for a 0.1-cm lump having the same linear attenuation coefficient as water in fatty breast tissue for (c) 20 keV and (d) 60 keV x-rays. Note which cases would be detectable for a film-screen image receptor sensitive only to contrasts greater than 2%.

P5.6. Compute the contrast between soft tissue (approximated as having the same attenuation coefficient as water) and a 1-mm-diameter artery filled with an iodine contrast medium at a density 10 milligram/cm^3. Use photon energies just below and just above the iodine K absorption edge. Use values of: μ/ρ_{water} = 0.36 cm^2/g and $\mu/\rho_{iodine\ contrast}$ = 8.42 cm^2/g for 30 keV and: μ/ρ_{water} = 0.26 cm^2/g and $\mu/\rho_{iodine\ contrast}$ = 22.38 cm^2/g for 40 keV x-rays with (a) no scattering and (b) 50% scattering fraction. (Only consider absorption by the widest part of the artery.)

P5.7. For Problems 5.3 through 5.6, calculate the smallest number of gray-scale bits necessary to resolve the contrasts in each problem. Comment on the helpfulness of digital imaging to each of the exams in question.

X-ray sources and detectors

P5.8. Figure P5.8 shows an emission spectrum for an x-ray tube. Explain your reasoning in answering the following questions: (a) What is the operating voltage of the tube? (b) What is the anode material? (c) Explain which features of the curve correspond to brehmsstrahlung and which to characteristic x-rays. (d) How would the curve be changed qualitatively if the operating voltage of the tube were halved? If the operating current were doubled?

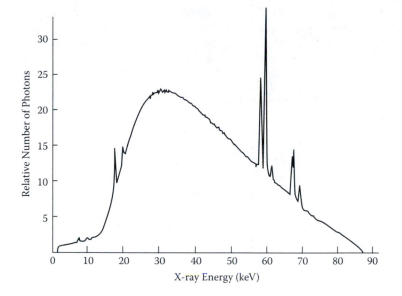

X-ray Energy (keV)

P5.9. Phosphors used in diagnostic x-ray imaging enhance the ability of film to detect x-rays by first converting the x-rays into photons of visible light. This is because the film is a better absorber of visible light photons than x-rays, and many photons result from a single x-ray photon. How many photons of visible light result if a 60-keV x-ray photon is converted into green visible light with 10% efficiency?

P5.10. Use geometry and Figure 5.16(d) to derive Equation 5.10, the relationship between image magnification M, source-patient distance d_1, and patient-receptor distance d_2.

P5.11. What would the blur and magnification be for the following values for focal spot size, source-patient distance, and patient-receptor distance: (as defined in Figure 5.16): d_1 = 39 cm and d_2 = 22 cm; focal spot size a = 0.1 mm. (These values are similar to those used in a high resolution followup mammogram. The breast actually would be several centimeters thick, but for this problem you can ignore its width.) Discuss how these numbers relate to the text's statements about how large an object within the breast can be resolved, and compare to typical intensifying screen blurs of 0.1 mm and greater.

P5.12. A digital imaging system has an FOV equal to 30 cm, and an imaging matrix with 512 × 512 pixels. (a) What is the blur, p, due to the pixel size alone? (b) Note that the blur due to the x-ray focal spot size, a, and pixel size are equal for choices of d_1 and d_2 where:

$$M = 1 + \frac{p}{a}$$

This is the optimal magnification for the system. Discuss why this last statement makes sense. (You don't have to derive the result mathematically. Hint: Consider what would happen for larger and smaller magnifications.) (c) For a point near the center of a CT scanner's aperture, d_1 and d_2 are nearly equal. For this region, how small would the focal spot size have to be to give a blur no greater than that due to the pixel size?

P5.13. For the film characteristic curves shown in Figure 5.17(b), what are the latitudes (dynamic ranges) for exposures that give useful contrast? Express in terms of the ratio of the lowest to highest exposure in the useful range.

6 Images from radioactivity

Radionuclide scans, SPECT, and PET

6.1 INTRODUCTION: RADIOACTIVITY AND MEDICINE

Until recently, researchers could only study the living brain indirectly, often by observing malfunctions caused by disease or accident. The workings of the normal brain were next to impossible to see in detail because the brain is protected by the skull, enveloped in a tough membrane and cushioned in fluid, making it difficult to access for measurements or observation. Now, nuclear medicine techniques such as single photon emission computed tomography (SPECT) and positron emission tomography (PET) imaging are making dramatically visible the actual biochemical and metabolic activity of the brain. (Another important technique, functional magnetic resonance imaging (fMRI), will be covered in Chapter 8.) These techniques have been used to study clinical depression, Alzheimer's disease, schizophrenia, and numerous other mental illnesses. Even more striking, these imaging methods have made it possible to study brain function in normal persons to determine, for example, which parts of the brain are involved in processing vision or understanding speech. Information from such imaging techniques can also be used to map out the brain's functioning prior to surgery, resulting in operations with a reduced likelihood of causing serious damage.

PET imaging works by using radioactive versions of common body chemicals to illuminate the workings of the brain. Radioactivity also plays a role in other low-cost, commonly used diagnostic techniques. These **radionuclide imaging** techniques give physicians an important tool for visualizing the functioning of many organs. For example, radionuclide "bone scans" can be used to detect inflammation due to arthritis, and radionuclide procedures for cardiology can measure the effectiveness with which the heart pumps blood. Specific radioactive chemical labels also can vividly highlight the presence of tumors (Figure 6.1).

Why is there a need for other imaging technologies, when radiography, ultrasound imaging, and fiber optical scopes offer so many possibilities for detecting disease? Fiber optic scopes can be used anywhere there is a cavity, but they cannot see inside solid structures—they cannot be used for imaging the brain, or for seeing within solid organs such as the kidneys, liver, or spleen. By contrast, ultrasound offers an extremely safe way of gaining

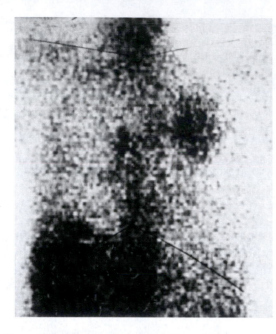

Figure 6.1 Radionuclide image made using gallium-67-citrate to image a tumor in the upper left lung. The image shows the chest, with the person's neck at the top of the image. Shades of gray are used to indicate the distribution of the radioactive tracer that targets the tumor, which is visible as a darker gray region visible near the upper right corner of the image. (Used with permission courtesy of R.J. Ott, M.A. Flower, J.W. Babich, and P.K. Marsden in Steve Webb, ed., *Physics of Medical Imaging*, Institute of Physics Publishing, Bristol, U.K., 1992.)

a detailed picture of even solid organs. However, important limitations prevent it from being universally useful. For example, the adult brain still cannot be imaged because the skull poses a barrier to sound, and many tissues remain indistinguishable in an ultrasound scan because they do not generate acoustic echoes. X-ray imaging is an excellent tool for many tasks, but it has a restricted ability to image body function and inherently low contrast for resolving soft tissues.

In Chapters 6 and 8 we study alternative imaging techniques that overcome these problems: radionuclide imaging, including SPECT and PET, and magnetic resonance imaging (MRI). All radionuclide images, including SPECT and PET, have relatively poor spatial resolution: details much smaller than a centimeter are blurred in images formed this way. However, a comparison of a typical chest x-ray (Figure 5.1) and radionuclide image (Figure 6.1) shows that, while radionuclide techniques generally have poor spatial resolution, their *contrast* is excellent. Also, all types of radionuclide imaging can be used to determine body *function* rather than merely anatomy.

This means that diseases that alter a physiological function can be detected sensitively, even in cases where there is no anatomical abnormality.

Much of the necessary science behind this technique has been developed already in Chapter 5. However, to understand fully how radionuclide imaging can have these capabilities, we must begin with a brief review of the physics within the atom.

6.2 NUCLEAR PHYSICS BASICS

To understand radioactivity, we must first understand the fundamental structure of the subcomponents of atoms. While chemistry describes the interactions *between* atoms, there can exist structure *within* the subatomic particles that make up atoms. In particular, the nucleus of the atom has proven to be a complex and fascinating entity in its own right, meriting its own field of study called **nuclear physics**.

The nucleus of an atom is composed of two sub-atomic species, called generically **nucleons**: the **proton** and the **neutron**. Protons have a positive electrical charge, equal in magnitude but opposite in sign to the charge of the electron, while neutrons are electrically neutral (that is, they have no charge). This means that the electrical forces that bind electrons to the nucleus, and bind atoms together into molecules, are affected only by the number of protons and electrons. The chemical element to which an atom belongs is given by the number of protons in its nucleus. For example, carbon (C) always has six protons in its nucleus, hydrogen (H) always has one, oxygen (O) eight, etc. The nucleons are packed into a tiny volume roughly 100,000 times smaller than that of an atom.

The reason that the nucleus sticks together in the first place has to do with the **strong nuclear attractive force** between nucleons. While the electrical force between two charged particles is present at all separations, the strong nuclear force only operates at extremely short distances. That is, two charged particles always exert an electrical force on each other no matter how far apart they are, but two nucleons only one atom's width apart exert essentially *no* force on each other. The short-ranged nuclear force creates a generally attractive interaction between the nucleons within a nucleus. Nuclear forces are felt or exerted only by nucleons, never by electrons. In addition to the nuclear forces, the protons in a nucleus also experience electrical forces that occur, because many particles of like charge (the protons) are confined to a small volume. The protons repel one another strongly, so they could not be confined to the nucleus without the balancing effect of the attractive nuclear forces between *all* nucleons. The field of nuclear physics has been developed to understand how these two competing effects (the repulsion between protons vs. the attraction between all nucleons) cause the observed organization of nuclei in nature. We will look at a few consequences of this competition shortly.

The nuclei of many chemical elements can be found in several different forms in nature. For example, the element hydrogen can be found in three forms, all of which have one proton but different numbers of neutrons. These alternate versions of a single element are called **isotopes**; each isotope has the same atomic number Z, but different total numbers of nucleons. Since changing the number of neutrons in a nucleus leaves its charge unaltered, different isotopes have virtually identical chemical properties. The different isotopes of a particular chemical element are indicated either by noting the number of nucleons or by adding a superscript to the letter symbol for the element. The superscript refers to the *total number of nucleons* (called the **mass number**) in the isotope's nucleus. For example, the three forms of hydrogen are: normal hydrogen, hydrogen-1 or ^{1}H (1 proton); deuterium, hydrogen-2 or ^{2}H (1 proton + 1 neutron); and tritium, hydrogen-3 or ^{3}H (1 proton + 2 neutrons). Any one of these isotopes can play a chemical role similar to that of normal hydrogen. For example, normal water consists of one oxygen and two hydrogens, while "heavy water" is made of one oxygen and two deuterium atoms. The various isotopes occur in nature in varying abundances; for example, seawater contains a small fraction of heavy water.

The stability of a particular nucleus is determined by the competition between attractive nuclear forces between all of the nucleons, and repulsive interactions between only the protons. Particular combinations of proton and neutron number are quite stable and exist indefinitely. In general, most light (low Z) stable isotopes have nuclei with *roughly* equal numbers of protons and neutrons. For example, carbon has two stable forms: the most common being carbon-12 (6 protons + 6 neutrons) and carbon-13 (6 protons + 7 neutrons), and several unstable forms: carbon-11 (6 protons + 5 neutrons) and carbon-14 (6 protons + 8 neutrons). Other nucleon combinations will resemble an atom with an electron in an excited state: such a configuration can be tolerated for some period of time, but it will eventually decay to a more stable state (Chapter 3). An unstable nucleus can rearrange its nucleons, shedding some particles to achieve a more energetically favorable configuration. Similar to the case of the excited atom, this rearrangement may result in the emission of a very high energy photon, a nucleon, or other particles.

The stabilization of the nucleus by particle emission is termed **radioactive decay**, and the emitted particles are called **decay products**. These phenomena in general are referred to by the term **radioactivity**. Radioactivity occurs in artificially produced laboratory samples, but also in our bodies and many naturally occurring ores. Those isotopes of a particular element which exhibit radioactivity are referred to as **radioisotopes**; when we discuss radioactive versions of different elements, we use the term **radionuclides**. Several different particles can be given off during radioactive decay, depending upon the isotope under consideration:

- **Alpha radiation.** This particle is a helium atom nucleus, consisting of two protons plus two neutrons. Alpha particles have twice the positive charge of a proton. The radioactive radon gas found in the natural environment emits alpha particles when it decays.
- **Beta radiation.** Either an electron is ejected, or the nucleus emits a particle called the **positron**. The positron is identical to the electron in all respects except that it has positive electrical charge. Iodine-131, a radionuclide used to treat cancer of the thyroid, emits electrons when it decays, while fluorine-18, which is used in PET imaging, emits positrons.
- **Gamma radiation.** The emission of a very high energy photon, either an x-ray or gamma ray. Technetium-99m, a radionuclide commonly used in medical imaging, emits gamma rays.
- **Neutrons.** The nucleus sheds one of its neutrons while stabilizing.

Many naturally occurring radionuclides do not immediately become stable after one decay. Indeed, many, like radon gas, undergo a chain of radioactive decays before finally reaching a stable state. The processes by which particular unstable isotopes decay can be determined from published tables; a few examples are listed in Table 6.1.

We describe the energies carried off by radioactive decay products using the unit of the electron-Volt (eV) introduced in Chapter 5. Particles emitted by a radioactive decay process have energies measured in MeV (Mega-eV or 10^6 eV). By comparison, the energies of biologically important chemical bonds and the energies of photons of visible light are typically several eV. Thus, a single radioactive decay product in theory has enough energy to break millions of chemical bonds. The term **ionizing radiation** is used to describe both energetic photons (x-rays and gamma rays) and particles of matter such as energetic neutrons, protons, electrons, positrons, and alpha particles. A particular form of ionizing radiation has the same properties whether produced by radioactivity or by some other process.

Table 6.1 Some examples of radionuclides that emit alpha, beta, or gamma emission on undergoing radioactive decay

Isotope	Decay product (type of particle emitted)
radon-222	alpha
strontium-90	beta (electron)
oxygen-15	beta (positron)
technetium-99m	gamma

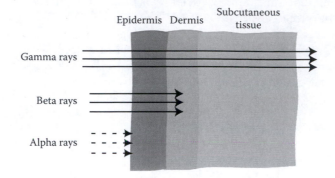

Figure 6.2 Ranges in the body of various forms of ionizing radiation.

Charged particles—alpha particles, electrons, or positrons—can inter-act with atoms by electrical forces all along their pathway. As a result of this strong interaction, they have a greater probability of being absorbed by atoms in human tissue than do gamma ray photons. This also results in their having a much shorter **range**—distance of travel before absorp-tion occurs—than a gamma ray, since their energy is absorbed much more quickly. For example, 5 MeV alpha particles have a range of a few cm in air and less than 0.01 cm in water, while 1 MeV electrons and positrons have ranges of 0.4 cm in water. By contrast, a gamma photon of energy 1 MeV has a range of many cm in water. Since most tissues are largely water, these values describe the particles' approximate ranges in the body also (Figure 6.2). However, these numbers do not tell the whole story in understanding the utility of each particle for imaging and therapy. The range of alpha and beta particles can be defined as the dis-tance beyond which *all* particles have been absorbed. However, gamma rays do not have such a hard limit beyond which they have been entirely absorbed. As explained in Chapter 5, their range instead is the distance at which some fixed fraction have been absorbed, so many gamma rays penetrate farther than the range. For imaging purposes, the particles emitted by radioactive decay must escape the body to be detected outside. Therefore, gamma rays are our principal interest in this chapter, since they are the only decay product that will be able to penetrate appreciable thicknesses of body tissue.

6.3 RADIOACTIVITY FADES WITH TIME: THE CONCEPT OF HALF-LIVES

All radioactive nuclei eventually decay and become stable elements, given enough time. One might expect that each radionuclide would have something like an average lifespan, akin to what is observed for plants and animals as well as many mechanical processes. For example, we can say how long a lifetime a car part typically has before it wears down. However, we cannot characterize how long a sample of radioactive material stays radioactive in this simple way. Instead, we describe its behavior using a time called the **half-life, $T_{1/2}$**.

To understand this concept, consider what happens after a certain number of radionuclides has been prepared for a medical procedure. Rather than having an approximate lifetime for stability, after which it is in danger of decaying, each particular nucleus in the sample *always* has a fixed probability of decaying. Every period of time, starting from the moment of its creation, there is the *same* probability of radioactive decays occurring. The number of decays occurring each moment (and hence the number of emitted particles) is proportional to the total number of radioactive nuclei remaining in the radioactive sample. After a nuclei decays to a stable state, it can no longer emit particles.* This means that there is a steady erosion with time of the radioactivity, from the greatest value at the sample's creation to increasingly smaller values.

The time behavior of radioactive decay leads to the following rule for predicting how many radioactive nuclei, $N(t)$, will be left after a time, t. If the sample starts out with a number N_{start} nuclei, then after one half-life, $T_{1/2}$, the number of nuclei remaining is $(1/2) N_{start}$. After two half-lives, one-half of that, $(1/2) \times (1/2)$ or one-fourth $(1/4) N_{start}$ remains; after three half-lives $(1/2) \times (1/2) \times (1/2)$ or one-eighth $(1/8) N_{start}$. A plot of the number of radioactive nuclei remaining in the sample as a function of time would look like Figure 6.3, which shows the characteristic time behavior of the decline of radioactivity. This distinctive behavior, in which a fixed fraction of the sample decays in a given period of time, is the hallmark of exponential decay. We have seen several manifestations already of this common phenomenon in the absorption of sound in Chapter 4, and photons in Chapter 5.

Because the half-life rule gives a method for determining how many radioactive nuclei are left after a certain period of time, it also determines how much radiation is emitted by the sample at any time. Therefore, the number of particles emitted by a source also decreases by one-half every half-life, and a plot of its time variation also would look like Figure 6.3.

The radioactivity of a certain quantity of a radionuclide is described by the **source activity** (or just activity): how many radioactive decays occur every second. The unit for source activity is the **becquerel (Bq)**, equal to one decay every second. An older conventional unit, the **curie (Ci)**, is much larger:

---

* For some nuclei, reaching a stable state requires several successive decays, a complication we are ignoring here. In such a case, each decay process would have a distinct half-life.

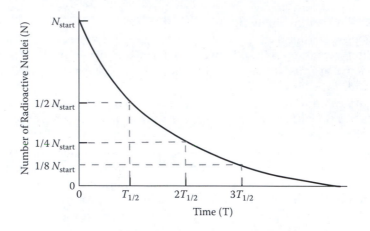

Figure 6.3 The decline with time of the source activity of a sample can be characterized by a time known as a half-life. After one half-life has elapsed, half of the radioactive nuclei in a sample have decayed, leaving half of the original level of source activity.

$$1 \text{ Bq} = 1 \text{ decay/sec} \tag{6.1}$$

$$1 \text{ Ci} = 3.7 \times 10^{10} \text{ decays/sec}$$

If a radioactive source has a source activity of 2 MBq (mega, million, or 10^6 Bq), then it is undergoing 2×10^6 decays/sec and consequently emitting 2×10^6 decay particles per second. The source activities used in medical imaging vary over a wide range, from less than one MBq to hundreds of MBq. For example, a typical scan performed with the radioisotope thalium-201 might employ about 75 MBq. Much larger source activities are used in radiation therapy, as discussed in Chapter 7.

The exact mathematical expression for radioactive decay involves an exponential falloff of source activity, $A(t)$. If we call the starting source activity A_o and the half-life $T_{1/2}$, then the equation that governs radioactive decay is:

$$A(t) = A_o e^{-0.693\, t\, /T_{1/2}} \tag{6.2}$$

where t is time, measured in the same units as the half-life. While this equation may look complicated, it is merely a mathematical version of the statement, "The number of nuclei that decay at any instant is always equal to a constant fraction of the number of nuclei present." In other words, Equation 6.2 describes the same mathematics as the earlier discussion of half-lives.

Sample calculations: The factor of 0.693 in Equation (6.2) is necessary because, when $t = T_{1/2}$, we have:

$$A\left(T_{1/2}\right) = A_o e^{-0.693\, T_{1/2}/T_{1/2}} = A_o e^{-0.693} = \frac{1}{2} A_o \qquad (6.3)$$

Now, let's work out some examples of the radioactive decay law. For example, in nuclear medicine imaging, the radioactive nuclei used must have half-lives appropriate to the length of the imaging procedure, since it would be undesirable to have appreciable amounts of radioactive waste remaining in the body or excreted into the environment. The most commonly used radionuclide for imaging, technetium-99m, has a half-life of 6.02 hours. How much of the original source activity of this isotope remains one day after the procedure? Since one day is equal to approximately four half-lives:

$$1 \text{ day} = 24 \text{ hours} = 4 \text{ (6 hours)} \simeq 4T_{1/2} \qquad (6.4)$$

The remaining source activity is diminished by four factors of $(1/2)$, to $(1/2) \times (1/2) \times (1/2) \times (1/2) = 1/16$ of the original value.

However, it is also necessary for the half-life to be large enough for the radionuclide to be administered to the patient and the scan performed before the radioactivity diminishes to an undetectable level. Let's estimate that an hour would suffice. How much of the original technetium-99m remains one hour after the original source activity has been administered? Since the time is not an even multiple of the half-life, we must use the exponential decay formula, Equation 6.2, to compute the remaining source activity:

$$A\left(t = 1 \text{ hour}\right) = A_o e^{-0.693\,(1\text{ hour})/(6.02\text{ hours})} = A_o e^{-0.115} = 0.89 A_o \qquad (6.5)$$

Approximately 89% of the original source activity remains after one hour, so this isotope's half-life represents a good compromise between presenting a long-term source of radioactivity and rapid decay, which would make imaging difficult.

Table 6.2 illustrates how widely the half-lives of different radionuclides vary. Even the same chemical element can have radioisotopes with extremely different half-lives. The half-life sets a firm limit on how long radioactive wastes remain dangerous: once created, a radionuclide will lose its radioactivity according to exponential decay and there is no known way to hurry this process along. As discussed above, this consideration

Table 6.2 Half-lives of various isotopes

Radionuclide	Half-life $T_{1/2}$	Particle emitted
carbon-11	20.4 minutes	positron
iodine-123	13 hours	gamma
iodine-131	8.05 days	gamma
strontium-90	28.7 years	beta (electron)
carbon-14	5600 years	beta (electron
plutonium-239	24,000 years	alpha
uranium-238	4.5 billion years	gamma

Table 6.3 Some properties of several isotopes used in nuclear medicine

Radionuclide	Half-life $T_{1/2}$	Particle emitted
technetium-99m	6 hours	140 keV gamma ray
gallium-67	78.3 hours	93, 184, and 300 keV gamma rays
iodine-123	13 hours	159 keV gamma ray
xenon-133	5.27 days	81 keV gamma ray
thallium-201	73 hours	68–80.3 keV gamma rays

and the constraint that the sample must retain appreciable source activity throughout the imaging procedure limit those radionuclides used for medical imaging to those with half-lives of minutes to days (Table 6.3). On the other hand, radiation therapy sources that can be carefully maintained in a hospital are chosen to have long half-lives. This reduces the need to create and transport new sources frequently.

In medicine, radionuclides usually are introduced into the body attached to a molecule or drug, a process called **radiolabeling**. The time for which the body retains a radiolabeled chemical may be very different from the half-life of the isotope used to produce the chemical, since the radioactivity can be cleared by excretion. We can also define a **biological half-life**, T_B, which describes the time required for the body to expel one-half of the chemical. The exact value of T_B depends on the chemistry and physiology of body processes, but it will be the same for all isotopes of a chemical element. For example, iodine is cleared from the thyroid with a T_B of roughly 130 days, while strontium-90 absorbed into bone has a T_B of 45 years.* To keep matters straight, $T_{1/2}$ is sometimes called the **physical half-life** to indicate that it is determined only by nuclear physics phenomena. These two very different processes combine to give an **effective half-life**, T_E, with which a radionuclide will clear from the

---

* Slightly different values of the biological half-life are quoted in various sources, reflecting variations between individuals.

body by one-half. The effective half-life is less than either the biological or physical half-lives, because the isotope's presence is being reduced *both* by excretion and by radioactive decay. For example, the effective half-life for clearance of iodine-131 from the thyroid is roughly seven days and the effective half-life for strontium-90 in the bones is roughly 17 years.

The effective half-life, T_E, which replaces $T_{1/2}$ in computing doses from radionuclides within the body, can be computed mathematically by:

$$\frac{1}{T_E} = \frac{1}{T_{1/2}} + \frac{1}{T_B} \tag{6.6a}$$

or

$$T_E = \frac{T_B \times T_{1/2}}{T_{1/2} + T_B} \tag{6.6b}$$

Sample calculation: Equation 6.6(a) can be derived by noting that the source activity drops by two exponential factors, one due to the physical exponential decay, the other due to biological excretion of the radionuclide, which is also described by an exponential decay law:

$$
\begin{aligned}
A\left(T_{1/2}\right) &= A_o e^{-0.693\,t\,/T_{1/2}} \times e^{-0.693\,t\,/T_B} \\
&= A_o e^{-0.693\,t\,/T_{1/2} - 0.693\,t\,/T_B} \\
&= A_o e^{-\left(0.693\,t\,/T_{1/2} + 0.693\,t\,/T_B\right)} \\
&= A_o e^{-0.693t\left(1/T_{1/2} + 1/T_B\right)} \\
&= A_o e^{-0.693\,t\,/T_E}
\end{aligned}
\tag{6.7}
$$

Thus, the decrease due to both these factors is itself an exponential, with half-life given by Equation 6.6(b).

Sample calculation: Iodine-131, a radionuclide used in cancer therapy and treating thyroid disease, has a physical half-life of $T_{1/2} = 8.05$ days, but a biological half-life of $T_B = 130$ days. What value of half-life does one use in computing how long the body is exposed to radiation? We can compute this with the help of Equation 6.6(b):

(continued on next page)

$$T_E = \frac{T_B \times T_{1/2}}{T_{1/2} + T_B}$$

$$= \frac{(130 \text{ days}) \times (8.05 \text{ days})}{(8.05 \text{ days}) + (130 \text{ days})} \qquad (6.8)$$

$$= 7.6 \text{ days}$$

Thus, a value of 7.6 days for the effective half-life, T_E, describes how long it will take iodine-131 to be reduced to half its original source activity in the body.

6.4 GAMMA CAMERA IMAGING

In **radionuclide imaging** (Figures 6.4 and 6.6), the source of ionizing radiation is located *within* the body. The person being scanned ingests, breathes in, or is injected with a molecule labeled with a radionuclide. Such **radiopharmaceuticals** are designed to be incorporated into some physiological process the physician wishes to study, or to concentrate preferentially in a particular organ or a pathological structure such as a tumor. In a typical scan, after the radionuclide has been administered the patient is positioned near a large area detector called a **gamma camera** or **Anger camera** (Figure 6.4). This device registers the position at which gamma rays are emitted by radionuclides in the person's body. The gamma camera detects both the number of gamma rays absorbed and their position on its planar face. Thus, the gamma camera measures a *projection* of the locations in the body where the radiopharmaceutical has concentrated (Figure 6.4a). This concept is quite similar to the way radiographs are obtained, with a few crucial differences (compare Figure 5.2 in Chapter 5). First, the source of gamma rays in radionuclide imaging is *within* the body, not external to the body, as is the case for x-ray imaging. Another major difference is that the body has a low background level of radioactivity compared to the source activity of the radiopharmaceuticals administered. This means that radionuclide images have the potential for extremely high contrast compared to radiography, which generally detects relatively small variations in x-ray transmission.

A gamma camera consists of four parts (Figure 6.5a). The first piece, called a **collimator**, is a flat sheet perforated with hollow channels and made of a gamma-absorbing metal such as lead. Gamma rays hitting the collimator are absorbed, not detected. The dimensions of the holes defines the paths of the gamma rays that can penetrate the collimator to be detected, restricting them to those that originate directly below each hole

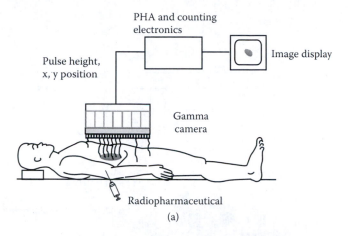

Pulse height,
x, y position

PHA and counting
electronics

Image display

Gamma
camera

Radiopharmaceutical

(a)

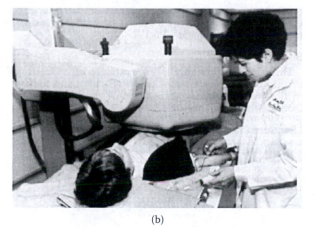

(b)

Figure 6.4 Radionuclide scan with a planar gamma camera (a) Schematic diagram
of a scan. (b) Actual scan in progress. (Reproduced with permission
courtesy of Siemens Medical Systems.)

(Figure 6.5b). This ensures that the detector above measures a projection of
the radionuclide distribution below. Although the collimators help define
the origin of gamma rays, and hence improve the spatial resolution (blur)
of the image, they also cut down drastically on what fraction of the emitted
gamma radiation actually gets detected. Thus, there is an inherent tradeoff
between high sensitivity (detecting a greater number of emitted gamma
rays) and good spatial resolution/low blur (excluding gamma rays which
do not follow exactly the right path to penetrate a channel). In practice,
gamma cameras can have several interchangeable collimators to allow for
different imaging conditions.

The actual detection of gamma rays occurs in a large, flat scintillation
crystal of the type discussed in Chapter 5. Single crystals can be produced

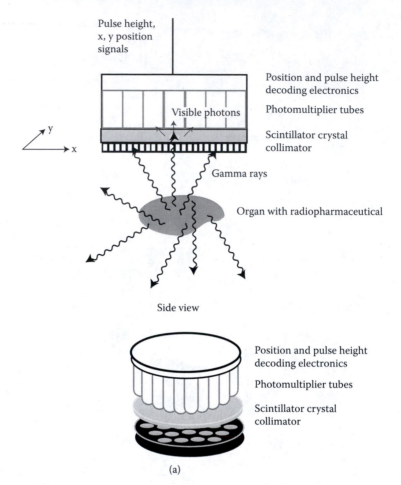

Pulse height, x, y position signals

Position and pulse height decoding electronics

Photomultiplier tubes

Visible photons

Scintillator crystal collimator

Gamma rays

Organ with radiopharmaceutical

Side view

Position and pulse height decoding electronics

Photomultiplier tubes

Scintillator crystal collimator

(a)

Figure 6.5 (a) Construction of a gamma camera. (b) Illustration of the tradeoff between blur and sensitivity in selecting gamma camera collimator channel dimensions. (c) Illustration of how energy windows can be used to accept only photons with energies close to the original emitted gamma ray energy, and exclude those due to scattering and other undesirable processes.

large enough that their field of view permits imaging the entire chest at one time. Just as in the scintillation detectors described in Chapter 5, the scintillation crystal absorbs gamma rays and re-emits some of their energy as flashes of visible light. Just as in radiographic intensifying screens, the image blur is determined in part by the scintillation crystal thickness, due to the spread of the visible light photons in a thick crystal. Thicker crystals give greater sensitivity because there is a higher probability of gamma ray absorption, at the cost of greater blur.

Several photomultiplier tubes (PMTs) located behind the crystal intercept visible photons produced by each gamma ray (Figure 6.5a). By summing the

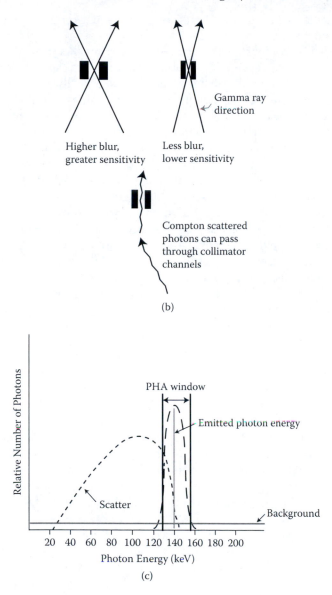

Gamma ray
direction

Higher blur,
greater sensitivity

Less blur,
lower sensitivity

Compton scattered
photons can pass
through collimator
channels

(b)

PHA window

Emitted photon energy

Relative Number of Photons

Scatter

Background

20 40 60 80 100 120 140 160 180 200

Photon Energy (keV)

(c)

Figure 6.5 (continued).

PMTs' detected intensities, the energy of the gamma ray can be measured since the total number of visible photons emitted is proportional to the original gamma ray's energy. In addition, different PMTs detect greater or lesser light intensities depending on how close they are to the location of the gamma ray absorption. A mathematical model can be used to reconstruct the point on the crystal at which the gamma ray was absorbed, using this variation in the intensity of visible light measured by each detector.

Electronics attached to the PMTs keep track of gamma ray energy and x and y position on the detector face, and pass on this information to a computer. The computer compiles an image from this information about how many gamma rays each location on the gamma camera detects. The final image can be stored and manipulated electronically and displayed on a computer screen, using all the digital image processing capabilities described in Chapter 5. In addition, different designs now exist for creating small gamma cameras for specialized applications and imaging geometries.

In general, radionuclide images have more noise and greater blur than those produced with x-rays. So many gamma rays are excluded from image formation that radionuclide scans are made up from fewer photons on average than comparable x-ray images, resulting in greater statistical variations in image intensity. As a result, the main source of noise is quantum noise or mottle, as discussed in Chapter 5. Many trade-offs, including the competition between blur and sensitivity, and the desire to keep patient doses low, determine these relatively high noise levels. Even so, useful images are achievable because there frequently is enough intrinsic contrast between the source activities of the region of interest and neighboring areas.

Several sources of photons can degrade this contrast. Naturally occurring radioactivity and cosmic rays (high energy photons from outer space) contribute an overall background level of radioactivity. More significantly, the gamma rays emitted by radionuclides can undergo processes that change their direction (Chapter 5). Compton scattering of the emitted photons can result in a high level of scattered x-rays, while characteristic x-rays can be emitted after the original photon undergoes the photoelectric effect. In either case, collimators are useless in scatter reduction (Figure 6.5b). This is because, unlike radiography, there is no single direction of the original photons to screen for. The original gamma rays and other photons are equally likely to be emitted in any direction in radionuclide imaging. However, the *energy* of scattered photons and characteristic x-rays is lower than that of the emitted photon. Thus, a technique called **pulse height analysis (PHA)** can be used to accept only the emitted gamma ray energy (Figure 6.5c).

PHA works in the following fashion. Figure 6.5(b) shows a plot of the number of photons detected during radionuclide imaging vs. photon energy. Recall that any gamma ray photon detected by the gamma camera has an energy that can be computed by adding up the total light intensity registered by the PMTs. This signal is called the pulse, and its height is a measure of gamma photon energy. The plot is generated then by counting up how many detected photons have energies near each value plotted. The original emitted gamma rays have energies that all lie very close to a value called the **photopeak** (the large peak in Figure 6.5b); the peak value shown of 140 keV corresponds to technetium-99m. The background level of radioactivity and cosmic rays contribute a low number of photons at all energies. Compton scattering and other processes result in a broad distribution at energies up to the photopeak value. If all of the photons in this distribution were summed together (corresponding to the total area under the curve in

Figure 6.5b), the desired photopeak would be only a small fraction of the entire signal measured at each point on the image. However, if the detector electronics are set to accept only a range of energies—called an energy **window**—(shown in gray in Figure 6.5b) around the photopeak, this greatly reduces the signal that the scattered photons and background contribute to the image. Thus, PHA accepts only photons with energies near the emitted value to send on to the computer for image reconstruction.

Another limitation of radionuclide imaging is that the emitted photons are attenuated by photoelectric absorption and Compton scattering, just as occurs in x-ray imaging (Chapter 5). However, whereas radiography *measures* this attenuation directly, radionuclide imaging merely *fails to record* the attenuated photons. If not corrected for, this effect can give an erroneous map of source activity throughout the body. For example, assume that the body's attenuation coefficient for photons, μ, is uniform. Then, a gamma ray is more likely to be attenuated if it is emitted by a region of the body farther from the detector than one directly underneath the gamma camera. As a result, the source activity of regions farther from the detector would be systematically underestimated without attenuation correction. A mathematical model can be used to correct for attenuation, assuming some average value of μ characteristic of body tissues and the photon energy used. However, in reality the value of μ varies appreciably throughout the body. In the chest, for example, the lungs attenuate photons much less than do soft tissues, which in turn have lower values of μ than the ribs. A region of low attenuation might show up as having a pathologically high uptake of the tracer if this variation is not corrected for (Figure 6.6).

In practice, a technique similar to radiography can be used to compile a map of attenuation coefficients, μ, throughout the body to be used in performing corrections to the gamma camera image. Radioactive sources *external* to the body can be used to accumulate a transmission image of the same region being imaged by emission. The geometry is similar to that for radiography, with the external radioactive source replacing the x-ray generator and the gamma camera acting as the image receptor. Just as in Chapter 5, this transmission data then can be analyzed to provide the required information at the appropriate photon energy range. The additional radiation risk is small, since the radiation dose from exposure to the external sources typically is several orders of magnitude smaller than that due to the radionuclide itself.

As discussed earlier in the chapter, the choice of decay product for imaging depends upon the particle's range in various materials. For example, the particles used for imaging ideally should be transmitted by the body, but they should also be detectable by the gamma camera's scintillators and stopped by collimators and shielding. In practice, the best compromise between these ideals occurs for gamma rays with energies between 50 and 200 keV. For example, technetium-99m emits 140 keV gamma rays, which can be blocked effectively by relatively thin lead collimators within the gamma camera and by lead barriers for shielding healthcare workers.

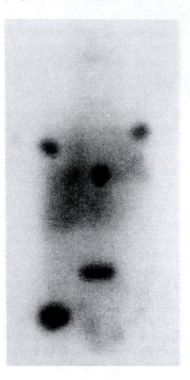

Figure 6.6 Radionuclide image of lung and bone tumors that have spread from a thyroid tumor. The outline of the entire torso and upper body can be visualized as a light gray region with low source activity. The tumors show up as darker masses because they have preferentially taken up iodine-131, the radionuclide used. (Reproduced with permission from J.R. Williams and D.I. Thwaites, *Radiotherapy Physics in Practice*, Oxford University Press, Oxford, U.K., 1993.)

One half of these gamma rays are transmitted through body tissues 4.6 cm thick, but about 90% are absorbed by detector scintillator crystals 1 cm thick—enough particles escape the body to provide a large signal for imaging and yet they can be readily detected by scintillation detectors.

It was also mentioned earlier that alpha and beta rays are absorbed before they can exit the body because charged particles have such short ranges. Thus, radionuclides for imaging should not emit charged particles, since beta or alpha rays will add to the undesirable effects of the radiation dose without providing a useful signal for imaging. For example, the isotope iodine-131 is useful for therapy, but less useful for imaging alone because it emits both gamma and beta rays. By contrast, a different isotope of iodine, iodine-123, emits only gamma rays and is much safer for use in imaging the thyroid.

The creation of effective imaging agents is not only dependent on favorable properties of the radionuclides themselves, but on the creation of radiopharmaceuticals specific to body chemistry and processes. The evolution of imaging technologies such as nuclear medicine imaging, ultrasound, and MRI (Chapter 8) to encompass the investigation of molecular, biochemical, cellular, and metabolic processes within the body has become known as **molecular imaging**. The fundamental idea behind molecular imaging is that knowledge of the body's biochemical processes can be used to create target molecules that selectively bind to receptor sites particular to disease or metabolic processes; these same agents then can be used either to image the process of interest, or to deliver drugs selectively using the same high specificity of interactions that make labeling possible.

Many radionuclides have been identified which both emit an appropriate gamma ray energy and form a chemical compound of interest. Technetium-99m can now be attached to so many useful compounds that it is extremely widely used in nuclear medicine imaging. Gamma camera scans with technetium-99m and other radionuclides are used to image the skeleton, urinary tract, lungs, heart, liver, and thyroid gland, among other applications. For example, the distribution of technetium-99m-labeled red blood cells can be used to trace the flow of blood and indicate the quality of circulation throughout the body. Others radiopharmaceuticals are taken up preferentially by a particular organ or by tumors. For example, a chemical compound called technetium-99m-HIDA normally is concentrated in the gallbladder. Thus, an abnormal absence of radioactive tracer compound could indicate impaired circulation in a region of the body (in the first case) or blockage of the gallbladder (in the second). In **scintimammography**, a technetium-99m tracer compound can be used to image tumors in breast cancer.

More than 70% of nuclear medicine imaging is performed with technetium-labeled compounds, but a variety of other useful radionuclides exist. Xenon-133 is a gas that can be used to image the lungs and respiratory system. Gallium-67 is used in cancer imaging; for example, the compound gallium-67-citrate preferentially segregates to tumors and abscesses, marking their locations (Figure 6.1). Both gallium-67 and indium-111 can be attached to **antibodies**, molecules of the immune system which recognize foreign (and hence possibly disease-causing) materials. Researchers are seeking antibodies that will bind to tumors for even more specificity in radiolabeling. In imaging the heart, several different kinds of information about blood flow and heart function can be determined. Thallium-201, rubidium-81, and rubidium-82 can substitute for the potassium that heart muscle needs to function properly. The distribution and amounts of thallium-201 taken up by the heart muscle are therefore an indication of muscular activity. Similarly, red blood cells tagged with technetium-99m spread throughout the bloodstream and indicate the volume of blood present in the chambers of the heart. Measurements also can indicate the blood volume per heart beat using this technique.

By taking successive images a fixed time apart, changes of the radioactive tracer's distribution over time also can be measured quantitatively. The time-behavior of the tracer molecule in the body can be mathematically modeled, allowing physicians to extract the rate of important physiological processes. For example, scans of the kidneys and urinary tract can determine how effectively radionuclides introduced into the bloodstream are properly filtered out and excreted. The filtration rate of the radioactive tracers gives a measure of kidney function for detecting blockages, monitoring the organs' general health, or seeing whether transplanted organs are working properly.

These procedures can provide a lower-cost alternative to more expensive imaging techniques such as MRI. A large signal for imaging can be achieved with extremely small amounts—typically billionths of a gram—of the radiolabeled tracer. Since these minute amounts correspond to concentrations too small for drug activity, the radiopharmaceuticals do not affect body function, although they still must meet federal standards for drug purity and safety. Chapter 7 addresses in more detail how to determine safe levels for the radiation doses resulting from radionuclide imaging.

6.5 EMISSION TOMOGRAPHY WITH RADIONUCLIDES: SPECT AND PET

A major drawback of radionuclide imaging with a gamma camera is that it only offers a single projection of the body's structures, rather than giving a three-dimensional picture. Every point on the gamma camera image corresponds to an entire *line* within the person being imaged (Figure 6.7a). Radionuclides at many different depths within the body cause only one detector above to respond. This means that planar gamma camera images contain no depth information, and so cannot resolve overlapping structures. This also means that the shape of a structure can be very unclear in a gamma camera image (Figure 6.7). Just as in radiography, a projection also can have relatively low contrast if background source activity is significant. For some types of scans, a planar image provides a complete and accurate picture image, but for others this effect can seriously impair the image's usefulness.

Just as CT imaging can remedy these problems in radiography, **emission computed tomography** (ECT) provides three-dimensional information about the distribution of radionuclides within the body. As explained in Chapter 5, computed tomography refers to the mathematical techniques by which projections of an object can be reassembled into cross-sectional images. While we only considered the applications of these ideas to x-ray imaging in Chapter 5, these same ideas can also be adapted to radionuclide imaging, as we will now see.

The basic idea behind SPECT imaging is shown in simplified form in Figure 6.8, analogous to Figure 5.29. In Figure 6.8(a), a schematic cross section of the body is shown, along with two detector arrays. Just as in gamma camera imaging, each detector in the array measures a projection of the emitted gamma ray distribution. In addition, collimators restrict the

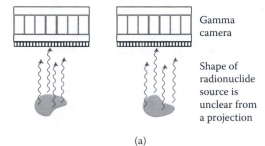

(a)

Figure 6.7 Illustration of loss of depth information in gamma camera imaging. (a) Gamma rays emitted at different depths will register in the same detector, and the two different emitter shapes shown will both result in the same detectors registering the same pattern. This means that the spatial location and shape of regions where radionuclides are concentrated cannot in general be determined from planar gamma camera images alone. Gallium-67 radionuclide scans of the head and torso (b) indicate tumors in a lymph node (large arrow) and near a vertebra (small arrow), but the exact positions of the tumors is unclear and their contrast relatively poor. (c) A series of axial SPECT images through the upper abdomen of the same patient. The SPECT images show more clearly the location and distribution of gallium-67 near the vertebra. Higher uptake is present in the upper images (solid arrow) compared with the normal uptake in the lower images (open arrow), indicating the vertical extent of the tumor. Also note the improved contrast of the SPECT images compared to part (b). (Used with permission courtesy of Paul C. Stomper, *Cancer Imaging Manual*, J.B. Lippincott Company, Philadelphia, 1993.)

gamma ray's directions so that only gamma rays that originate from the cross section shown can reach the detectors. When corrected for attenuation and scattering, the photon intensity measured by each detector is a measure of the body's distribution of radionuclides along one line within the body. The two different arrays shown detect projections at right angles to each other (Figure 6.8a). Because they detect gamma rays emitted at different angles, the two projections determine both the radionuclides' position left to right (top array) and top to bottom (left-hand array). These are called forward projections, in analogy to the forward projections measured in x-ray CT (Chapter 5). A computer records the number of intercepted gamma rays in each detector for each position of the array as it is rotated around the patient. This information is used to reconstruct the radionuclides' source activity by back projecting—crudely speaking, tracing inward along the gamma ray's apparent pathway– from the positions along each array where gamma rays were registered (Figure 6.8b). Just as in x-ray CT, regions that overlap upon back projection correspond to areas within the body with high source activity. Information collected from detectors oriented at a series of angular positions helps refine the actual reconstructed distribution further. Finally, just as in x-ray CT, for accurate image reconstruction

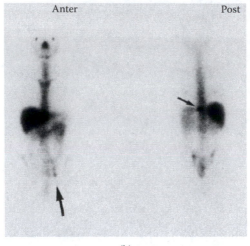

(b)

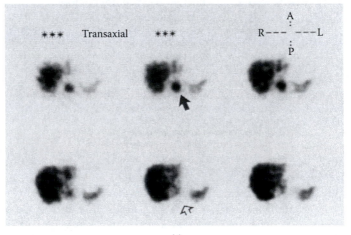

(c)

Figure 6.7 (continued).

emission CT forward projection data requires an additional mathematical process called filtering before backprojection is performed.

Actual SPECT scanners either can use rings of detectors surrounding the patient or rotating gamma cameras (Figure 6.8c and d). Either geometry permits cross sections to be taken either in an axial plane or other orientations if different sets of opposing detectors are used. SPECT scanners make use of the same basic detector design and the same radionuclides as gamma camera imaging since both have the same requirements for particle type and energy. While this contributes to SPECT being a widely available and

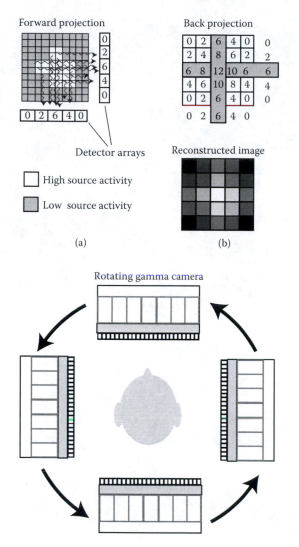

Figure 6.8 Schematic representation of the actual experimental forward (a) and the computed back (b) projections used in SPECT. (c) Photograph of a patient preparing to undergo a SPECT scan in a scanner. (d) Illustration of how a rotating gamma camera can be used to perform SPECT. (Used with permission courtesy of Siemens Medical Systems.)

commonly used technique, it also means that SPECT also shares many of the same problems as gamma camera imaging. SPECT scanners have inherently poor spatial resolutions, with typical blurs of 10 mm or more, with small values achievable for specialized head and small animal scanners. In addition, SPECT makes very inefficient use of radionuclides since only a very small fraction of all gamma rays emitted are actually intercepted by

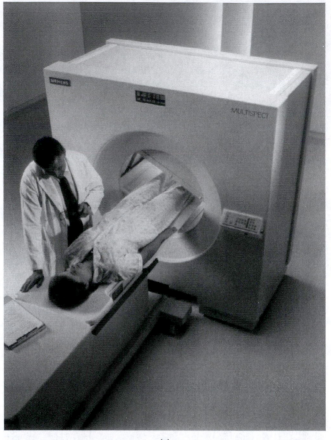

(c)

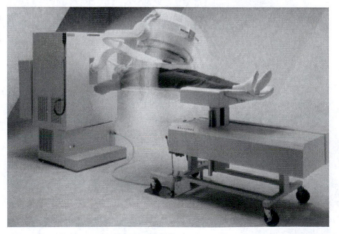

(d)

Figure 6.8 (continued).

detectors. This results in images that are noisy compared to typical CT images. However, SPECT scanners are often effective in helping to diagnose brain conditions, to image the heart and major blood vessels, to locate tumors and to image bone diseases. These capabilities result because, just as with planar gamma camera imaging, SPECT images have high contrast and can detect function in three dimensions. As with gamma camera imaging, radioactive tracer chemicals can be used to measure blood flow and a variety of important biochemical activity within the body, as well as the interactions of drugs. The kinetics of the radiolabeled tracer molecule can be modeled mathematically, and its abundance reconstructed using SPECT to allow the rate of the biological process itself to be determined.

An idea similar to SPECT is used in the related technique of **positron emission tomography (PET)**. Certain radionuclides decay by emitting positrons, the **antimatter** twin of electrons. By antimatter, we mean that positrons have the same mass and many of the same properties as electrons. However, they have exactly opposite electrical charges: the electron has one negative and the positron one positive elementary unit of charge. When a radionuclide in the body undergoes beta decay by releasing a positron, the positron travels only a short range before interacting with one of the electrons bound to atoms within the body (Table 6.4). Now, when a particle and its antimatter partner are brought together, they are attracted to each other because of their opposite electrical charges. This attraction causes the electron and positron pair to bind briefly into an atom-like system called **positronium**. This state is itself unstable, however, and the pair eventually undergoes a second reaction in which the electron and positron are said to **annihilate** each other (Figure 6.9). No particle with mass remains after this encounter; instead, two high energy photons are observed exiting. Each photon created has an energy of exactly 0.511 MeV, but no mass and no electrical charge. This is consistent with the conservation of charge, since the positive and negative charges of the electron and positron add to zero total charge. What about conservation of energy? Phenomena such as this led to the hypothesis that the mass that disappeared has been converted into the energy of the two photons. In fact, this loss of mass is also observed in nuclear decay and in **nuclear fission**, a process in which nuclei are bombarded by energetic particles to force them to fracture into pieces. In every

Table 6.4 Some of the radionuclides used in PET imaging

Positron emitting radionuclide	Positron range in water (mm)	Half-life (min)
Fluorine-18	1.0	110
Gallium-68	1.7	68
Carbon-11	1.1	20
Rubidium-82	1.7	1.3

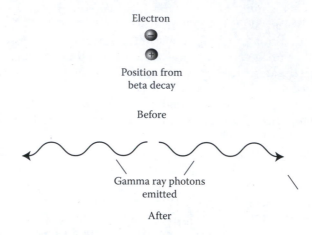

Figure 6.9 View of annihilation of a positron decay product and an electron from
body tissue, generating two oppositely directed gamma rays

case, a new amount of energy appears in association with the observed loss
of mass.

Albert Einstein postulated that a mass, m, is equivalent to an amount
of energy, E, by the famous equation $E = mc^2$. In this equation, E is called
the **rest mass energy** and c the speed of light in empty space. The rest mass
energy of an electron or positron, for example, is 0.511 MeV. This relation explains numerous specific experiments on nuclear decay, fission, and
particle annihilation. In particular, when the electron and positron annihilate, their rest mass energy reappears in a new form: the two 0.511 MeV
photons. If the positron and electron were at rest, the two photons are
emitted traveling in exactly opposite directions (Figure 6.9). If the original
decay happened in an isotope within the body, these high energy photons
can exit the body to be detected.

Figure 6.10 shows how a PET scanner makes use of this phenomenon.
The person to undergo a PET scan ingests or is injected with a chemical labeled with a positron-emitting radionuclide. These chemicals course
through the body, and are taken up preferentially in specific tissues or during specific metabolic processes. For illustration, in Figure 6.10(b) they
are shown as having accumulated in a region of the brain, shown in axial
cross section. The radionuclides decay with some characteristic half-life by
emitting positrons. Each positron travels through the body, meeting with
an electron within the range of a few millimeters of its place of creation;
their annihilation results in two high energy photons traveling in opposite
directions. The person to be scanned is placed at the center of a stationary detector array, consisting of many rings of many separate scintillation
detectors. (For simplicity, only one ring is shown in the figures, but modern

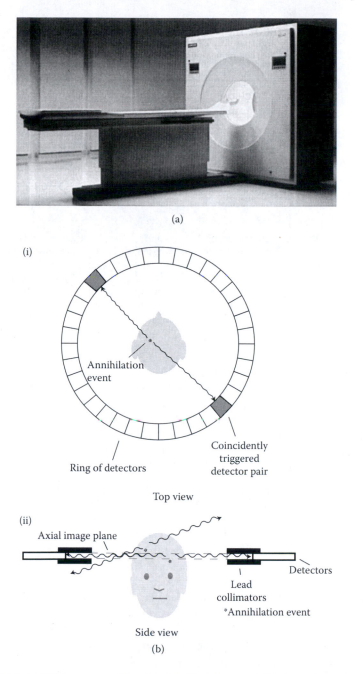

(a)

(i)

Annihilation event

Ring of detectors

Coincidently triggered detector pair

Top view

(ii)

Axial image plane

Detectors

Lead collimators

*Annihilation event

Side view

(b)

Figure 6.10 (a) PET scanner. (Siemens Medical Systems) (b) Detection scheme for PET imaging. The side view shows how only radionuclides in a particular cross-sectional plane will be detected by the rings of detectors.

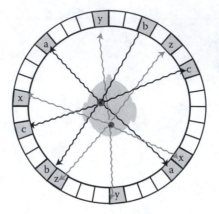

Figure 6.11 Detectors surrounding the patient being imaged by a PET scanner register the number of coincidentally detected gamma rays emitted. A computer records the line of response (LOR) connecting each coincidently triggered detector pair (indicated by like letter labels). As in other forms of computed tomography, an idea of the technique's basis can be seen by noting that radiolabeled regions (dark gray) coincide with the intersection of multiple LORs, and the number of LORs contributing to the image will indicate that region's relative source activity.

PET scanners use 3D detection and can perform entire body scans during a procedure. Research is also ongoing to develop direct solid state detectors similar to those discussed in Chapter 5.) When a positron-emitting decay occurs, two detectors fire: one for each gamma ray photon. The location of the radionuclide that emitted the positron must lie along a straight line between the two detectors, called the **line of response (LOR)**. A computer can compute the LORs followed by each coincident pair of photons (Figure 6.11). Just as in SPECT, this information is used as the input to filtered back-projection calculations for reconstructing a cross-sectional map of source activity.

How does the detector know that the two photons came from the same positron annihilation? An electronic method called **coincidence detection** looks for two photons so close together in time that they very likely came from the same annihilation. Each detector in the array is connected with other detectors in the array so that it will only record a count if another detector also records a count within a **coincident timing window** of 15 to 4.5 nanoseconds (10^{-9} s or billionths of a second). It is possible that gamma rays from two separate decays could hit two detectors close enough in time to be mistaken for a single beta decay. However, such **random events** are unlikely if the source activity administered is kept low.

As in SPECT, each detector directly measures a projection, since photons from various points along the line will register in the same detector. Like SPECT, the attenuation of photons by intervening body tissues is a problem that must be corrected for. However, unlike SPECT, the requirement that coincident counts be recorded allows for additional rejection of Compton scattered photons and those due to background radiation. The rejection of scattered photons can be improved further by several other techniques similar to those used in SPECT. For example, collimators placed before the detectors can be configured to enhance contrast by accepting only back-to-back photons from true decay events. This helps exclude cases where gamma rays traveling at oblique angles coincidentally hit two detectors within a timing window. However, this also reduces the number of photons detected and restricts the LORs the scanner can detect. Just as in gamma camera imaging, electronic PHA methods can be used to reject Compton scattered photons that would give erroneous LORs. In addition, the coincident timing techniques discussed above can be modified so as to reduce the counts due to random events and background. This can be accomplished by screening for coincident events using both (1) the usual coincident timing window and (2) a timing window that requires a long delay between detection of the two gamma rays. The signal due to the second timing window cannot be due to true decay events, so it represents only random events and background gamma ray emission. Hence, the signal from (2) can be subtracted from the coincident timing window signal (1) to give the signal due only to true decays.

It is possible to compute *where along the line* the nuclei decayed if the *differences* in detection times are measured in what is called **time-of-flight-PET**, using an idea very similar to the pulse-echo technique used in ultrasound (Chapter 4). Some modern scanner integrate this information into the image reconstruction algorithms, although time-of-flight in itself offers only coarse spatial resolution because of timing limitations in the detection electronics.

PET also has a significant advantage in the types of positron-emitting radiolabels available. The radionuclides used include oxygen-15, carbon-11, nitrogen-13, fluorine-18, gallium-68, and rubidium-82 (Table 6.4). This list includes elements—carbon, oxygen, and nitrogen—that are major constituents of the body's organic compounds. Thus, it is possible to synthesize radiolabeled versions of naturally occurring body chemicals, drugs or other molecules with their biochemical properties intact. Fluorine can be readily incorporated into many drugs and naturally occurring molecules as a substitute for hydrogen. For example, the fluorine-18-labeled sugar fluoro-deoxyglucose (FDG) is metabolized by brain cells in place of the naturally occurring sugar glucose, so PET can detect the distribution of the radioactive sugar in the brain to show which regions are most metabolically active, and hence using the greatest amount of energy. Similarly, blood flow to the brain can be visualized either by using carbon dioxide labeled with oxygen-15 or carbon-11, or water labeled with oxygen-15 incorporated into the bloodstream. The brain's use of oxygen also can be monitored using oxygen-15. Since changes in the blood supply locally within the brain are assumed to reflect variations in its activity, these measurements give clues to which regions are most active at any moment. While they are not native to the body, the more exotic elements on the list are used as chemical labels for interesting molecules. For example, rubidium-82 is used in cardiac imaging to map the health of heart muscle, while gallium-68 is a useful label for drugs.

The spatial resolution of PET scans is limited in practice to 4 mm for current scanners for humans. This is appreciably worse than the best resolutions achievable by CT, MRI, and ultrasound, but an improvement over SPECT. PET's spatial resolution is inherently limited by the positron's range in body tissue, in addition to the usual imaging geometry limitations (Table 6.4). This is because emitted positrons travel within the body before annihilating, corrupting information about the position of the original decay site. With improvements in detector design, or confining the field of view to smaller volumes for the brain or small research animals, higher spatial resolutions are being achieved, but the fundamental limits are not appreciably smaller than current values.

PET images can be displayed either in a gray-scale image or using false color maps to display source activity within a cross-sectional plane or reconstructed three-dimensional image. Since both SPECT and PET measure function rather than anatomy, it is useful to use them in combination with other imaging modalities such as CT or MRI, which are sensitive probes of body anatomy. Techniques have been developed to put images obtained from multiple techniques in registry so they can be combined into single images.

Just as with other radionuclide imaging procedures, in PET the person being scanned must ingest a low dose of a radiopharmaceutical. Because of their short half-lives, these radiopharmaceuticals must be artificially produced and the desired tracer molecule synthesized. Most of the radionuclides used in PET must be produced onsite using an expensive particle physics accelerator called a **cyclotron** (Figure 6.12a). Cyclotrons use electrical fields that alternate in polarity to accelerate ions of hydrogen to extremely high energies. These nuclei are confined to a circular orbit by magnetic fields while they are boosted to high energies on the order of several MeV. The very energetic charged nuclei then are allowed to exit the cyclotron toward a target. The target contains stable nuclei that can undergo a nuclear reaction when bombarded with excess protons from the very energetic hydrogen. This process transforms them into heavier, positron-emitting radioisotopes. Carbon-11, nitrogen-13, oxygen-15, and fluorine-18 all require a cyclotron for their production. The resulting radioisotopes can be transferred to a dedicated **biosynthesizer unit**, which swiftly performs any chemical reactions required to produce the desired radiopharmaceutical. The expense and complexity of a dedicated cyclotron facility once restricted the availability of PET. However, fluorine-18 has the additional significant advantage that its half-life is long enough to allow it to be distributed commercially, rather than produced onsite with a cyclotron. This fact, and the wide utility of fluorine-18 labeled radiotracers, has greatly expanded the scope of PET scanning.

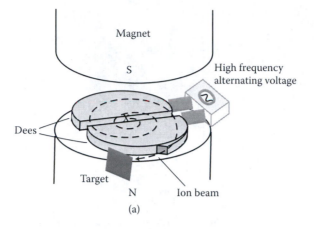

Magnet

S

High frequency
alternating voltage

Dees

Target

N   Ion beam

(a)

Figure 6.12 Illustration of the production of radionuclides for nuclear medicine imaging using (a) cyclotrons and (b) generators. (a) Simplified illustration of the operation of a cyclotron for producing radioisotopes. An ion source (X) emits a stream of charged nuclei, in this case hydrogen ions. These ions are subjected to a voltage between the two halves (Dees) of the cyclotron. As they gain energy, the moving ions' paths are bent into a circle by the poles of a magnet enclosing the Dees. Once they have completed half a circuit, the polarity of the voltage between the Dees is switched, so the ions are once again accelerated toward the next Dee. The increase in velocity results in a spiral orbit, as the Dee's voltages continue to alternate in polarity and the ions gain energy. The ions finally are directed toward a target of stable nuclei, which become radioisotopes after undergoing nuclear reactions with the bombarding hydrogen nuclei. (b) In a radionuclide generator, a long half-life "parent" radionuclide (in this case, molybdenum-99) is immobilized on a column packed full of a material that binds it via chemical attachment. Over time, radioactive decay gradually transforms the bound species into the desired, shorter half-life "daughter" radionuclide (technetium-99m). However, this daughter has a different atomic number (Z), so it is chemically different from its parent. This means the daughter is no longer bound to the column, so it can be eluted (washed off) by rinsing the column with a saline solution.

One of the advantages of the radionuclides gallium-68 and rubidium-82 is that they can be produced by a smaller, cheaper **generator** (Figure 6.12b). In a radionuclide generator, a long half-life "parent" radionuclide is immobilized on a column packed full of a material that binds it via chemical attachment. Over time, radioactive decay gradually transforms the bound species into the desired, shorter half-life "daughter" radionuclide. However, this daughter has a different atomic number (Z), so it is chemically different from its parent. This means the daughter is no longer bound to the column, so it can be eluted (washed off) by rinsing the column with a saline solution. Technetium-99m is one example of a generator-produced radionuclide. Research into performing labeling chemistry with generator-produced

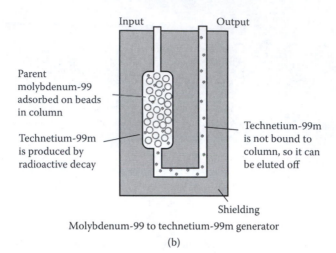

Input   Output

Parent
molybdenum-99
adsorbed on beads
in column

Technetium-99m
is produced by
radioactive decay

Technetium-99m
is not bound to
column, so it can
be eluted off

Shielding

Molybdenum-99 to technetium-99m generator

(b)

Figure 6.12 (continued).

radionuclides and methods of manufacturing inexpensive, compact cyclotrons are contributing to making PET ever more widely used.

These ECT techniques are useful in a variety of diagnostic applications in cardiology. For example, PET can be used to measure the extent to which the blood supply to a region of heart muscle is intact by measuring the source activity of a blood perfusion agent. The absence of the radioactive tracer can be used to map out regions of impaired blood flow. At the same time, the same region's metabolism can be assessed using FDG scans since the heart muscle can utilize glucose as a fuel. If the heart muscle is viable, then it should exhibit high rates of FDG metabolism. This information can be combined to determine, for example, whether a region of tissue is viable enough to benefit from an interventional procedure to re-establish blood flow. SPECT and PET can be used in cancer imaging to determine the blood supply to a tumor, to probe tumor metabolism, or to measure the distribution of radiopharmaceuticals specifically targeted to tumors. This information can help track the spread of tumors within the body or probe for their recurrence after surgery to remove the cancer.

6.6 APPLICATION: EMISSION COMPUTER TOMOGRAPHY STUDIES OF THE BRAIN

Because gamma rays easily penetrate the skull, radionuclide imaging is a useful tool for probing the brain. Physicians can both diagnose and study neurological diseases using SPECT and PET. Until recently, what little was known about the physiological causes of brain disorders had to be surmised from various sources, including studies of animal models, studies of persons with brain tumors or other lesions, autopsies of the brains of disease sufferers, and the study of the psychological effects of drugs. Researchers could not directly measure how human brain function was altered by disease, or probe the effects of drugs on the brain in a living subject. Now PET and SPECT allow physicians to monitor blood flow and blood volume, glucose use, and oxygen metabolism within the brain. Ordinarily the blood–brain barrier ensures that only nutrients can pass from the circulatory system to the brain and excludes many drugs and toxins. ECT methods can look for breeches in the integrity of this system indicative of serious injury or disease, such as tumors, hemorrhages, or blood clots.

How do these brain scans work? Using PET or SPECT, a cross-sectional image of the brain is produced which shows the source activity of tracer radionuclides. For example, Figure 6.13 shows SPECT images obtained with radiolabeled tracers that distribute according to the flow of blood within the brain. Thus, this image gives a map of regional blood flow, which is uniform in a healthy person's brain (Figure 6.13a). Damage due to disruptions in the blood supply due to a stroke, for example, clearly appear in such images (Figure 6.13b). Figure 6.13(c) shows an image taken of the brain of a person with Alzheimer's disease, a degenerative disease that causes senile dementia. Damage to the brain is dramatically indicated by the absence of blood flow to large regions called the parietal lobes (shown at the bottom of the image). Thus, a SPECT or PET image can indicate changes in brain function which an anatomical study could easily miss. If it is desired to combine this information with detailed anatomical scans, images from MRI can be combined in registry with the SPECT or PET information to provide a correlation between structure and function.

These nuclear medicine imaging techniques can play a role in diagnosing brain cancer, differentiating between different kinds of dementia, assessing

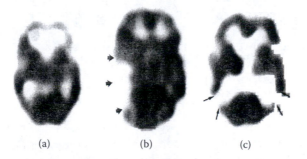

(a) (b) (c)

Figure 6.13 SPECT images of axial cross sections through the brain showing the distribution of a radiolabeled tracer drug which shows blood flow in (a) a normal subject, (b) one with brain damage due to an acute cerebral infarction (the authors note that a CT scan of the same person showed no damage); and (c) a patient with Alzheimer's disease. (Reproduced with permission courtesy of F. Leonard Holman and Sabah S. Tumeh, "Single-Photon Emission Computed Tomography (SPECT)," *Journal of the American Medical Association*, Vol. 263, 1990, pp. 561–564.)

stroke, and diagnosing and planning treatments for some forms of epilepsy. They are also being used to explore the causes of conditions such as speech disorders, depression, learning disorders, and drug dependency. Using PET, functional MRI (Chapter 8), and electrical imaging techniques, brain metabolism in living patients afflicted with psychiatric disorders such as schizophrenia and depression can be studied. In addition, PET and functional MRI have opened new frontiers in basic research into mental processes. It is important to be clear about what can be measured in this research. PET cannot really allow researchers to literally see thoughts, emotions, or memories, although such analogies often are used in the popular media. The brain works as a network, and most mental processes cannot be neatly localized into a specific part of the brain that "lights up" during a scan. Scientists *can* use PET to measure quantities that reflect the brain's metabolic activity—its use of energy and biochemicals—in broadly defined regions. PET also has important limitations. Each scan takes much longer than the time required for nerve cells to send a signal. Since PET has such a poor spatial resolution, typically several mm at best, it may miss altogether essential, small-scale details in the brain's activity. However, when researchers bear in mind problems such as these, PET brain scans can yield important clues to outstanding problems in neuroscience.

PET images can be taken during different mental tasks to determine which regions of the brain are active, and more than one radioactive tracer can be employed to trace blood flow and glucose and oxygen metabolism. While the maps of brain activity ascertained by these methods are fairly coarse in spatial detail, they can show regions of activity clearly. In addition, a variety of psychoactive drugs can be radiolabeled, and their distribution throughout the brain traced. Important naturally occurring chemicals also yield important clues to brain function and give feedback to researchers working at developing new drugs. The transmission of signals throughout the nervous system takes place by two processes. Within nerve cells, or **neurons**, the signals travel electrically, like an electrical signal passing down a electrical cable. However, when signals need to be transmitted from one neuron to another, they are conveyed by special chemicals called **neurotransmitters**. The transmitting neuron releases these neurotransmitters, which are sensed by the receiving neuron using special receptor molecules specific to the neurotransmitter encountered. Examples of neurotransmitter molecules include **dopamine** and **serotonin**. Some models of psychiatric disease postulate a difference in either the number or the functioning of a specific neurotransmitter, leading to an abnormal sensitivity, which can create disturbances in mental functioning. One example involves the investigation of causes of Parkinson's disease. Patients suffering from this disease exhibit symptoms such as tremors, muscular weakness, and rigidity. The underlying cause of Parkinson's disease involves a reduction in the number of cells that release dopamine. A drug called L-DOPA can help alleviate this problem by increasing dopamine synthesis within the brain. PET allows the abnormal dopamine uptake in Parkinson's disease to be studied in living patients using radioactively labeled L-DOPA. In another example, drug abuse has been observed to cause changes in dopamine release and substitute drugs observed to bind to receptors for opiates.

A serious complication in such studies is that persons suffering from neurological diseases are often taking psychoactive drugs, which may themselves alter brain activity. Thus, differences in brain function may be a result of the treatment, rather than an underlying cause. These studies can also be difficult to reproduce, in part because individual variation in brain function is substantial, so researchers must devise ways to distinguish which differences are truly related to abnormalities. Often, a composite "average" brain scan for healthy and diseased patients is compiled, with the remaining differences assumed to result from the disease. Thus, while tomography of the brain offers unprecedented opportunities for diagnosis and research, they must be interpreted carefully and used in combination with other research tools.

In basic research, PET has played a major role in mapping the locations of brain activity during various cognitive or perceptual tasks. For example, look carefully at another person for a moment, then close your eyes and bring to mind a mental picture of that person. The two experiences feel very similar—are the same parts of the brain involved in "seeing" the actual visual image and the imagined visual image? With PET, scientists can study brain activity during both processes to determine that, indeed, some of the same regions of the brain are active during both: you generate the imagined image using the visual processing regions of your brain.

These studies also clearly show shifts in the location and efficiency of brain activity as novel mental tasks are learned. Using PET, researchers have shown that reading a word excites different parts of the brain more than reading nonsensical strings of consonants, demonstrating how even subtle differences in processing are detectable using these methods. Indeed, much of the research into brain activity has concentrated on learning tasks and processing words.

PET has played an important role in unraveling some of the greatest mysteries of the mind, but a newer technique, functional MRI, allows yet faster and higher resolution images of many of the same processes. Chapter 8 explores how these techniques are further expanding the possibilities for neuroscience.

6.7 HYBRID SCANNERS

SPECT/CT and PET/CT scanners have become commercially available recently, combining the unique capabilities of each imaging modality into one integrated package. Not a single new technology, these so-called **hybrid scanners** simply combine two separate scanners in a single device, arranged so their openings coincide along a central axis. By lying upon a single, movable table, a patient can be rapidly, successively scanned for anatomy with superior spatial resolution with CT at one location in the hybrid scanner and for functional imaging with radioactive contrast media with SPECT or PET at a different location, enabling combined whole-body scanning in minutes. (One important time savings is that the CT scan can be used to correct the emission tomography scan for attenuation, saving the lengthy time usually devoted to doing a transmission scan with a radioactive source.) The integrated scanner design allows images to be taken in quick succession, minimizing patient motion and enabling the creation of combined images that coregister (align and overlap) the same features on a computer. These combined images can display both CT and SPECT or PET image information by using different visual cues, such as showing the CT data as grayscale and the SPECT or PET data as color maps (Figure 6.14). For example, CT can be used to delineate the location of a suspicious mass in anatomical detail relative to organs, while PET can determine whether it has the functional signatures of a malignant tumor. These technologies are

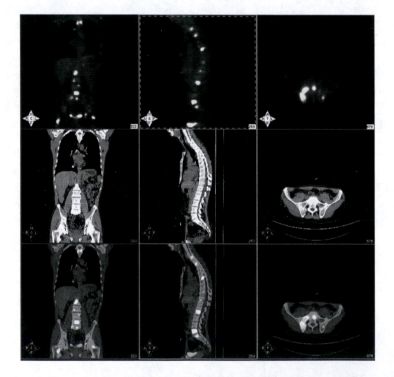

Figure 6.14 (See color figure following page 78.) Hybrid PET/CT imaging in oncology, showing how PET images (top row) can be combined with CT (middle row) by "coregistering" color maps from PET onto the grayscale CT images (bottom row). These hybrid images allow regions of enhanced contrast in PET to be compared to the anatomical information from CT for enhanced diagnostic accuracy. (Images courtesy of Drs. Daniel Appelbaum and Yonglin Pu, University of Chicago.)

already in wide use in cardiology, neurology, and oncology applications. For example, whole body PET/CT scans with the commercially available, radiolabeled sugar FDG can be used in diagnosing and in planning the course of treatment (surgery, radiation therapy, or chemotherapy) for many common cancers as well as in monitoring the progress of therapy and long-term follow-ups. These scans work by making use of the fact that malignant tumors use more glucose then normal tissues. The complementary information from the two different scanning modalities can make diagnoses more accurate, since CT can find tumors that might not show up on PET as actively metabolizing glucose, reducing the number of false negatives, while PET can distinguish between malignant and benign tumors that have the same appearance in CT, reducing the number of false positives. For radiation therapy planning (Chapter 7), the addition of PET information to CT anatomical images provides details about the spatial distribution of the biological activities of tumors, so that their metabolic features can be understood and targeted in planning detailed radiation dose distributions, not just their morphology. In cancer therapy, hybrid scanning can monitor the progression of the response of individual tumors to the treatment, identifying whether some might be unresponsive, so alternative therapies can be tried earlier for selected tumors. Hybrid scanners have been shown to improve the accuracy of diagnoses in approximately 50% of patients, while also providing information that influences the course of therapy in an estimated 10 to 20% of cases.*

Chemicals are currently under investigation to provide radiolabeled markers that would indicate biological states relevant to diagnosis and treatment planning, such as cellular proliferation, cell death, low oxygen levels (using oxygen-13), patterns of gene expression, and specific hormone receptors. Other radiopharmaceuticals can serve as markers for imaging bone metabolism, or the synthesis of DNA (as a way of determining tumor proliferation), proteins and membrane lipids. We will visit such molecular medicine innovations that combine molecular biology and biochemistry with imaging and therapeutic applications again in the context of radiation therapy in Chapter 7 and magnetic resonance imaging in Chapter 8.

SUGGESTED READING

Internet and multimedia

There are numerous rapidly changing web resources available through the radiology departments of almost all major medical schools. Many of

---

* See "PET scanning and functional anatomic image fusion" and other articles in *The Cancer Journal*, Vol. 10(4), pp. v–vi ff. (2004).

these feature radiology teaching files that display sample images for a variety of procedures. One particularly helpful site is the program "Let's Play PET," maintained by the UCLA School of Medicine Crump Institute for Biological Imaging at http://www.crump.ucla.edu/lpp/lpphome.html and the BrainMap website at http://brainmap.org/.

Books and articles

Russell K. Hobbie, *Intermediate Physics for Medicine and Biology*. John Wiley & Sons, New York, 1988, p. 623.

Michael I. Posner and Marcus E. Raichle, *Images of Mind*. Scientific American Library, New York, 1994.

Perry Sprawls, Jr., *Physical Principles of Medical Imaging*. Medical Physics Publishing. Madison, WI, 1995.

Steve Webb, ed., *Physics of Medical Imaging*. Institute of Physics Publishing, Bristol, U.K., 1992, p. 633.

Articles

Michel M. Ter-Pogossian, Marcus E. Raichle, and Burton E. Sobel, "Positron emission tomography," *Sci. Am.* (Oct. 1980), pp. 171–181.

Timothy J. McCarthy, Sally W. Schwartz, and Michael J. Welch, "Nuclear medicine and positron emission tomography," *J. Chem. Ed.*, vol. 71 (Oct. 1994), pp. 830–836.

QUESTIONS

Q6.1.   Explain why radioisotopes that produce gamma rays are used for imaging applications, and why those that produce beta or alpha particles would be poor choices.

Q6.2.   Discuss why the effective half-life of a radionuclide in the body can differ from the physical half-life. Can the effective half-life ever be longer than the physical half-life? Can it be shorter? Explain your answers.

Q6.3.   Explain in detail the operation of a PET (positron emission tomography) scanner, illustrating your points by using more than one drawing, appropriately labeled. Give one application of PET and describe why PET works uniquely well in this case. What are the limitations of this technique, compared with other imaging modalities discussed in the text? Compare PET with SPECT, explaining the differences between the two techniques.

Q6.4.   Explain why coincident timing windows help PET scanners detect only gamma ray pairs emitted by a positron annihilation event. Discuss why, conversely, introducing a delay time between the detection of the two gamma rays ensures that the pair could not have been produced by a positron annihilation.

PROBLEMS

P6.1. A worker is preparing a radiopharmaceutical containing a radio-active isotope of iodine to be used in a procedure requiring a source activity of 2.0 MBq. If the procedure will be performed approximately 2 days in the future, what source activity should initially be prepared if the isotope is: (a) iodine-123, with a half-life of 13 hours? (b) iodine-131, with a half-life of 8.05 days?

P6.2. Cobalt-60 has been used as a gamma ray source in radiation therapy procedures. Its half-life is 5.3 years. (a) Roughly, what fraction of the original source activity is left after 11 years? (b) Would you need to correct for radioactive decay over the course of a treatment lasting days or a few weeks? (Assume you wish to know the source activity to within a few percent.)

P6.3. You have been administered 100 MBq of technetium-99m for a radioisotope scan. About how long must you wait until your source activity falls to 25 MBq?

P6.4. If the physical half-life of sulfur-35 is 87.1 days, and the biologic half-life in the testicle is 632 days, what is its effective half-life in this organ?

P6.5. The effective half-life of plutonium-238 is 62 years, and its physical half-life is 90 years. (a) What is the biologic half-life of plutonium? (b) If the physical half-life of plutonium-239 is 24,000 years, what is its effective half-life? (c) In a early radiation experiment conducted by the U.S. Government, a man was administered a dose of both isotopes of plutonium. The man lived for an additional 21 years after receiving the plutonium. By how much did the source activity in his body from each isotope diminish in this time?

P6.6. A person participating in a study of male/female differences in brain function receives a dose of 185 MBq of a radiopharmaceutical before undergoing a PET scan. After 3 hours, a source activity of only 59.3 MBq remains. Assuming that the biologic half-life is much longer than the physical half-life, which of the radioisotopes in Table 6.4 was administered?

P6.7. Figures 6.4 and 6.5 show a gamma camera collimator that has parallel holes. For this collimator design, the image formed is the same size as the actual distribution of radionuclides. Design collimators that instead (a) magnify or (b) minify (make smaller) the images. For both cases explain what the advantages and dis-advantages of these designs would be.

P6.8. To understand the effect of attenuation on the measured gamma camera signal for 140 keV photons, compute the amount by which the actual count rate is attenuated for gamma photons that must travel through: (a) 1 cm and (b) 10 cm of soft tissue. (Use information from Chapter 5 regarding the attenuation of x-ray photons in water.)

P6.9. Time-of-flight PET scanners work by detecting the difference in times required for two coincidentally detected gamma rays to travel to two detectors. The location of the positron that generated these gamma rays is then reconstructed using a calculation similar to that used in echo ranging in ultrasound imaging. (a) Explain how this information is used to compute distances. (Recall that gamma rays travel at the speed of light.) (b) The spatial resolution of such a device is limited by the smallest difference in time its detector electronics can distinguish. If such an instrument has a resolution of 3 cm, how well can it distinguish coincident times? If a PET scanner can distinguish times as small as 300 picoseconds (10^{-12} s), how well can it detect position?

USEFUL SOURCES OF PROBLEMS

Joseph John Bevelacqua, *Contemporary Health Physics*. John Wiley & Sons, New York, 1995.

Joseph John Bevelacqua, *Basic Health Physics*. John Wiley & Sons, New York, 1999.

Herman Cember, *Introduction to Health Physics*. McGraw-Hill, New York, 1992.

Russell K. Hobbie, *Intermediate Physics for Medicine and Biology*. Springer AIP Press, New York, 1997.

7 Radiation therapy and radiation safety in medicine

7.1 INTRODUCTION

The National Cancer Institute estimates that half of all U.S. cancer patients now are treated with ionizing radiation in **radiation therapy** (or **radiotherapy**), while enormous numbers of lifesaving medical exams (see Chapters 5 and 6) make routine use of small doses of radiation. In spite of this, a widespread perception exists that any amount of radiation represents a serious hazard. The truth is complicated: ionizing radiation can be used to diagnose and treat cancer and other illnesses, and yet itself can be a **carcinogen** (cancer-causing agent), or cause an illness called radiation sickness. In this chapter, we review the risks and benefits involved in using ionizing radiation in medicine. We will see that the radiation doses used in medical imaging have been lowered over time, until the benefits of proper medical care usually outweigh the risk. In fact, the compromise between risk and benefit in modern medical imaging is more favorable than that presented by many common drugs, few of which are absolutely complication free and some of which cause lethal reactions in an extremely small number of cases.

It helps to begin by clarifying what the term *radiation* means in this context. Visible, infrared and ultraviolet light, microwaves, radio waves, x-rays, and gamma rays are all different types of electromagnetic radiation (Chapter 3). All transport energy in packets called photons, and this energy can be deposited in human tissue under the right circumstances. Some of these forms of electromagnetic radiation have photons with energies too small to permit them to disrupt chemical bonds. This category includes radiowaves, microwaves, infrared radiation, visible light, and the radiation emitted by electrical appliances and power lines. These, instead, can damage human tissue primarily by heating, although only at extremely high-power densities. The discussion of laser surgery in Chapter 3 hinges on this phenomenon. Microwave ovens also operate on this principle: they heat water molecules within food, and the spread of heat to the rest of the dish cooks the meal. Conversely, higher energy photons have enough energy to actually break chemical bonds. This allows ultra-violet radiation, x-rays, and gamma rays to create chemical damage within the body.[*] In Chapter 6 we explained how this distinction is used to establish a category called ionizing radiation, which encompasses energetic particles of matter (alpha rays, neutrons, electrons, and protons), as well as gamma rays and x-rays. Ionizing radiation is produced by medical x-ray generators, CT scanners, radioactive materials (including radionuclides for nuclear medicine imaging), nuclear reactors, nuclear waste, and fallout from nuclear weapons, but *not* by diagnostic ultrasound, MRI scanners, microwave ovens, visible lasers, or electrical appliances.

To understand the risks and benefits of ionizing radiation, we must first ask how ionizing radiation and its effects are measured, and what the typical radiation doses are for common medical procedures. Next, we review the effects of radiation on biological systems, and relate dose levels to radiation sickness, cancer, and genetic risk. After reviewing our present understanding of the genesis of cancer from aberrations in normal cell development, we will see how radiation can contribute to causing cancer and cell death. With this background in place, we can understand how safe levels for radiation exposure in imaging are established, and how radiation can be utilized for cancer therapy.

7.2 MEASURING RADIOACTIVITY AND RADIATION

An obvious starting place for describing the effects of radiation exposures is to draw analogies with drug doses and drug-toxicity levels. Describing drug doses is easy: one merely gives the amount—the volume or mass—administered. Ordinarily, the toxicity of a drug is described using the **LD** (for **lethal dose**) **50/30**: the amount of the drug required to kill 50% (one-half) of the population receiving it within 30 days. This grim measure uses the figure of 50% because normal variation between individuals results in a spread of the lethal doses. Thirty days is an arbitrary number, chosen to take into account longer-term effects of the drug.

Unfortunately, the radiation equivalent of a drug dose is more complicated than just describing, for example, the amount of radioactive material administered for a gamma camera scan or radiation therapy. The real quantity of interest must describe how much radiation the body is subjected to, how much of it is absorbed by the body, and what physiological effects result. In addition, the ordinary measures of a drug's toxicity do not suffice for describing radiation's effects. Extremely high exposures can quickly cause death, but many of the risks of radiation (such as an increased risk of cancer) do not manifest themselves for years. Because of these complexities,

---

[*] We will not discuss ultraviolet radiation in this chapter because it is not utilized widely in medicine. Also, because ultraviolet radiation is absorbed by the outermost layers of the skin, it plays a role in inducing skin cancer, but not other types of cancer.

it is helpful to define several quantities, each of which is useful in quantifying radiation exposures in medical applications.

As described in Chapter 6, a source's level of radioactivity is described by giving the source activity: how many nuclear decays occur every second. Source activities for characteristic amounts of radioisotopes used in imaging applications range from a fraction of a MBq to hundreds of MBq. By contrast, many *thousands* of MBq can be administered every session during radiation therapy for cancer. Once it has been created, a radioactive source of any sort begins to lose its source activity according to the half-life rule (Chapter 6). For determining the actual physiological effect of a source, the effective half-life must be used since it takes into account both the isotope's half-life and its persistence in the body.

However, just knowing the source activity does not specify the radiation's physiological effect. How do we compare the radiation absorbed during a diagnostic x-ray, a PET scan, and a radiation therapy treatment? To do so requires determining the energy of the particles of radiation used and the likelihood of each particle depositing its energy in an absorbing tissue. Along with the source activity, this information determines a *power*: the source activity describes how many radioactive decays happen each second, and each radioactive decay produces a particle with energy. A certain amount of energy passes from the radiation source to the absorbing tissue every second, but only a fraction of this power actually gets absorbed within the body. The quantity of radiation absorbed also must depend on the exposure time. We will now discuss the quantities used to quantify the total energy absorbed by body tissue.

One measure commonly used in radiology and medical physics is the **exposure**, defined as the amount of ionization produced in air by x-rays and gamma rays. Exposures are measured in units of roentgens (**R**). A roentgen is given by the amount of charge created in one kilogram of air; 1 roentgen is equal to 2.58×10^{24} coulomb/kg. The exposure is used, for example, to determine the correct conditions for producing a diagnostic radiograph. However, by itself it is only a measure of the amount of radiation that reaches the body, not the amount actually absorbed by body tissue. Another limitation is that the exposure is not defined for ionizing radiation other than high-energy photons.

A different unit, the **absorbed dose** (or **dose**), is used to measure the radiation energy absorbed during radiation therapy and imaging procedures. It also gives a useful means for evaluating radiation safety levels. The absorbed dose characterizes how much energy was deposited into each kilogram of tissue exposed to ionizing radiation of any kind. (Note that the absorbed dose does *not* distinguish between different types of radiation.) The reason the mass of tissue is taken into account is that the absorbed dose measures how concentrated a dose was received: if a given number of gamma rays, for example, were concentrated into a tumor, then the dose is higher than if the same amount were spread throughout the entire body. There are two units for measuring absorbed dose, the **gray** and the **rad**.

The gray (**Gy**) is equal to one joule of radiation energy per kilogram of body mass (1 J/kg). (All doses mentioned in this chapter are given in Gy. To express the same dose in rads, multiply the dose in Gy by 100.) As an approximate rule of thumb, a 1-roentgen exposure to x-rays or gamma rays results in a dose of about 0.01 Gy (1 rad) to soft tissue.

The absorbed dose really does give an idea of how much damage the body might incur. Doses of roughly 1 to 10 Gy to the whole body or vital organs can cause radiation sickness. Many doses of several Gy are typically delivered to tumors during radiation therapy for cancer, while the absorbed doses for frequently performed x-ray examinations are typically several mGy (milli Gray—thousandths of a gray) or lower, and dental x-rays deliver even smaller doses. For example, a diagnostic chest x-ray delivers a dose of about 0.01 to 0.15 mGy, while each view of the breast in a mammogram corresponds to a dose of about 1 mGy. Because CT requires a series of x-ray exposures at varying angles to make up a complete scan, doses are higher, in the range of 10 mGy or more. Radioisotope imaging delivers doses to the entire body in the range of several mGy or less, with somewhat higher doses resulting in the organ where the radioisotope concentrates. Fluoroscopy results in doses as high as 0.05 Gy per minute of exposure, so it is used more sparingly than other imaging technologies.

The absorbed dose does give some information on the effects of different types of radiation. For example, iodine is concentrated in the thyroid gland, so the radioisotopes iodine-131 or iodine-123 can be used to image or to treat this organ. The biochemical properties of compounds containing these radioisotopes are the same, but iodine-123 produces only gamma rays while iodine-131 emits both electrons and gamma rays. If similar source activities of the two radioisotopes are administered, the thyroid dose for iodine-131 that results is much higher than that for iodine-123. This is in part because beta particles (electrons) are strongly absorbed in a very short range compared to the gamma rays, hence they account for over 90% of the total dose for iodine-123. However, even though some information about biological effects is contained in the dose, the question still remains: how do we compare the damage due to the same dose from different particles?

A quantity called the **linear energy transfer** (**LET**) describes how much energy is deposited on average every unit of distance along a particle's path. The particle's range is related to its LET, since a short range means the particle rapidly disperses its energy (that is, has a high LET). The LET varies greatly between high LET neutrons and alpha particles, and low LET x-rays, gamma rays, and electrons. For reasons we will discuss later in the chapter, the same dose of particles with different LETs results in different amounts of biological damage; for example, a given dose of alpha rays is more likely to result in long-term damage than the same dose of x-rays. However, because the high LET alpha particles have ranges much shorter than low LET, they can only exhibit their greater potential for damage in a thin layer of tissue nearest the source.

One attempt to measure and define the effects of various forms of radiation on living tissue involves a quantity called the **relative biological effect** (**RBE**). The RBE of a particle is the ratio of the dose of a standard particle required to cause the same amount of biological damage as a dose of the radiation under consideration. The standard particle is chosen to be 200 keV photons typical of those used in radioisotope imaging. (Adding to the already daunting terminology of this field, similar quantities called the **quality factor** (or **radiation weighting factor**) are often used instead of the RBE.) Effects due to exposure to any other form of ionizing radiation are then quoted in terms of how damaging they are compared to these standard x-ray photons. For RBE = 2, the radiation is twice as damaging, for RBE = 0.5, it is half as damaging. X-rays, gamma rays, and beta particles (electrons and positrons) are all defined as having RBEs of 1.0; alpha particles have an RBE of about 20; and neutrons have values ranging from 5 to 20, depending upon energy. Thus information about LET is included in the definition of RBE. The **dose equivalent** takes into account the biological effect of an absorbed dose by multiplying the absorbed dose by the RBE for the particles encountered. Its units are the **rem** or the **sievert** (**Sv**). The dose equivalent in Sv is equal to the dose in Gy multiplied by the radiation's RBE.

$$\text{Dose equivalent (Sv)} = \text{dose (Gy)} \times \text{RBE} \qquad (7.1)$$

(All dose equivalents mentioned in this chapter are given in Sv. To express the dose equivalent in rem, multiply the value in Sv by 100.) Most medical applications use beta particles, x-rays, or gamma rays with RBE of 1.0, so the doses in Gy are interchangeable with the same values in Sv. On the other hand, the radioactive gas, radon, and its decay products emit alpha particles. This means that a dose of 1 Gy due to radon exposure equals a dose equivalent of: RBE × 1 Gy = 20 × 1 Gy=20 Sv.

Although the sievert is widely used, it is almost certainly not the case that one can compare the biological effects of different forms of radiation in so simplistic a way. For example, the relative effects of a dose due to two different particles actually depends upon the actual magnitude of the dose received; the relative effects are almost certainly very different for small doses and large ones. It's also often not the case that the same dose delivered to different organs has the same biological effect. Two quantities that try to account for these variations are the **organ dose** (the dose equivalent for a specific organ) and the **effective dose** (which sums together the dose equivalents for various organs, multiplied by a **tissue weighting factor**, an estimate of relative radiation risk).

The absorbed dose cannot be measured directly, but it can be inferred from other measurable quantities. **Radiation dosimetry** involves methods developed to assess and control the doses delivered during therapeutic and diagnostic imaging procedures. For beam sources of radiation used in radiography and therapy, the exposure in roentgens can be measured directly, using an ionization detector. This then can be converted into an absorbed dose, using appropriate correction factors to go between the measured quantity (ionization of air) to the desired one (the absorbed dose). For imaging or therapy performed with radio-nuclides, the absorbed dose from a procedure (the **dose commitment**) must be computed from the administered source activity, half-life, and exposure time.

For determining the absorbed dose, it is necessary to know the net number of radioactive decays over time, a quantity called the **cumulative activity** $\tilde{A}$. The source activity gives the number of radioactive decays per second, so for times very short compared to the half-life, it is possible to compute this by multiplying the source activity administered, A_0, by the exposure time, T. (Note that throughout this discussion, one must make use of the correct half-life for each particular application. For example, if the goal is to measure the number of decays from a sample of radioactive material in the laboratory, one would use $T_{1/2}$; however, if the source is in the human body and the goal is to compute quantities relating to radiation exposure, then T_E is the correct choice (Chapter 6).)

$$\tilde{A}=1.443\ A_0 \times T \qquad \text{in units of Bq-s for } T \ll T_{1/2} \qquad (7.2)$$

The cumulative activity has units of Bq-s, so the units of time cancel out, since this quantity measures a total *number* of decays: Bq-s = (decays/s) × s. However, in general, the source activity decreases significantly with time, so it is necessary to compute the cumulative activity using exponential decay. This results in a calculation of the area under the curve in Figure 6.3, beginning at the time the radionuclide was introduced into the organ and ending when the exposure ended. For times long compared to the half-life, we can use as an approximation the following relation in computing the dose commitment, D, which holds for exposures starting at t=0 and ending for times much greater than the half-life:

$$\tilde{A}=1.443\ A_0 \times T_{1/2} \qquad \text{in units of Bq-s for } T \gg T_{1/2} \qquad (7.3)$$

For example, this approximation is good to 3% for 5 half-lives or longer.

It is necessary to know other information for computing the dose commitment, including the mass, m, of the organ of interest. If the radioactive decay produces more than one particle, or if additional radiation results from absorption and re-emission processes, then we need to know the *average* energy per decay, E, in joules. This can be found in many published tables for various radionuclides of medical interest. Not every particle emitted is absorbed by the body, so it is also necessary to compute the **absorbed fraction**, Φ, of the emitted radiation. Since the source of radiation can generally be a different organ from the target organ for which the dose is computed, we have:

$$\Phi = \frac{\left(\text{radiation absorbed by target organ}\right)}{\left(\text{radiation emitted by source organ}\right)} \qquad (7.4)$$

Finally, these quantities are combined into an equation for the dose commitment, D:

$$D = \tilde{A} \, E \, \Phi/m \tag{7.5}$$

For some simple cases, Φ can be computed exactly. For example, electrons and other charged particles are totally absorbed within a short range of their emission, so $\Phi = 100\%$ in those instances. However, to compute Φ for photons, which are absorbed in a probabilistic fashion, a more complicated calculation must be performed. It is usually necessary to use a computer to model the distribution of the radionuclide throughout the body and the photon absorption properties of different tissues. Computer programs have been developed for dosimetry calculations that incorporate realistic models of the human body. These use probabilistic methods to compute Φ. (That is, a computer is used to compute a likely distribution of radionuclides throughout the body. The computation then follows the history of a computer-generated photon emitted during a radioactive decay. At each position in the body, the computer calculates the probability of absorption of a photon of given energy, then generates a random number to use along with the computed odds to decide whether the photon is absorbed there.) Values of Φ generated in this fashion have been compiled, and consequently can be used to compute absorbed doses accurately.

Sample calculation: One study of the effects of radiation follows patients receiving iodine-131 for diagnostic reasons.[*] The average administered source activity was 1.9 MBq, and the average uptake was 40%. Estimate the average thyroid dose for the typical radioisotope imaging procedure in this study, using a typical thyroid mass of 0.020 kg.

First, we need additional information about the radioactive decay pathways that iodine-131 undergoes. This radionuclide produces both beta and gamma particles, and the average energy per beta decay is $E_\beta = 0.192$ MeV, while the energy of the principal gamma photon emitted is $E_\gamma = 0.364$ MeV; the respective values of the absorbed fraction for the two particles are $\Phi_\beta = 1$ and $\Phi_\gamma = 0.026$.[†] We will assume that the radioisotope is uniformly distributed throughout the thyroid, so the entire organ gets a uniform dose. The effective half-life for iodine must be computed from the physical half-life, 8.05 days, and the biological half-life of 74 days in the thyroid. We will break the calculation into several steps:

(continued on next page)

---

[*] Per Hall and Lars-Erik Holm, "Late consequences of radioiodine for diagnosis and therapy in Sweden," *Thyroid*, Vol. 7(2) (1997), pp. 205–208.

[†] J.R. Williams and D.I. Thwaites. *Radiotherapy Physics in Practice*. Oxford University Press, Oxford, U.K., 1993; Table 11.2, p. 255.

1. How much energy (in joules) is emitted per decay? This requires us to convert from units of eV to joules:

$$E_\beta = 0.192 \times 10^6 \text{ eV} \times 1.60 \times 10^{-19} \text{ J/eV} = 3.07 \times 10^{-14} \text{ J} \quad (7.6a)$$

$$E_\gamma = 0.364 \times 10^6 \text{ eV} \times 1.60 \times 10^{-19} \text{ J/eV} = 5.82 \times 10^{-14} \text{ J} \quad (7.6b)$$

2. What is the effective half-life? From Equation 6.6(b) we have:

$$T_E = \frac{T_B \times T_{1/2}}{T_B + T_{1/2}} = \frac{74\,\text{days} \times 8.05\,\text{days}}{74\,\text{days} + 8.05\,\text{days}} = 7.3 \text{ days} \quad (7.7)$$

3. What is the cumulative activity? First we need to compute the starting source activity, taking into account the fact that only 40% of the radioactive iodine is taken into the thyroid:

$$A_0 = 1.9 \times 10^6 \text{ Bq} \times 40\% \quad (7.8)$$

It is appropriate to use Equation 7.3, using the appropriate effective half-life, if we assume the dose is delivered over a time long compared to the effective half-life:

$$\tilde{A} = 1.443 A_0 \, T_{1/2} \text{ Bq} - \text{s}$$

$$= 1.443 \times \left(1.9 \times 10^6 \text{Bq} \times 40\%\right) \times 7.3\,\text{days} \times \left(24 \text{ hr/day}\right)$$

$$\times \left(60 \text{ min/hr}\right) \times \left(60 \text{ s/min}\right) \quad (7.9)$$

$$= 6.9 \times 10^{11} \text{Bq} - \text{s}$$

$$= 6.9 \times 10^{11} \text{decays}$$

4. We can now compute the thyroid dose commitment using Equation 7.4, corrected for the fact that two species of decay products are emitted:

$$D = \tilde{A}\left(E_\beta \Phi_\beta + E_\gamma \Phi_\gamma\right)/m$$

$$= 6.9 \times 10^{11}$$

$$\times \left(\left(3.07 \times 10^{-14}\,\text{J} \times 1\right) + \left(5.82 \times 10^{-14}\,\text{J} \times 0.026\right)\right)/0.020\,\text{kg} \quad (7.10)$$

$$= 1.1 \text{ J/kg} = 1.1 \text{ Gy}$$

which agrees with the estimated average dose assumed in the reference.

Several methods exist for monitoring radiation exposures for safety purposes. **Dosimeters** are worn by workers who are exposed as part of their occupation; these can take the form of badges, rings, cards, or other convenient shapes. Modern dosimeters incorporate a material that interacts with ionizing radiation in such as way that the resulting energy transfer results in electrons being promoted into higher orbitals and trapped there (Chapter 3). Two versions of this idea, **optically stimulated luminescence** and **thermoluminescence**, measure the original ionizing radiation dose by releasing the stored energy as visible light when exposed to visible light or heat, respectively. Visible light detectors then can be used to determine the magnitude of the wearer's radiation dose. Traditional film badges contain x-ray film that changes its optical density when exposed to ionizing radiation. Typically, after the worker has worn the badge for a month, the film's optical density is read by a machine that then computes the total radiation dose. Obviously, these devices cannot alert a wearer of exposures immediately, but they can indicate long-term problems.

One way to place radiation doses in context is to consider the values one encounters in daily life. If you were to take a Geiger counter (a type of portable ionizing radiation detector) and measure radiation levels around your home and workplace, you might be surprised to learn that your environment exposes you to ionizing radiation every day. Table 7.1 lists the dose

Table 7.1 Annual ionizing radiation doses for U.S. population

Source	Average annual dose (mSv)
Natural	
Radon	2.0
Cosmic rays	0.27
Terrestrial (soil, rocks, etc.)	0.28
Internal (radioisotopes in the body)	0.39
Total natural (sum of four preceding items)	**3.0**
Artificial	
Medical x-ray diagnosis	0.39
Nuclear medicine	0.14
Consumer products	0.10
Occupational	<0.01
Nuclear fuel cycle	<0.01
Fallout	<0.01
Misc. (government labs, transportation, etc.)	<0.01
Total artificial (sum of seven preceding categories)	**0.63**
Total natural and artificial	**3.6**

Source: National Council on Radiation Protection and Measurements [NCRP], *Ionizing Radiation Exposures of the Population of the United States*, Report No. 93, Washington, D.C., 1987.

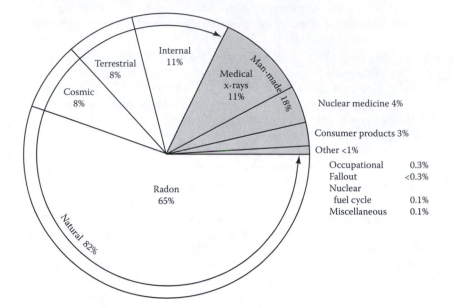

Figure 7.1 Annual ionizing radiation dose to average member of the U.S. population: breakdown by source. Data from National Council on Radiation
Protection and Measurements (NCRP), *Ionizing Radiation Exposures
of the Population of the United States*, Report No. 93, Washington,
D.C., 1987.

equivalent received by the average U.S. citizen each year, while Figure 7.1
displays this same information graphically. The average radiation dose per
person in the U.S. from all sources, averaged over the entire population, is
roughly 3.6 mSv per year. Of that total dose, 82% is due to natural sources,
and over half of that is due to radon gas (55%), a radioactive gas present
in many homes (Figure 7.1). The remaining 18% due to human-produced
sources primarily results from medical x-rays (11%), nuclear medicine
uses (4%), and consumer products containing small amounts of radioactive materials (3%). Only 1% of the total annual dose per capita is due to
occupational exposures, fallout, and nuclear power plants. It is notable that
the typical additional dose from a standard medical imaging procedure is
actually small compared to the environmental radiation levels we are all
exposed to every year.

7.3 ORIGINS OF THE BIOLOGICAL EFFECTS
OF IONIZING RADIATION

To understand the role of radiation in therapy, we need to first understand the microscopic mechanisms by which radiation damage can bring
about genetic changes and cell death. Each cell of the body has a central

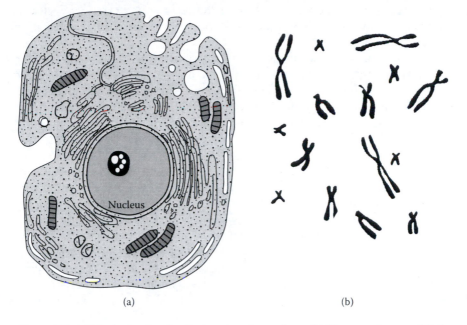

(a)   (b)

Figure 7.2 (a) Typical animal cell, showing the nucleus. (b) The genetic materials in humans is contained in structures called chromosomes located within the nucleus.

compartment called the **nucleus** in which the gene-carrying **chromosomes** are stored (Figure 7.2a). These chromosomes are structures that carry instructions for producing proteins (Figure 7.2b). Parents pass on their genetic information to their offspring through the transmission of chromosomes in **germ cells** (eggs or sperm). Humans have two copies each of 23 types of chromosomes in the **somatic** (nongerm) cells of the body, for a total of 46. Until recently, it was believed that only ionizing radiation that passes directly through a cell's nucleus causes lasting damage. For example, for certain cells it is possible to remove the nucleus temporarily, then deliver an otherwise lethal dose of radiation to the remaining cell material, or **cytoplasm**. When the nucleus is replaced, the cell can function and reproduce normally. In another line of experiments, chemicals that specifically enhance the damage received by the cell's genetic material increased the overall damage to the cell in proportion to the amount of the chemical present. This indicates that the only lasting damage to the cell occurred as a result of events relating to the genetic material contained only in the cell's nucleus and nowhere else. Since the nucleus takes up only a small fraction of the cell body, it is unlikely to be struck by particles of ionizing radiation. This partly explains the resistance of living organisms to radiation damage: only in the unlikely event of a direct hit to the nucleus can a long-term problem emerge. It should be noted, however, that a variety of experimental studies on cells show that damage targeted to selected cells can induce radiation effects in neighboring cells; this "bystander" effect is not yet well understood, and its implications for radiation risk estimation in humans are unclear.

The mechanism by which genetic damage is induced involves damage to the chromosomes' **DNA** (deoxyribonucleic acid) molecules, which contain the actual hereditary information. DNA is an example of a **polymer,** a molecule composed of many similar repeating units linked together like beads on a string. In this case, the units are called **nucleic acids.** They are distinguished by four chemical groups called **bases: adenine (A), guanine (G), cytosine (C),** and **thymine (T).** The bases are attached to a backbone structure to make up a strand. Two such polymer strands make up the complete DNA molecule, each winding about the other in a double helical structure resembling a spiral staircase (Figure 7.3a).

In this double helix, the two bases meet and associate in the middle of the staircase to stabilize the molecule. Only certain pairs of bases can associate in this fashion: adenine must pair with thymine (A with T), and guanine must pair with cytosine (G with C). This means that by describing one strand of the DNA molecule, you have also defined the other strand as well. In fact, the body can use one strand of DNA to make a new copy by matching a **complementary** set of new bases with the existing strand as a template (Figure 7.3b).

The complete collection of information stored in an organism's DNA is called its **genome;** in humans, this comprises roughly six billion base pairs. The sequence of base pairs in DNA specifies the construction of the body's proteins. Proteins are another variety of polymer, which form the basis of the body's functional and structural organization; proteins are chains of chemical groups called **amino acids. Triplets** (sets of three bases in a row) code for one of the twenty amino acids that are the building blocks of proteins; for example, the three nucleic acids, AAA, code for the amino acid lysine, while TAC codes for the amino acid tyrosine. Thus, the **sequence** of base pairs along a strand of DNA is a blueprint for constructing proteins (Figure 7.4a). A stretch of DNA sufficient to describe the construction of a protein is called a **gene.**

Mutations are changes to the base pair sequence of a DNA molecule, and hence the protein it encodes. Mutations can result, for example, from insertions of extra base pairs, a substitution of a different pair for an existing pair, chemical changes to the bases, deletions of existing bases, or rearrangements within the original DNA (Figure 7.4b). Most mutations are lethal, and inhibit protein production altogether. Others allow the cell to make an impaired version of a necessary protein. For example, the disease sickle cell anemia results when a single altered base pair results in a modified version of the important blood protein, hemoglobin. Similarly, cystic fibrosis is caused by mutations within a particular gene. Mutations that cause gross changes in the chromosomes can also cause genetic disease; for example, Down's syndrome results from an additional copy of a particular chromosome.

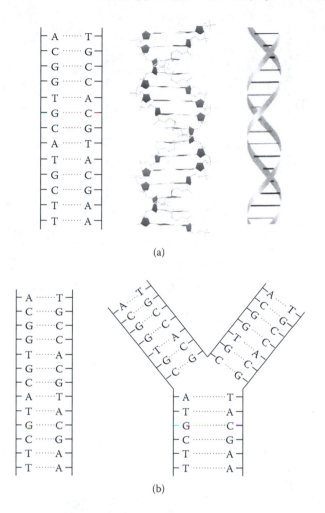

Figure 7.3 (a) The double helical structure of a DNA molecule, shown schematically (left) and in representations (center and right) which make apparent the chemical structure and double-helical nature of the molecule.
(b) A starting strand of DNA (left) can be replicated by matching complementary base pairs to make two strands of DNA (right).

Chemicals and viruses can enhance the rate of mutations by chemically
altering DNA molecules; substances with this property are called **muta-
gens**, and are said to be **mutagenic**. These include many potent carcinogens,
such as benzene and nicotine. Radiation can cause mutations, and we will
now see how and why this effect occurs.

When ionizing radiation enters the body, there is a probability that it
may be transmitted without transferring any of its energy. However, those
particles that do interact can cause the ionization of atoms along the path.
Some ionized atoms harmlessly recombine with their electrons, but the

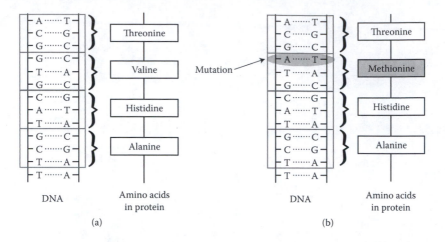

Figure 7.4 (a) DNA molecules encode the information necessary for the production of proteins as triplets of base pairs, which correspond to the code for specific amino acids. (b) Mutations change the information in a gene and thus, the protein it codes for. The sequence of bases shown in (a) has been altered (arrow) so that A has been substituted for G in the genetic code, leading to a change in the amino acid coded for. While GTG codes for the amino acid valine, ATG codes for a different amino acid, methionine. Such a change can radically alter the biochemical properties of the proteins produced using the mutated DNA.

ionization also has the potential to break a chemical bond. The freed electron produced in this fashion can go on to ionize further atoms, potentially wreaking further chemical damage. Those ionizations that do result in immediate chemical harm to important body chemicals are referred to as the **direct effect**. Ionizing radiation primarily directly affects water, because water makes up a larger fraction of the cell's volume than do proteins or DNA. When water is ionized, it can form many reactive chemical species, called **free radicals**. These species last only a very short time, during which they can break chemical bonds in other nearby molecules. This secondary ionization of other molecules by reactive water is called the **indirect effect**, and it is hypothesized to be the dominant mechanism by which ionizing radiation harms cells. In this case, the body can fight back by using special chemicals that quickly deactivate the free radicals formed.

Since only those direct or indirect interactions that affect DNA are important, most ionizing radiation is relatively innocuous. Cells appear perfectly able to function normally after sustaining damage to proteins, sugars, and fats, presumably because many copies of each of these molecules exist. Since only about 1% of the ionizations due to a 1-Gy dose happen in the genetic material, most radiation has no lasting effect. However, even when DNA is hit, almost all of this damage is quickly repaired. Genetic damage frequently occurs spontaneously from errors in cell metabolism, and to a much lesser extent from dangerous chemicals, ultraviolet light, and natural

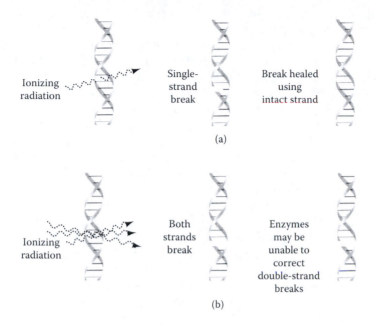

Figure 7.5 Two types of damage to DNA molecules. (a) When ionizing radiation produced a break in only one strand of DNA, the complementarity of base-pairing can be used to heal the broken strand using proteins called repair enzymes. (b) If both strands of DNA are broken, base-pairing cannot be employed to heal the break. As a result, either the break may not be repaired or attempts at repair may result in incorrect DNA sequences.

background radiation. Consequently, highly efficient natural mechanisms have evolved for repairing damaged DNA, using special-purpose proteins called **repair enzymes.**

Ionizing radiation can cause roughly four basic injuries to DNA: **single-** or **double-strand breaks** in DNA, damage to the bases without breakage of the backbone, and cross-links formed between the DNA and itself or another molecule. The last two defects can be healed by DNA repair enzymes, so it is not clear if they cause lasting genetic damage. A single-strand break involves the cleavage of a bond along the backbone of one strand of the double helix (Figure 7.5a). Since the other strand is left intact, it is possible to reconstruct the original sequence perfectly, using repair enzymes that match the unharmed strand base for base. The repair time proceeds rapidly, with a half-life of several minutes, so single-strand breaks are relatively innocuous. Double-strand breaks occur when chemical bonds are cleaved along both backbones, so that the entire DNA molecule has been split in two (Figure 7.5b). This destroys the pairing needed to complete the destroyed sequence of bases. Even if repair enzymes heal the break, the strands may be improperly joined, or the joined ends may suffer lasting damage. Should this occur, additional layers of the body's DNA surveillance system exist to find such errors and either prevent the cell from dividing or trigger cell death.

Double-strand breaks are less likely than single ones, since two separate chemical events are needed to cause them. This helps explain why high LET radiation is more damaging than low LET radiation, since high LET particles such as alpha particles can cause an entire series of closely clustered ionizations that could result in a trail of damage. The incidence of double-strand breaks is thought to be low (around 40 per genome per gray). However, because of the difficulty of properly repairing double-strand breaks, they have been proposed to be the main cause of damage to living organisms by ionizing radiation. In addition, ionizing radiation is capable of producing entire closely spaced clusters of DNA damage, a feature that may play a role in its carcinogenic properties. However, the actual mechanisms by which damage to DNA is converted into mutations and then long-term genetic damage are only now being fully explored. One of the "colon cancer genes" referred to in Chapter 2 actually corresponds to mutations causing the disruption of a repair enzyme that can repair single-strand breaks. Because the repair enzyme is not working properly, other mutations persist rather than being repaired, predisposing persons carrying the gene to enhanced cancer risk. A rare disease called *xeroderma pigmentosum*, associated with high rates of skin cancer, occurs when other DNA repair enzymes are defective. Results such as these suggest that the genetic risks due to radiation may be concentrated largely in individuals with such genetic defects.

When the cell attempts to repair broken chromosomes by reattaching broken ends, abnormal structures can result. Using light microscopy, one can observe these abnormalities in the white blood cells of patients undergoing radiation therapy and workers exposed to high levels of radiation in occupational settings; about 1 in 10 cells are observed to have such aberrations for every Sv. From experiments performed on mice, the acute radiation dose required to cause a doubling of the natural rate of mutations is estimated to be 1 Sv; chronic doses are roughly one-third or less effective in causing visible mutations. These experiments are used to estimate the increase in genetic defects due to radiation exposure in humans, since there are no data for human populations. However, the relevance of such animal studies to human beings is not clear, because different species have different responses to radiation due in part to differences in DNA repair mechanisms. Also, until recently, only chromosomal defects and large-scale genetic changes could be detected, but modern DNA biotechnology promises to elucidate the effect of radiation at the level of individual genetic mutations.

How is such genetic damage related to the causes of cancer? In a healthy body, an extraordinary variety of different types of cells live in equilibrium, each present in the necessary numbers to promote the body's activities. In cancer, the unchecked division of one cell type leads to tumor formation. Cells also can lose the natural programming that causes them to die on schedule. Worse still, if they become malignant and **metastasize**, tumor cells can enter the bloodstream and invade distant parts of the body with new secondary tumors. This proliferation of secondary tumors is what makes cancer particularly deadly and hard to treat.

Cell growth and division, as well as programmed cell death, are all regulated by an elaborate system of checks and balances only now being unraveled by science. Some of the players in this system serve to promote the reproduction of cells. For example, genes called **oncogenes** (or **tumor promoters**) code for proteins that promote the reproduction of cells. Conversely, ordinarily cell proliferation is usually held in check by the opposing action of **tumor suppressors**, which limit cell division. Both tumor promoter and tumor suppressor genes are beneficial when present in the normal balance: the tumor promoters are often compared to the accelerator pedal of a car, and the tumor suppressors to the brakes. However, defects in either gene can predispose the cell to uncontrolled division: a car with a stuck accelerator or brake failure is equally out of control. A mutation can inactivate or prevent the production of tumor suppressors in any of a number of ways, while causing a tumor promoter to promote unchecked cell division requires a more specific alteration. Consequently, most of the genetic defects associated with cancer discovered thus far involve tumor suppressor genes.

If ionizing radiation causes a tumor suppressor gene to mutate, this does not necessarily lead to cancer. In general, the body's defenses are adequate to protect against individual failures in the system. For instance, scientists have proposed that in colorectal cancer, over three tumor suppressor genes must fail, and more than one oncogene must go wrong. However, there are many additional sources of mutations that can contribute to inducing cancer. Mutated genes can be inherited, caused by viral infections, or result from exposure to carcinogenic chemicals. Thus, while ionizing radiation alone may not cause cancer, exposures can occur in concert with other insults to the body, and the combination may then result in the disease. The existence of repair mechanisms for genetic damage and the requirement for other contributing factors in the multistep process of cancer induction help explain the relatively low incidence of harmful effects from radiation.

7.4 THE TWO REGIMES OF RADIATION DAMAGE: RADIATION SICKNESS AND CANCER RISK

Understanding how ionizing radiation affects living organisms involves comprehending two very different regimes in which damage occurs. Extremely high **acute** (rapidly delivered) doses have a very different effect compared to **chronic** (slowly delivered) doses, both in the type and degree of damage. The consequence of high acute doses is a syndrome called **radiation sickness**, which sets in within hours or weeks of the initial exposure. By contrast, no special disease results from low chronic exposures; instead, the main consequence is a predisposition toward developing cancers of all types. Grasping this distinction is essential to understanding how radiation can both cause and treat cancer.

Extremely high acute doses to the entire body, or to certain vulnerable organs, can result in severe radiation sickness. Acute doses of many Gy can produce the symptoms characteristic of this syndrome, including nausea and vomiting, fatigue, and hair loss; the resulting high levels of radiation damage to the blood-producing tissues, gastrointestinal tract, and the central nervous system can prove deadly. As noted earlier, these doses are comparable to those delivered during radiation therapy, but are many orders of magnitude lower than those encountered during diagnostic medical procedures. The LD50/30 for gamma rays is roughly 4 Gy, so doses this high delivered to the entire body can result in the death of the exposed individual.

The response of body tissues to high, acute doses of radiation exhibits a **threshold** of damage: the damage is irreparable for doses greater than the threshold, but below the threshold dose, complete recovery is possible. This can be illustrated graphically with a dose-effect curve, such as that shown in Figure 7.6(a); the dose-effect curve plots how an effect (number of cells killed, incidence of cancer, etc.) depends upon the radiation dose administered. Single doses below 0.25 to 0.50 Gy usually do not generate the symptoms of radiation sickness, although some effects have been observed for doses as low as 0.14 Gy, well above the doses from any modern imaging procedure. The *rate* at which the dose of radiation was delivered is essential in producing this damage. A single high dose of several Gy results in radiation sickness, but not if the same dose is delivered gradually over the course of a lifetime. The mechanism by which most of the damage in the deterministic regime occurs is presumably due to mutations left uncorrected by repair enzymes. These may completely disrupt the ability of the cell to reproduce itself, or to produce the proteins it needs to function. This effect exhibits a threshold, because the cell populations within the tissues can reproduce to replace those killed or damaged by radiation during low chronic exposures, but not if too high a fraction are rapidly destroyed. In addition, cells have repair mechanisms for coping with radiation damage. High, acute doses may be able to overwhelm these defenses, while the same dose delivered slowly permits the cell to recover. This explains why lifetime accumulations of small doses from diagnostic x-rays, CT, and radioisotope imaging do not cause radiation sickness.

Our bodies contain both stable, nonreproducing cell populations like nerve cells as well as cells that must be replaced regularly. Examples of the latter include the lining of the gastrointestinal tract, blood cells, skin cells, and hair cells. The threshold for damage is lower for these cells than for stable types. Consequently, radiation sickness preferentially results in trauma to the fast-growing cell populations, which explains why side effects of radiation therapy for cancer can include nausea, damage to bone marrow, and hair loss.

There is a clear cause-and-effect relationship between high acute radiation doses and radiation sickness: the severity increases predictably as the dose increases. High doses of radiation are called **deterministic** to indicate this direct link between radiation dose and resulting illness (Figure 7.6a).

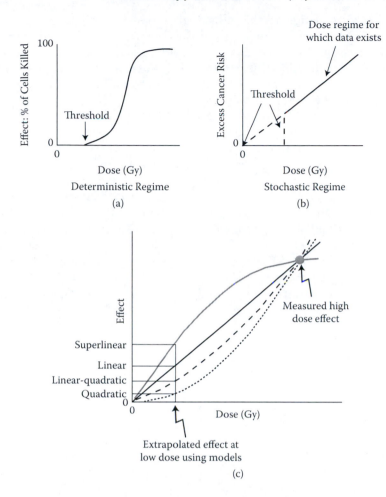

Figure 7.6 (a) Dose-effect curves for the deterministic regime, showing a clear threshold for damage. (b) Dose-effect curve for the stochastic regime for effects such as excess cancer risk from radiation. Data typically are not available for very low doses, so it is not possible to directly measure whether or not a threshold is present. (c) Different models for extrapolating measured high-dose effect data (circle) to lower doses. The measured data point is consistent with various models, including a straight line or linear model (solid black), linear-quadratic (dashed), quadratic (dotted), or superlinear (light gray). The extrapolated effect at low doses is greater for the linear model than it is for the linear-quadratic or quadratic models, but less than for the superlinear model. See discussion in text.

The deterministic regime can be compared to the predictable effects of a drug. For example, drunkenness reliably results from exposure to alcohol, and the degree of drunkenness varies predictably with the amount of alcohol consumed. However, with both radiation and alcohol, there is considerable variation in the individual response. Similarly, a threshold exists in ultrasound imaging for damage by heating and cell disruption, which is determined by the intensity of sound used and the exposure time. The FDA seeks to reduce the risk from exposure to zero by regulating the intensity and exposure times of diagnostic ultrasound imaging devices to lie well below these threshold values.

Alternatively, if a person receives a low, chronic exposure to radiation, no immediate disease results. Instead, that person accumulates an increased lifetime risk of eventually developing cancer. The effect of low doses of radiation is called **stochastic**, meaning probabilistic, or statistical. Cancer induction by radiation can be compared to a perverse kind of lottery in which many people draw lots for a penalty (getting cancer) rather than a prize; there is no way to predict if a particular individual will "win." Another analogy compares radiation with smoking, which increases one's risk of developing lung cancer—but most smokers do not develop lung cancer, and some nonsmokers (rarely) do. The likelihood of developing radiation-induced cancer increases with the total dose received, so the stochastic risks are present for high acute doses of radiation. However, it is an "all-or-nothing" effect—that is, the probability of developing cancer increases with dose, but not the severity of the disease. Lifetime exposure in the stochastic regime is cumulative: a person incurs the same cancer risk from the same total dose, whether it is broken into three parts or delivered all at once. The net cancer risk appears to vary in proportion to the dose (twice the dose gives twice the risk, etc.) (Figure 7.6b), with possible departures from this rule to be discussed shortly. Because these long-term risks of the stochastic regime are so much harder to gauge than the immediate damage due to high acute doses, it is much more difficult to establish the magnitude of the risk and to determine if a threshold exists for this regime as well.

Our present understanding gives a plausible interpretation of how low radiation doses can induce cancer. For low doses in the stochastic regime, so few mutations occur that cells are not likely to die. However, unrepaired mutations may reprogram these surviving cells to function somewhat incorrectly, or they may create genetic instabilities that result in further changes. In combination with other contributing factors, this may cause a cell to lose its ability to regulate its growth and development and become malignant. The uncertainty in the timing and degree of stochastic radiation damage comes about from many accumulated uncertainties: will the ionizing radiation interact with molecules in the body, will the ionization cause chemical damage, will that damage harm DNA, will the damage go unrepaired, will the resulting mutation contribute to carcinogenesis, and will the other predisposing factors necessary for tumor formation occur?

A massive body of evidence exists that shows that high acute radiation doses cause cancer. The chief resource used in estimating radiation risks is the study of 86,500 survivors of the atomic bombs dropped on Hiroshima and Nagasaki during World War II in 1945. Publicly available data from this study have been analyzed by various groups to estimate the effects of radiation on the incidence of cancer, birth defects, and other conditions. This grim data is especially valuable as the atomic bomb survivors were exposed to widely varying doses, making it possible to study how cancer risk increases with increasing dose. Scientists have sought to supplement these population studies by studying cells grown in culture and animals (usually mice) exposed to radiation, which are the chief source of information on genetic risks such as birth defects. Basic research into molecular genetics, cell biology, developmental biology, and the causes of cancer play an increasingly important role in elucidating the relation between radiation and carcinogenesis. Other studies have followed persons exposed during medical procedures, those occupationally exposed in mining, radiology, and the nuclear industry, persons living with high natural rates of radioactivity, and those exposed as a result of accidents.

For example, other studies follow the consequences of the severe nuclear accident at the Chernobyl nuclear power plant in the Ukraine in 1986. While about 30 people died from the accident itself and over a hundred were injured by radiation sickness, several million people were exposed to radioactive fallout. So far, increases in thyroid cancer in children have been confirmed for several countries most affected by the releases; this population was at risk because iodine-131 radionuclides in milk and food preferentially lodge in the thyroid. The evidence of increases in other cancers reveals no overall increase in cancer mortality or incidence in the affected regions; however, these results remain tentative, since the latent period for many cancers is long and these population studies are limited by the difficulty of distinguishing even a large estimated number of increased cancers from the even larger number that would occur naturally with no extra exposure.

Sample calculation: How valid is a population study? The issue of statistical significance. All cancers occur naturally in the population at large, and there is no test to determine whether or not a particular case was linked to radiation exposure. In general, all that can be determined is the amount by which the *observed* cancer mortality in an exposed group exceeds the *expected* cancer mortality for an unexposed control group. In addition, cancer induction occurs with a **latent period**, a pause of from several years to over a decade before any radiation damage actually leads to cancer. Thus, studies must follow populations for a very long time after the dose has been received to be meaningful. Population studies can also give misleading results if they are poorly designed. For example, the mere act of carefully screening a group for cancer may "increase" the apparent cancer rate through better detection, so both the control and study groups should be treated equivalently. Studies of radiation-induced cancer should account for

(continued on next page)

Table 7.2 Observed solid cancer cases from the Japanese atomic bomb survivor study

Dose category (Gy)	Cases	Background	Fitted excess
<0.005	9,597	9,537	3
0.005–0.1	4,406	4,374	81
0.1–0.2	968	910	75
0.2–0.5	1,144	963	179
0.5–1	688	493	206
1–2	460	248	196
2–4	185	71	111
Total	17,448	16,595	853

Source: Data reproduced from Preston, D.L., Ron E., Tokuoka S., Funamoto S., Nishi N., Soda M., Mabuchi K., Kodama K., "Solid cancer incidence in atomic bomb survivors: 1958–1998," *Radiation Research*, Vol. 168(1), pp. 1–64, 2007.

the population's age distribution, nationality, health status, smoking history, and exposure to other carcinogens. Needless to say, such careful matching has been achieved only in a small fraction of all studies. Even in the largest of studies, the total increase in cancer is small. For example, radiation exposures apparently caused 428 out of 4863 total deaths due to cancer (that is, 9% of the total) between 1950 and 1990 for the Japanese atomic bomb survivors. How do we assess whether this increase is significant—that is, genuinely due to radiation—or just a chance occurrence?

In ordinary conversation, the word "significant" denotes a value judgment, but in science it takes on a quantitative meaning: **statistical significance**. To understand this, consider actual numbers for the Japanese atomic bomb survivor study (Table 7.2). This table summarizes the *incidence* of solid tumors (cancers other than leukemia) for all of the study population for the period 1958 to 1998. The actual number of observed cases is given for groups that received varying radiation doses. The background number of cases is generated from a model that includes similar but unexposed populations. Notice that for all dose levels, the number of observed cancers *exceeds* that for the background. The scientists who performed this analysis also used a model to compute the difference between the observed and expected cases of cancer; this difference is listed as the fitted excess and it is based on a model designed to compensate for differences in the baseline risk between populations.

(continued on next page)

In reality, even a perfect study comparing two identical unexposed groups will exhibit departures from the expected cancer rates, due simply to chance variations. That is, assuming we know the true average cancer rate for the entire U.S. population, if we studied a group of 100,000 persons perfectly representative of the population at large, they would likely have a cancer rate somewhat different from the average. By repeating this experiment (choosing different groups of the same size, determining their cancer rate), we would get a *range* of cancer rates clustering around the average value. Using statistics, we can find that the actual cancer rate will lie within a range of values called a **confidence interval** for 95% of the measurements. However, a 5% chance still exists that greater or lesser values will be observed. The size of the confidence interval depends strongly on the number of observed cancer cases. For a perfectly conducted study with no biases, we can estimate this 95% confidence interval to be equal to 2 times the square root of the average number of cancer cases.

We can apply this reasoning to find out the chance variations anticipated for Table 7.2. For the group receiving 0.1–0.2 Gy doses, 968 people actually developed cancer; the study's authors computed that 75 of these were in excess of what was expected. Let us assume that all of the uncertainty derives from the observed number of cancers: 968. To find the 95% confidence intervals, we compute the range of variation for the number of observed cases: $2 \times \sqrt{968} = 2 \times 31 = 62$. This means that a range of (968 + 62) = 1030 cases to (968 – 62) = 902 cases would be expected due to chance alone, 95% of the time. For 0.1–0.2 Gy, this range of variation (62) is smaller than the fitted excess (75)—the increase at this dose level is said to be "statistically significant." Note that other sources of uncertainty can come into play: the background number differs from the observed number by a value different from the fitted excess, which corrects for other sources of variation between those populations. When repeating the same calculation for the numbers for 0.005–0.1 Gy, we see that the confidence intervals exceed the fitted excess—the increase could have been due to chance.

Thus, a population study must observe a large enough number of excess cancer deaths to suppress fluctuations in the death rate due to chance. Significant increases can be detected only when either the risk is very high (for example, from high doses) or the study population is very large. The small size of the risk and the difficulty of finding and following up on large numbers of people subjected to well-known, similar doses of radiation are the major limitations in radiation risk assessment.

(continued on next page)

For example, to establish the predicted increase in cancer mortality due to one diagnostic x-ray, over 10 million cancer deaths would have to be observed, for both the exposed and the control groups. Another example is the inconclusive results (so far) for elevated cancer rates from the Chernobyl accident. While thyroid cancer incidence has risen after Chernobyl, no *overall* increase in cancer incidence has been detected in Europe. Sometimes this result is used to argue that low levels of exposure to ionizing radiation carry no cancer risk. In reality, only an estimated 25,000 cases of non-thyroid cancer are predicted to occur due to this accident—a large number, but one hard to see in comparison to the expected *several hundred million* cases expected in its absence.* How large a fluctuation would be expected if, for example, 200 million cases of cancer ordinarily occurred? Our rule above estimates that we would see variations as large as $\pm 2 \times \sqrt{200,000,000} \approx \pm 28,000$ even without radiation exposure. It would be impossible to say with any confidence whether the expected additional 25,000 were due to Chernobyl or just random fluctuations. The reason that elevated childhood thyroid rates were confirmed is the extreme rarity of this disease and its large value post-Chernobyl.

---

* Cardis, E., Krewski, D., Boniol, M., Drozdovitch, V., Darby, S.C., Gilbert, E.S. et al., "Estimates of the cancer burden in Europe from radioactive fallout from the Chernobyl accident," *Int. J. Cancer*, Vol. 119, pp. 1224–35, 2006.

While data exist for both high and low LET radiation, most of the studies involve exposures to low LET x-rays and gamma rays. The accumulated evidence from human population studies is in general agreement on risks for acute doses greater than 0.15 Sv. The references at the end of this chapter list two standard sources that thoroughly review this information: the 2006 report of the National Academy of Sciences, *Biological Effects of Ionizing Radiations* (BEIR VII) and the 2000 report of the United Nations Scientific Committee on the Effects of Atomic Radiation (UNSCEAR, 2000). In particular, BEIR VII gives an estimate of 1000 additional cancer deaths for every 100,000 persons exposed to 0.1 Sv (100 mSv) of radiation dose to the whole body above background, with smaller doses corresponding to proportionately lower risks. In the U.S., about 42,000 of every 100,000 people (given the makeup of the present population) would eventually die from cancer not caused by radiation. For a medical exam delivering a 1 mSv dose to the whole body, an application of this risk estimate would give an increase of 10 deaths per 100,000 people in addition to the 42,000 cancer deaths ordinarily expected. This constitutes a 0.024% increase in lifetime risk for cancer. These studies also show that some organs are more susceptible than others, so that the most significant increases appear to be in certain cancers, such as leukemia, breast, thyroid, bone, and skin cancers. The age at exposure also matters, with radiation doses at earlier ages tending to cause greater cancer risks in general.

If the Japanese atomic bomb survivor data and other major studies showed that the statistically significant risks were observed down to doses in the range of 1mSv, then estimating the risk from diagnostic medical procedures would be less ambiguous. In fact, the smallest dose for which statistically significant increases exist is about 0.15 Sv. On the other hand, observations of the observed effect as a function of dose can indicate whether linear models that describe statistically significant trends at large doses are consistent with the observed risk at low doses. Indeed, although the risk at the lowest observed doses is not statistically significant, it too is consistently nonzero and all observed values agree with the linear model (Figure 7.7a and b).

To explore the low dose regime, researchers have looked at numerous other populations exposed to low doses of radiation, often accumulating to significant doses in time. The evolving understanding of carcinogenesis indicates that one issue is how important the *dose rate* is in causing cancer. For example, a very large dose delivered at low-dose rates does not cause radiation sickness because of the existence of a threshold. If a threshold exists for low-level exposures, then stochastic risks could be reduced to zero by delivering low enough doses at a low enough rate. Another argument arises because some laboratory studies of radiation effects in laboratory systems have found a dose-effect curve with a curvilinear dependence on dose (illustrated in Figure 7.6c); indeed, the radiation-induced cancer risk for leukemia also agrees with this model. Some scientists argue that data from all population studies should be extrapolated to low doses using this method, which would indicate that low doses are less effective at causing cancer than the linear model indicates. However, analyses by BEIR VII and UNSCEAR agree that most population studies correspond best to a linear model with no threshold, even at low doses and low dose rates. The risk estimates quoted above already factor in an estimate of reduced risk due to low doses and low dose rates corresponding to medical exams or other low dose chronic exposures; BEIR VII estimates a reduction in risk of a factor of 1.5 for low compared to high doses.

Further complicating the picture, researchers have uncovered evidence that low doses of radiation actually stimulate the body's repair mechanisms. This phenomenon, called the **adaptive response**, has been observed to occur when either mice or human cells in culture have first been subjected to relatively small doses of radiation before being exposed to a very large dose. The smaller dose seems to provide a short-term reduction in harm due to the later large dose, presumably by activating DNA repair mechanisms. The BEIR VII concluded from the present evidence that it is impossible at this point to extrapolate from studies in cells to risk estimates for humans, pointing out that in any case, there is no evidence of a *net* benefit from small doses of radiation being protective against later small chronic doses. This effect is being investigated especially in connection with radiation

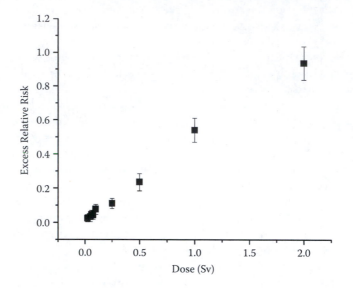

Figure 7.7 (a) Incidence of solid cancer as a function of radiation dose in Gy for the Japanese atomic bomb survivor studies. The quantity plotted vs. dose to the colon is the Excess Relative Risk (ERR), defined as ERR = (observed cases – expected cases)/expected cases. Solid circles represent datapoints from the study. (Adapted from Figure 3 in Preston, D.L., Ron E., Tokuoka S., Funamoto S., Nishi N., Soda M., Mabuchi K., Kodama K., "Solid cancer incidence in atomic bomb survivors: 1958–1998," *Radiation Research*, Vol. 168(1), pp. 1–64 (2007), which also contains more details of the analysis.) (b) Similar results from the atomic bomb survivor study, but plotted for only the low dose regime <100 mSv. (Data replotted from Figure 1 in David J. Brenner and Carl D. Elliston, "Estimated radiation risks potentially associated with full-body CT scanning," *Radiology,* Vol. 232, pp. 735–738, 2004.)

therapy, which must factor in cellular changes induced by prior radiation exposure that might cause tumors to be resistant to radiation or protect normal cells from damage. Conversely, *hyper*-radiation sensitivity has also been observed at low doses in cellular studies, but again the results to date were deemed by BEIR VII to have no relevance to human risk estimates.

Several studies of radiation exposures due to diagnostic imaging techniques are reviewed in BEIR VII.* For example, a statistically significant elevated risk for breast cancer was seen in women tuberculosis patients exposed to repeated fluoroscopy exams; although their cumulative dose was appreciable, each individual exam delivered a dose in mGy comparable

---

* Committee to Assess Health Risks from Exposure to Low Levels of Ionizing Radiation, National Research Council of the National Academies, *Health Risks from Exposure to Low Levels of Ionizing Radiation: BEIR VII Phase 2*, National Academy Press, Washington, D.C., 2006, pp. 170–172.

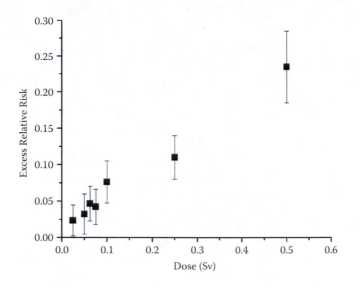

Figure 7.7 (continued).

to a modern CT scan so the dose rate and individual doses were in the low chronic dose range. Probably the largest study of the risk of low-dose rate radiation exposure has followed persons exposed to iodine-131 radionuclides internally for treatments of hyperthyroidism and for diagnostic imaging. In Sweden, very large numbers of such individuals have been followed for extremely long follow-up times with very careful record keeping. Importantly, the radiation doses in these studies were very carefully measured and controlled for, unlike most other studies in which exposures were estimated long after the fact. These data indicate a cancer risk lower than that extrapolated from the atomic bomb survivor study for radionuclide imaging procedures.

So far, we have only considered the consequences of radiation damage to somatic cells. However, radiation exposure to germ cells in the reproductive organs can lead to sterility. Acute doses of over one-tenth of a Gy can cause temporary sterility, and acute doses of several Gy, permanent sterility. In addition, radiation damage to the germ cells could lead to inheritable genetic defects. These increases have not been observed in humans, so studies on mice have been used to estimate a 1 in 250,000 risk of all inheritable defects over two generations for a 1-mSv dose. The use of a lead apron to shield the reproductive organs during diagnostic x-ray exams can reduce or eliminate these risks.

Because every human develops from one original cell that successively divides into multiple cells, genetic damage at an early stage of embryonic development can be carried through to subsequent stages. On the other hand, a badly damaged cell may sabotage the entire embryo if the damage occurs at an early enough stage, thus causing a miscarriage rather than a lasting birth defect. Animal studies show clear negative effects due to high levels of radiation exposure in the womb. In humans, enhanced rates of severe mental retardation, a reduction in IQ, and growth and developmental impairment have been observed in children of atomic bomb survivors exposed to high acute doses of radiation during gestation. No evidence exists to show that low chronic exposures during pregnancy cause birth defects, but physicians still exercise additional care in deciding whether or not to expose pregnant women to ionizing radiation. However, extrapolation from the high-dose data shows that the additional risk involved from inadvertently having even several diagnostic x-ray or radioisotope imaging procedures during pregnancy is at worst extremely low.

The principle presently governing the safe use of radiation is abbreviated **ALARA**, for *As Low As Reasonably Achievable*. This means that radiation should be used only when a net benefit results, and even then the lowest possible doses should be employed. To limit the impact of medical exposures on public health, physicians have worked hard over the past century to reduce the dose per procedure. The very first x-ray units delivered doses more than *1000 times* modern doses. The decreasing doses have come about from research into improved detector and x-ray source design and more careful selection of radioisotopes, so the quality of images has actually improved at the same time. Physicians also now have the option of choosing imaging techniques such as ultrasound or MRI, which do not use ionizing radiation. When possible, doses are limited to only the organs being examined by controlling the field of view irradiated and by eliminating scattering. Radiation risks to the rest of the body can be greatly lowered or eliminated by shielding with lead aprons or collars. Radiation therapies are used primarily for treating life-threatening diseases, and trivial uses of radiation have been outlawed. Healthcare workers protect themselves in a variety of ways: by using lead shielding, by minimizing their exposure times (often by leaving the room during patient exposures), and by maximizing their distance from the radiation sources in use.

Frequent CT scanning: a new source of concern for radiation exposure? CT has widely been hailed as the single more important advance in diagnostic radiology since the discovery of x-rays. However, the dramatic increase in the number of CT scans administered in the U.S. and elsewhere is generating concerns in the medical community because radiation doses for CT are higher than those for other exams, and they tend to be delivered to a large body volume. For example, an adult abdominal CT scan delivers a dose of approximately 10 mSv, while those used for children are typically higher. The risk per individual is

(continued on next page)

still low: we can convert the earlier risk factor of 1000 excess cancer deaths/100,000 per 0.1 Sv to the risk for a 10 mSv = 0.01 Sv whole-body CT scan by multiplying by a factor of 0.01 Sv/0.1 Sv = 1/10. This means the risk per individual is 1/10 (1000 excess cancer deaths/100,000) = 1/1000. Therefore 1000 whole-body CT scans are estimated to produce one excess death from cancer due to radiation, with scans of only parts of the body corresponding to lower risks.

The concern arises because of the large number of CT scans performed each year, at least 62 million in 2007 and rising, the large number prescribed in pediatric cases, the increase in the use of higher-dose helical CT procedures, and the growing list of uses for CT in, for example, screening for colon and lung cancer and routine whole-body scanning without medical indications. Concerned radiologists argue that there is epidemiological evidence for risks at these doses since the dose from mulitple CT scans is the order of the smallest doses corresponding to statistically significant increases in population studies.[*] However, physicians point out that even the increased radiation-associated risk due to more procedures needs to be balanced against the dramatic advantages of widespread use of CT in diagnosing various conditions such as traumatic head injuries, heart problems, cancer, appendicitis, etc. Cases that once would have been investigated by exploratory surgery, with its manifold associated risks, can now be quickly resolved using noninvasive CT scans; many potentially serious conditions can be identified and treated at an earlier stage. Thus, the argument runs that better medical care more than offsets this additional cancer risk. On the other hand, the case that radiation doses similar to those delivered by repeated CT scans carry a cancer risk is increasingly strong, since doses in this range have been shown to cause statistically significant cancer increases in population studies described earlier.

The approach to managing this concern thus devolves on finding ways to reduce unnecessary CT scans (such as those used purely for "defensive medicine"—to avoid the risk of malpractice lawsuits, for example, or those repeated unnecessarily due to inadequacies in communication), educating physicians about the radiation doses associated with CT so they can better gauge whether to use it or an alternative, and ensuring that the parameters for x-ray exposures are routinely selected for the lowest dose consistent with diagnostic needs. The last adjustment is possible because the settings of the CT scanner determine the radiation dose, and these can be tailored to suit the size of person being scanned without degrading image quality unacceptably.

---

[*] David J. Brenner, Eric J. Hall, "Computer tomography—An increasing source of radiation exposure," *N. Eng. J. Med.*, Vol. 357 (22), pp. 2277–2284 (2007).

Benefits and risks for mammography: How do the odds of disease detection and radiation-induced cancer risk balance out for a diagnostic x-ray procedure such as routine mammograms for breast cancer screening (Chapter 5)? No studies have shown a direct link between breast cancer and mammograms. However, the data from BEIR reports can be used to estimate the cancer risk caused by having women in the U.S. undergo annual mammograms for early detection of breast cancer. In a mammogram, four films are usually taken (two views per breast) and each corresponds to a dose of about 1 mSv. Thus, the entire procedure results in a typical total dose of 4 mSv. To convert this into an estimated increase in cancer rate, we cannot simply use the risk estimate mentioned earlier because that figure applied to whole-body doses and all cancers. In a mammogram, the radiation dose is concentrated in the breast, so only extra breast cancer risk should be considered. Risk factors for each type of cancer have been computed for a 0.1-Sv dose.* In addition, the radiation-induced breast cancer risk is greatest for exposures during adolescence and childhood. If mammogram screenings only begin in the 40s, then the estimated *lifetime* risk factor drops to 20 excess breast cancer deaths per 100,000 women per 0.1-Sv dose. We must correct this estimate, because the actual dose per mammogram is only 4 mSv (0.004 Sv). To convert this number to a worst-case risk per mammogram, we divide the risk by a factor that accounts for dose; this means dividing by 0.1 Sv/0.004 Sv = 25. If a woman receives mammograms annually for, e.g., 10 years, we need to multiply the risk by 10. As a result, the total risk estimate is: 20 × 10/25 = 8 excess breast cancer deaths per 100,000 women. The studies discussed in Chapter 5 estimate that that mammography reduces mortality from breast cancer (currently 25 deaths per 100,000 women in 2005) by 28% to 65%. By this reasoning, mammograms offer a net benefit, even without a resolution of the debates about the effects of low radiation doses.

---

* Committee on the Biological Effects of Ionizing Radiations, Board on Radiation Effects Research, Commission on Life Sciences, National Research Council, *Health Effects of Exposure to Low Levels of Ionizing Radiation: BEIR V*, National Academy Press, Washington, D.C., 1990, p. 175; Lawrence N. Rothenberg, Stephen A. Feig, Arthur G. Haus, R. Edward Hendrick, Geoffrey R. Howe, John L. McCrohan, Edward A. Sickles, Martin J. Yaffe, Wende W. Logan-Young, *Report No. 149—A Guide to Mammography and Other Breast Imaging Procedures*, National Council on Radiation Protection and Measurements, 2004; S.A. Feig and R. E. Hendricks, "Radiation risk from screening mammography of women aged 40–49 years," *J. Natl. Cancer Inst. Monogr.*, Vol. 22, pp. 119–124 (1997).

Table 7.3 Comparative risks for various activities

Whole-body exposure to 2 mSv (0.2 rem) of ionizing radiation has the same risk as:

- Smoking 150 cigarettes (Smoking 20 cigarettes a day for 20 years gives a 1 in 150,000 chance of dying from lung cancer.)
- Traveling 5000 miles by car
- Working in a factory for 4 years (due to risks of occupational accidents)
- Rock climbing for 2.5 hours

Source: After R.J. Wootton, ed. *Radiation Protection for Patients*. Cambridge University Press, Cambridge, U.K., 1993.

While the healthcare community continues to exercise caution in the use of ionizing radiation, it is important to bear in mind the magnitude of the risks under consideration for typical diagnostic imaging procedures. These can best be put in context by a comparison with ordinary activities that carry approximately the same risk as the doses of radiation encountered in such situations (Table 7.3).

7.5 RADIATION THERAPY: KILLING TUMORS WITH RADIATION

In radiation therapy for cancer, lethal doses of radiation are rapidly delivered to malignant tumor cells. Because the doses are clearly in the deterministic regime, a predictable fraction of the tumor cells die as a result. The dream of researchers in the war against cancer has always been a drug that acts as a "magic bullet," able to seek out and destroy only tumor cells. At the moment, radiation therapy fails to fill this bill since it exposes healthy tissues to high doses, along with the tumors. As a result, the treatments deliver at least a stochastic dose to the rest of the body, possibly creating an enhanced risk of cancer at some later time. However, in cancer therapy this small future risk is weighed against an existing life-threatening disease. In addition, cancer chemotherapy presents many of the same risks. Because many chemotherapy drugs work by altering DNA, or otherwise disabling cell metabolism, they, too, target quickly reproducing cells, and so they produce many of the same toxic or carcinogenic effects as radiation.

Most malignant tumor cells fall into the class of rapidly reproducing cells that are easily affected by radiation. However, destroying enough of a tumor to prevent its regrowth is still a difficult task. Since only one cell left behind is all that's needed to reseed the tumor, in theory, radiation therapy must achieve *total* extinction of tumor cells. Cancer cells are not necessarily confined in separate, compact masses, but are often spread throughout the body, infiltrating vital organs. Thus, treating a cancer often unavoidably entails

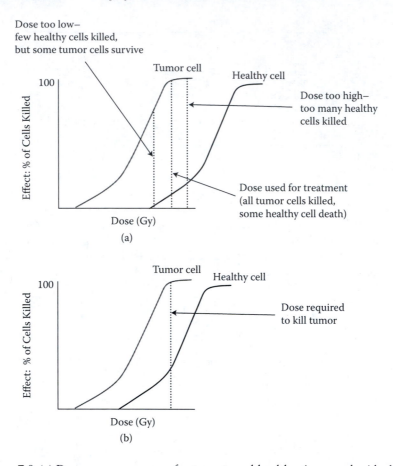

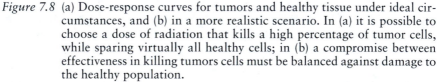

Figure 7.8 (a) Dose-response curves for tumors and healthy tissue under ideal circumstances, and (b) in a more realistic scenario. In (a) it is possible to choose a dose of radiation that kills a high percentage of tumor cells, while sparing virtually all healthy cells; in (b) a compromise between effectiveness in killing tumors cells must be balanced against damage to the healthy population.

treating an entire region of surrounding healthy tissue. This also means a compromise between effectiveness in killing the tumor and in sparing nearby healthy tissue to ensure the patient is able to recover after treatment.

To see how these two goals can be achieved in practice, consider the dose-response curves in Figure 7.8. The salient features of these curves are: (1) there is a threshold dose for cell killing, (2) the fraction of cells killed increases with dose via a characteristic S-shaped curve, and (3) there is a dose at which 100% of the cells are killed, so there is no effect of increasing the dose. If the threshold for the healthy tissue exceeds that for the tumor, treatments can use a dose that kills most—perhaps 90%—of tumor cells, yet affects relatively few—perhaps 5%—of the healthy cells (Figure 7.8a). However, the same plot shows that even small variations in this treatment dose lead to undesirable consequences: too high a dose kills too many healthy cells, while too low a dose spares tumor cells. Often, the treatment dose must be controlled to within several percent of the ideal value in order to avoid these two extremes. Worse still is the situation shown in Figure 7.8(b), where there is an appreciable overlap between the two curves, making the choice of dose size difficult. In this case, killing appreciable numbers of tumor cells necessarily inflicts great damage on the normal population.

In general, the form of the dose-response curve depends on the tissue from which the cells originate, the type of ionizing radiation, and its energy. The dose-response curve also depends on the rate at which the radiation dose is delivered, with more rapidly delivered doses causing more damage with a lower threshold. Since healthy cells tend to have better DNA repair mechanisms than do tumor cells, the latter effect can be taken advantage of by dividing the high dose required to kill tumor cells into many **fractions**. These smaller doses are delivered with a pause of a day or so between fractions, so that healthy cells have a chance to recover and repopulate. Other advantages of using fractions may include making the tumor cells more readily damaged by changing the point in the cell cycle at which the tumor cells are irradiated.

Tumors that respond readily to radiation therapy include those that are relatively localized, rapidly growing, and in a location accessible for treatment. For some regions of the body, radiation is especially effective (for example, in the treatment of superficial skin cancers). For others the responsiveness of tumor cells can differ little from that of neighboring healthy tissues. The cure rate, and the effectiveness of radiation as a cancer treatment, depends greatly on the type of cancer and specifics of individual cases.

Physicians treat cancer through a variety of approaches, including surgical removal, chemotherapy, radiation therapy, immunotherapy, and hormone therapy, several of which may be tried in combination or succession. In planning radiation therapy, physicians called **radiation oncologists** weigh all the information available to them about a specific case: the type of cancer, its history and location, the likely effectiveness of surgery and chemotherapy, other complicating conditions in the patient, and many other factors. Radiation therapy may be used as a **palliative** measure to reduce pain or deformation even if a cure is unlikely. Factors that can be controlled include the means of delivering the radiation, the type of radiation, total dose size, fractions into which the total dose is divided, and the time between fractions. The type of particle used and its energy are essential issues in radiation therapy. Since the main goal is to have the tumors absorb energy from radiation, high LET particles might seem like the obvious choice. However, the very short range of alpha particles (Figure 6.2) prevents them from reaching the entire diseased region. Neutrons have a longer range, but require a nearby nuclear reactor for their production. Even more exotic particles have been tested for radiation therapy, but presently, most therapy is performed with either high-energy photons or beta particles (electrons). Electrons with energies from 4 to 20 MeV have ranges of 1 to 6 cm. This short range allows them to be used to treat cancers of the skin, lip, chest wall, and the head and neck, while limiting the healthy tissue exposed. However, in most cases this short range does not suffice. For example, a deep-seated tumor in the abdomen might only be reachable by passing the beam through intervening tissue. This means that more penetrating photons with energies ranging into the MeV must be used in treating the majority of nonsuperficial tumors.

Three alternative approaches for delivering ionizing radiation for therapy exist: (1) **beam sources** external to the body produce a beam of ionizing radiation that is aimed at the tumor(s) during treatment sessions; (2) **brachytherapy sources**, sealed radioactive sources placed in proximity with the tumor; and (3) **unsealed sources**, radionuclides taken into the body in liquid form, either by injection or swallowing. Beam sources are the most widely used type. They provide beams of ionizing radiation, most commonly x-rays and electrons, which can be aimed at the malignant regions. The beam source must deliver a uniform, well-defined, and stable beam, with particles selected for the right choice of penetration depth for the job at hand. This ensures that the beam reaches only the regions intended and delivers the desired dose. Since the exact value of the dose delivered is so critical, dosimeters are used to monitor the dose received by the patient.

The most common beam sources are **linear accelerators** (**linacs**), which produce high-energy x-rays and electrons for treatment (Figure 7.9). These devices accelerate electrons to high energies using radiofrequency electromagnetic fields; these high-energy electrons can be used directly, or they can be used to generate x-rays in a fashion similar to the operation of an x-ray tube (Chapter 5). Linacs generate x-rays with energies in the range of 4 to 6 MeV and higher. Radioactive sources such as the gamma ray-emitting radionuclide cobalt-60 can also be used to generate beams for some applications. However, in general, the beam quality from radioactive sources is lower, the beam intensity diminishes with time, and they are limited to only one gamma ray energy. Neutrons have long been used in radiation therapy, although their use is limited by the extremely low number of facilities with this capability (only 3 in the U.S. and about a dozen worldwide) because their production requires a high-energy particle accelerator. Neutrons are particularly effective because of their high RBE and LET, leading to highly effective cell-killing, but they are used only for certain cancers resistant to treatment by conventional radiation therapy because of their scarcity and cost.

In planning treatment with a beam source, the physician must weigh in the factors described above, plus some additional practical considerations. The region to be treated must be clearly defined, usually by one or more imaging techniques. The region infiltrated by the tumor is referred to as the **target volume**, while the **treatment volume** is defined as the target volume plus a margin of several millimeters or more surrounding it. This additional region is treated to allow for a margin of error in defining the tumor's boundaries. With careful planning, the error in defining the location of

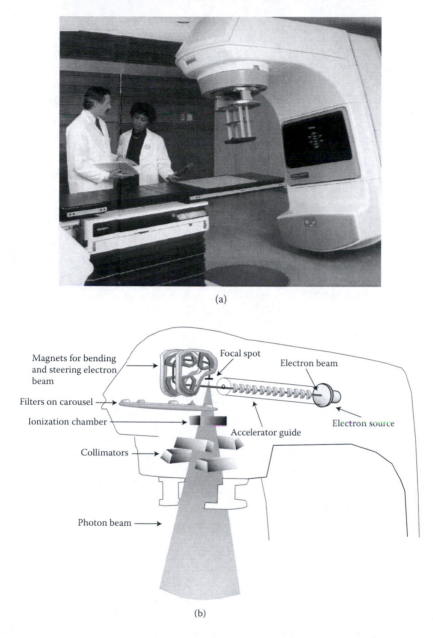

(a)

(b)

Figure 7.9 Photograph (a) and schematic drawing (b) of a linear accelerator x-ray
beam source (linac) used for radiation therapy. (Reproduced with permission courtesy of Varian Medical Systems.)

the treatment volume can be kept low enough to exclude large amounts
of healthy tissue. Ideally, a dose large enough to kill all tumor cells is delivered to the entire treatment volume, with zero dose falling outside.

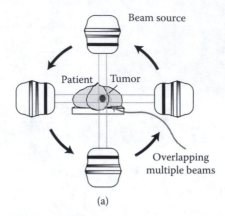

Beam source

Patient | Tumor

Overlapping
multiple beams

(a)

Figure 7.10 (*See color figure following page 78.*) (a) Multiple orientations of beam sources permit irradiation of the tumor from several angles, with the region of overlap chosen to correspond to the location of the tumor. In this scheme, the region receiving the highest radiation dose is not the point of entry (as would be true for a single beam), but the overlap. (b) In three-dimensional (3D), intensity modulated radiation therapy (IMRT) using stereotactic systems, gamma ray beams converge on a malignant tumor from all possible directions, using information from 3D CT image reconstructions to create a treatment that confines the dose to the contours of the tumor. The image shows a superimposed axial CT scan and radiation dose map from 3D IMRT planning for a case of prostate cancer. To target the prostate tumor, it is desired to confine the radiation dose so as to avoid the bladder and rectum (also shown as outlines.) Contour lines of the radiation dose in Gy indicate that the highest doses are indeed confined to the tumor, with little exposure to bordering normal tissues. (Image reproduced with permission courtesy of Robert Levine, Ph.D., Spectral Sciences, Inc.) (c) Actual beam source for delivering radiation therapy with multiple-beam orientations. Insets show how lead collimators can be used to shape the beam differently at each angle to more precisely target the actual region occupied by the tumor. (Reproduced with permission courtesy of Varian Medical Systems.)

A serious complication with beam sources is that healthy regions lying between the source and tumor are also exposed to high doses of radiation. Even worse, if the tumor is deep-seated, then the skin and superficially located tissues receive a higher radiation dose than the tumor itself if only a single beam is used. This is because the x-ray beam's intensity diminishes as it is absorbed by tissue along its path. One way to deal with this problem, **Intensity Modulated Radiation Therapy (IMRT)**, involves irradiating the tumor from many different directions, using multiple beams with varying intensities (Figure 7.10a). To give a simple example, the beams can be made to enter the body from four different directions. The four beams are directed to intersect at the tumor, so the total dose at the tumor is four times that at the nearby, nonoverlapping regions that pass through healthy tissue. Near the point where each beam enters the body the dose level is also

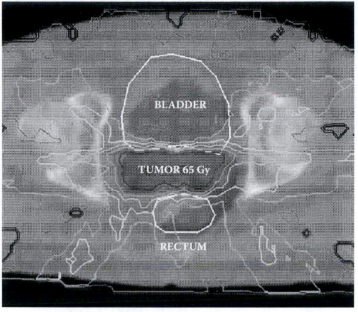

(b)

Figure 7.10 (continued).

high, but if numerous beams are used, the tumor receives by far the highest dose because it is in the region of overlap. In this fashion, the exposure received by healthy tissue can be kept below lethal levels, while very high doses are delivered specifically to the tumor (Figure 7.10b).

Another complication is that, ideally, the beam's **profile** (the variation of x-ray intensity across its width) should be adjusted to give a uniform dose to all treated regions. In IMRT, a set of computer-controlled metal leaves can be selectively inserted between the beam and the body, creating variations in intensity across the face of a beam by varying its absorption from side to side. The beam profile can be adjusted as needed for different orientations of the beam, and this information can be programmed into a computer controlling the multiple beam treatment. This "wedging" effect can be used to tailor the intensity profile so as to more precisely target the dose delivered by the multiple beams (Figure 7.10c). (Although our examples have assumed that the particle being delivered in IMRT is a high-energy photon, the same principles apply for other particles, such as electrons or protons, where shaping the targeted region is equally important for killing tumor cells while sparing normal tissue.)

One striking application of multiple beam technology is the **gamma-knife**, a helmet equipped with hundreds of cobalt-60 sources arranged so as to irradiate a brain or eye tumor from numerous directions. In combination with judicious positioning of lead collimators to shape the targeting of the

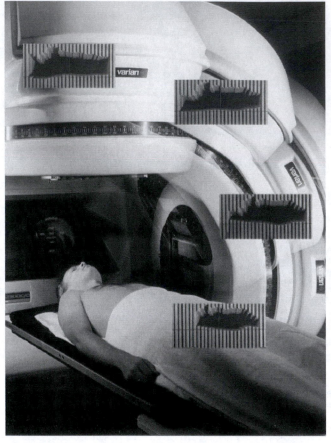

(c)

Figure 7.10 (continued).

multiple beams, the very large number of beams ensures that an extremely
large dose of photons can be delivered to the tumor while surrounding tissues are spared. Roboticized stereotactic radiosurgery and "Cyberknife"
technologies also implement this idea, but with steerable accelerator-based
beam sources that target only the tumor's volume.

As one can see from the preceding discussion, information technology
is playing an increasingly important and complex role in radiation therapy.
Hybrid CT/PET or CT/MRI scanners, or coregistered scans from varying imaging technologies, can be used to map out the tumor's boundaries
in three-dimensional detail. Computer models take this information and
calculate exactly how to aim numerous beams in order to precisely shape
the treatment volume, while minimizing the dose to surrounding healthy
regions. Since lowering the dose to nearby healthy tissue allows even higher
doses to be delivered to the tumor, this permits more effective therapies.

It also has the potential to seriously reduce side effects. By controlling the point of entry for each beam, its direction, the energy used, and the number of beams used, the actual volume receiving the highest dose of radiation can be carefully sculpted to conform to the tumor's location and shape. In **Helical Tomotherapy**, the idea behind spiral CT is used to provide an even more tailored three-dimensional beam profile. Similar to spiral CT, a rotating IMRT unit delivers intensity-modulated beams from many directions as the beam traces out a helical set of overlapping slices, enabling the target volume to be precisely sculpted in three dimensions.

The exact computation of the multiple beam directions and the doses delivered by each beam for a given number of beams can be performed using detailed information provided by CT scanners combined with other imaging modalities, such as PET, SPECT or MRI. Because the CT scanner also uses x-rays in imaging the body, it measures how x-ray absorbent different parts of the body are (Chapter 5). (By contrast, MRI can provide equally detailed images, but it does not measure x-ray absorption.) The CT cross-sectional data can be used to compute exactly how much of a dose each part of the body receives for a particular beam configuration. Computers are used to calculate and plot out the doses received by different regions in the body. These maps can be examined and different combinations of multiple beams and collimators manipulated to ensure that vital organs receive low doses while maximizing the dose to the tumor. CT scanners can be used subsequently to monitor the course of therapy by re-examining the treated tumor.

In order to check the exact alignment of the beams used for therapy, **radiation therapy simulators** are used. These devices have diagnostic x-ray devices or CT scanners mounted in a fashion identical to the actual beam sources used for therapy. The therapy can thus be mimicked while the patient's body is being imaged to make sure the beams are properly aimed. The patient receiving the therapy must be repositioned in exactly the same way each treatment session to ensure these carefully planned beams irradiate the intended regions. Laser beam indicators on the beam sources, along with marks on the body, tattoos, or special body casts, allow precise realignment of the treatment beam. Even better, CT scanning simultaneous with the radiation therapy can be performed at megaVolt energies that provide a good match to the properties of the photons being used for treatment, while identifying body anatomy at the time of the treatment. This avoids subtle internal rearrangements from distorting the locations of the targeted tissue. All of these techniques are encompassed by **Image Guided Radiation Therapy (IGRT)**, in which real-time imaging capability allows the radiation beam to track patient movements, while also instantly giving feedback on the progress of the treatment. Such techniques are especially important for prostate cancer or brain tumors, situations in which even small miscalculations could lead to serious medical consequences.

IMRT's rapid implementation does have its detractors, who argue that the adoption of this technology has been driven by hospitals competing for patients and higher insurance reimbursements, ahead of clinical studies of its effectiveness.* Others worry that because IMRT uses a higher intensity that it also can entail a greater radiation risk without proven benefits. It is hoped that ongoing clinical trials of IMRT will address these critiques. The high expense of *any* accelerator-based technique leads to radioactive cobalt-60 sources being more practical for radiation therapy in the developing world.

In contrast to external beam radiation therapy, in brachytherapy, a radioactive source can be directly applied to the neighborhood of the tumor, thereby greatly limiting exposure of healthy tissue. This method is mostly used for tumors accessible through natural openings, or those accessible via catheters or implanted needles. Brachytherapy sources are made from nontoxic radioactive materials encased in an ordinary metal and formed into a variety of shapes: needles, small pellets, fine wires, seeds, tubes, needles, etc. (Figure 7.11a); for example, iridium-192, with a half-life of 74 days, is a radioactive metal easily formed into many useful shapes. The radiation source is then implanted into, or placed directly against, the tumor (Figure 7.11b and c). Compared to beam sources, this technique can yield higher doses to the tumor, while limiting the irradiation of nearby healthy tissues. For example, implants can be used in treating cancer of the breast and prostate; brachytherapy can also be used to treat tumors accessible through body openings, like those in the female reproductive organs.

This method permits considerable control over the region to be irradiated and allows the treatment to be halted completely upon the removal of the sources. Unlike beam sources, brachytherapy sources can be left in place over a period of time to provide continual irradiation of cells with no intervening recovery periods. For implants left in place for long times, radioisotopes such as iodine-125 and palladium-103 are appropriate; with half-lives of 60 and 17 days, respectively, they deliver damaging doses of radiation over a defined period, then decay to a low activity in several months. Most brachytherapy sources emit both beta and gamma rays, but the beta rays are absorbed by the metal casing, leaving only the gamma rays to deliver the actual treatment dose. In another application, **High Dose Rate (HDR)** brachytherapy uses catheters inserted into a tumor as a pathway for introducing high activity radioactive sources temporarily. The movement of these sources is computer controlled as they are fed through the catheter into the tumor and then back out of the patient's body. By choosing the dwell time and positions of the sources, the radiation can be targeted precisely to the tumor, delivering very high doses in a short period of time, with no long-term radiation exposure.

---

* See the review of these issues in Steve Webb, *Contemporary IMRT: Developing Physics and Clinical Implementation*, Series in Medical Physics and Biomedical Engineering, Institute of Physics, Philadelphia and Bristol, U.K., 2005.

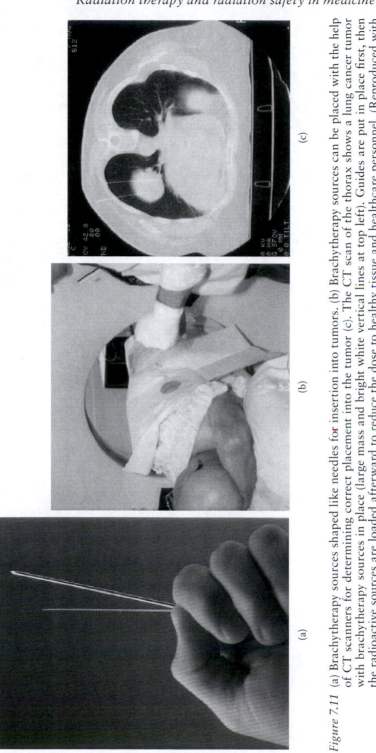

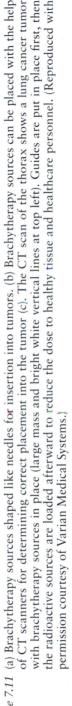

(a)　　　　(b)　　　　(c)

Figure 7.11 (a) Brachytherapy sources shaped like needles for insertion into tumors. (b) Brachytherapy sources can be placed with the help of CT scanners for determining correct placement into the tumor (c). The CT scan of the thorax shows a lung cancer tumor with brachytherapy sources in place (large mass and bright white vertical lines at top left). Guides are put in place first, then the radioactive sources are loaded afterward to reduce the dose to healthy tissue and healthcare personnel. (Reproduced with permission courtesy of Varian Medical Systems.)

Unsealed radionuclide sources, or systemic radiation therapy, are the least commonly used of all radiation therapy devices, yet they most closely approach the goal of "magic bullets" that specifically target certain tumors. They consist of radioactive fluids, or radioactive **colloids** (suspensions of large particles of radioactive materials), which can be either ingested by or injected into the person undergoing treatment. The radiolabeled drugs then remain in the body, concentrating in specific organs to which they deliver a high radiation dose. Beta emitters are best for these purposes, since the radionuclide penetrates the organ so thoroughly that the short range of electrons is not a problem. The half-life of an unsealed source radionuclide should be long enough to allow the drug to reach the organ to be treated and concentrate there, but not so long that it creates continuously radioactive human waste. These radiopharmaceuticals must meet stringent criteria before becoming a feasible method of concentrating ionizing radiation on the area of interest. Very few radionuclides measure up to these requirements, making this type of radiation therapy useful only in restricted types of cancer or other diseases.

Examples of radionuclides used in unsealed source therapy are iodine-131, with a beta range of 3 mm, and phosphorus-32, with a half-life of 14.3 days and a beta range of 10 mm. Because iodine is effectively partitioned into the thyroid gland and cleared from the rest of the body, iodine-131 administered orally is used for the treatment of thyroid cancer and hyperthyroidism (overactive thyroid gland). In the case of iodine-131, its emission of gamma rays allows gamma camera or SPECT imaging to be used to follow the course of treatment. Phosphorus-32 has a pronounced effect on blood-forming tissues, so it can be used in the treatment of leukemia and other blood disorders.

7.8 NEW DIRECTIONS IN RADIATION THERAPY

One emerging direction for radiation therapy is the use of protons as a superior—but expensive—choice of particle. As explained in Chapter 6, protons are positively charged hydrogen nuclei that interact strongly with other charged subatomic particles in the body because of their electrical charge. As a result, protons have high RBE and LET, and very different absorption properties from high-energy photons. In fact, their probability of transferring energy increases as they progressively slow down, leading to little energy transfer when they first enter the body, then a large energy transfer over a limited range (the Bragg peak) within the body. The depth of the Bragg peak within the body can be chosen by adjusting the proton's initial energy, and the usual tricks from IMRT can be applied to shape the direction and intensity profile of the proton beams used. As a result, protons can concentrate their radiation damage to a limited region within the body, with little energy deposition before or after (Figure 7.12a). By contrast, the

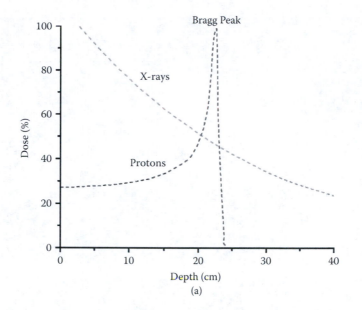

Figure 7.12 (*See color figure following page 78.*) (a) A plot of the percent of particle beams present as a function of depth within an absorber shows that protons follow a very different behavior from photons (gamma or x-rays). In particular, the vast majority of protons are absorbed by the Bragg peak depth, so tissues beyond this point in the body are not exposed to ionizing radiation. By contrast, photons have an exponential absorption, so x-ray beams have a much more gradual fall-off and hence expose a wider range of tissues to significant doses. (b) CT scan of the hips and prostate tumor, with superimposed color maps indicating radiation dose delivered at various points. The top image indicates the radiation dose (color map) from two proton beams incident from the sides of the body, while the bottom image shows the radiation dose due to two 18 MeV x-ray beams also incident from the sides. These images illustrate how for a fixed beam geometry, the radiation dose due to proton therapy (top) conforms much better to the tumor volume (green contour) than that for photon therapy (bottom). (Reproduced with permission courtesy of the National Association for Proton Therapy.)

distribution of photon intensity follows an exponential fall-off, necessarily being greatest near the surface and falling off only gradually with depth. This difference explains the desirability of protons for radiation therapy. Their absorption properties allow the targeted volume within the body to be more carefully defined than with photons, with limited radiation exposure before and after the tumor and greatly reduced collateral radiation damage even while greater radiation doses are delivered to the tumor itself (Figure 7.12b). This is especially important for pediatric applications, where reducing risks of radiation-related cancer is especially important because of the youth and sensitivity of the patients.

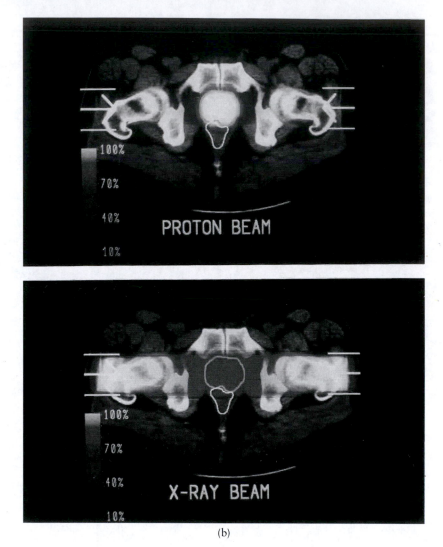

(b)

Figure 7.12 (continued).

Although these advantages have long been appreciated, proton radiation therapy facilities remain scarce because they require special cyclotron sources; as a result, even though major insurers and Medicare already cover the cost of treatment, it remains 20 to 30 times as expensive as conventional photon radiation therapy. Current research aims at finding ways to generate high energy protons using more compact and affordable devices, with the hope that protons may become the particle of choice.

Many other ongoing efforts aim at overcoming the limitations described in the previous section to improve the effectiveness of radiation therapy.

Modern genetic and biochemical research is constantly enhancing the understanding of radiation biology and its applicability to killing cancer cells. Studies now taking place on the interaction of chemotherapy agents and radiation therapy may eventually improve the overall efficacy of both. Many of the drugs now used for chemotherapy for cancer treatment appear to have an additional effectiveness in enhancing the sensitivity of malignant tissues to radiation or in blocking repair processes in between fractions. These potential **radiosensitizers** often work by increasing the oxygen levels available to tumor cells, which enhances radiation damage, although none is presently approved by the FDA for this purpose. If the susceptibility of cancers could be selectively enhanced over that of healthy nearby tissues, the same effectiveness could be achieved with lower, safer doses of radiation. The interaction between the two treatments is thought to occur because many chemotherapy drugs also damage DNA and inhibit repair processes, and hence can prevent the malignant cells from recovering from radiation-induced damage. An additional potential enhancement of radiation therapy is research into **radioprotectants**: drugs that preferentially *protect* healthy tissue, while not altering the response of the cancer to the ionizing radiation. The U.S. FDA has approved one drug, amifostine, for this purpose, and a variety of others are under investigation as ways of avoiding or alleviating damage to normal tissues.

Yet another frontier will be described in our final chapter, where we see how modern imaging techniques meet molecular biology and biochemistry in molecular imaging applications of MRI.

SUGGESTED READING

Radiation therapy

Eric J. Hall and Amato J. Giaccia, *Radiobiology for the Radiologist*, Lippincott Williams & Wilkins, New York, 2005.

William R. Hendee, Geoffrey S. Ibbott, and Eric G. Hendee, *Radiation Therapy Physics*, Wiley-Liss, New York, 2004.

Steve Webb, *Contemporary IMRT: Developing Physics and Clinical Implementation*, Taylor & Francis, London, 2004.

J.R. Williams and D.I. Thwaites (eds.), *Radiotherapy Physics In Practice,* Oxford University Press, Oxford, U.K., 2000.

Comprehensive summaries of the risks of ionizing radiation

Sources and Effects of Ionizing Radiation, Vol. 1 and 2, 2000 Report to the General Assembly, with scientific annexes and Hereditary Effects of Radiation, UNSCEAR 2001 Report to the General Assembly, with scientific annex. United Nations Scientific Committee on the Effects of Atomic Radiation (UNSCEAR), United Nations, New York.

Committee to Assess Health Risks from Exposure to Low Levels of Ionizing Radiation, National Research Council of the National Academies, *Health Risks from Exposure to Low Levels of Ionizing Radiation: BEIR VII Phase 2*, National Academy Press, Washington, D.C., 2006.

Peter M. Mauch and Jay S. Loeffler, *Radiation Oncology: Technology and Biology*. W.B. Saunders Company, Philadelphia, 1994.

QUESTIONS

Q7.1. Explain in your own words the present understanding of the biological effects of ionizing radiation. Which aspects are important to diagnostic medical applications? To therapeutic applications? To radiation safety?

Q7.2. If an individual received a dose of 1 Gy of radiation, what other information would you need to know about the circumstances of the exposure in order to judge the severity of the biological effects?

Q7.3. Persons exposed to radiation in the workplace are given radiation dosimeters to wear. Explain how you could add thin metal filters to the dosimeter in front of its detector to determine the type and energy of the radiation detected. (Hint: Think about the ranges of different particles with various energies.)

Q7.4. Discuss the advantages and disadvantages of different means of delivering ionizing radiation for therapeutic purposes.

Q7.5. Why are x-ray or gamma ray photons and electrons the most commonly used particles for cancer therapy? Give at least two reasons. Explain the advantages of the proton as a particle for radiation therapy.

Q7.6. Why are multiple beams now used in radiation therapy? What are the advantages of employing such a geometry?

Q7.7. What information do CT scanners provide for radiation therapy planning that PET, SPECT and MRI cannot?

PROBLEMS

P7.1. The typical dose to the whole body from a conventional thallium-201 study is estimated to be 0.65 mGy per 1 MBq dose. Perform a crude worst-case estimate of this quantity, using the following numbers: $T_{1/2} = 72$ hours; $\Phi = 0.8$ (for a simple model assuming a sphere with the same mass as a typical person [60 kg] with a point radioactive source located at its center);[*] $E_- = 68$ to 80.3 keV gamma rays. (Assume 100% uptake and retention.)

P7.2. One of the most important sources of internal radiation is the naturally occurring radioisotope, potassium-40, which makes

---

[*] Herman Cember. *Introduction to Health Physics*. McGraw-Hill, New York, 1992, p. 158.

up 0.012% of the potassium found in the body. These nuclei decay by emitting both beta particles and gamma rays. For the sake of this calculation, assume the radiation dose to the body is mostly due to total absorption of the beta particles, and that, on average, each radioactive decay deposits 0.39 MeV of energy. Assume an average source activity of potassium-40 in the body is 4630 Bq and a total body mass of 70 kg. Compute the annual radiation dose due to potassium-40, and find out how much it contributes to the average annual dose of 0.39 mSv due to internal radioisotopes.

P7.3. Would you expect to be able to detect the increase in cancer deaths due to the extra radiation dose received due to cosmic rays due to living at high altitudes? Assume the annual radiation doses due to cosmic rays are as follows:

Sea level: 41 millirem
Denver, Colorado (5000 ft.): 70 millirem
Leadville, Colorado (10,500 ft.): 160 millirem

Assume for this problem that the population of Denver, Colorado, is 1,600,000 and that of Leadville, 3900. (These are historical numbers, for reasons that will become apparent.) Assume for this problem that the BEIR risk estimates are valid. How many total excess cancer deaths would you expect due to the additional radiation exposure at high altitudes? Should this difference be detectable statistically in a study where you could somehow determine the cause of death of each one of the present residents over a long period of time? (Hint: Use the background cancer rates given in Chapter 7 to estimate the expected cancer deaths for exposures at sea level, and use the definition of statistical significance described in Chapter 7. Assume that you could control for all other possible influences on the cancer rate—an unlikely assumption at best.)

P7.4. Plot the data for cancer incidence from Table 7.2 in a fashion similar to that used in Figure 7.7. Use the excess relative risk, as defined in the caption for Figure 7.7, plotted vs. average dose, given in the table below. Use vertical lines to denote the range of the 95% confidence intervals (calculated in Table P7.1). Qualitatively speaking, which of the functional forms shown in Figure 7.6c do these data most resemble?

USEFUL SOURCES OF MORE ADVANCED PROBLEMS

Joseph John Bevelacqua, *Contemporary Health Physics*. John Wiley & Sons, New York, 1995.
Herman Cember, *Introduction to Health Physics*. McGraw-Hill, New York, 1992.
Russell K. Hobbie, *Intermediate Physics for Medicine and Biology*. Springer-Verlag, New York, 1997.

8   Magnetic resonance imaging

8.1 INTRODUCTION

Evolution has left us with hinge-like knee joints exquisitely vulnerable to damage. As a result, sports fans are familiar with the sight of a favorite athlete crumpled in agony from a knee injury, and many amateur athletes suffer similar injuries (Figure 8.1). None of the imaging techniques we have considered thus far can provide images with the combination of high spatial resolution and excellent soft tissue contrast required to permit the study of a wounded joint. However, **magnetic resonance imaging** (**MRI**) can image even soft tissues, with results as crisply detailed as drawings from an anatomy text. MRI collects its maps of the body noninvasively, so it can be used both to diagnose an injury and then monitor the process of healing and recovery that can determine an athlete's fate.

MRI scanners also excel at numerous other applications. Because MRI achieves the elusive goal of clearly distinguishing between different types of brain tissue, it has become an important tool for detecting brain tumors, for diagnosing strokes, and for revealing changes in the brain associated with multiple sclerosis, epilepsy, senile dementia, and AIDS (Figure 8.2). It can be used throughout the body since no structures are obscured by bone or air, and the spatial resolution of 0.5 mm or smaller is comparable to the best available with other tomographic techniques. The novel mechanisms that determine the contrast in MRI allow it to resolve different types of soft tissues and distinguish changes due to body metabolism, pathological conditions, and dynamic processes. MRI ordinarily permits the collection of cross sections in any anatomical plane (Figure 8.2). The reconstruction of three-dimensional images is now available for clinical use, allowing physicians to visualize the actual shape of an organ, as well as to image complex body cross sections. The ongoing development of new contrast media and MRI spectroscopic techniques promises to further extend the range of distinguishable tissues.

Dynamic MRI techniques, or **functional MRI** (**fMRI**), shrink the time required for scans to the point where MRI becomes capable of imaging body function at speeds superior to CT, SPECT, and PET. By enabling the creation of snapshots of the beating heart, this opens up the possibility of

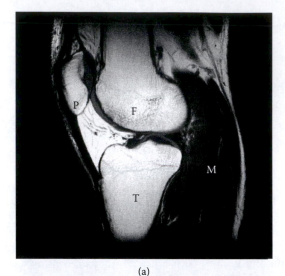

(a)

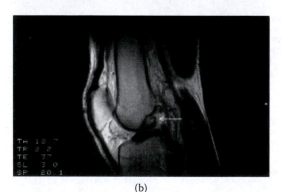

(b)

Figure 8.1 (a) Sagittal MRI scan of the knee, illustrating the technique's high spatial resolution and excellent soft tissue contrast. Anatomical features
that can be discerned easily include the femur (F, thighbone), tibia
(T, the weight-bearing bone of the lower leg), patella (P, kneecap), various muscles of the leg (M), and the detailed structure of cartilage and
other soft tissues within the knee joint itself. (Reproduced with permission courtesy of the National Library of Medicine's Visible Human
Project, at http://www.nlm.nih.gov) (b) Many common sports injuries
can be imaged with MRI, such as tears of the crucial ligaments (arrow)
that connect the femur and tibia. (Reproduced with permission courtesy of Siemens Medical Systems.)

MRI studies of the heart and circulatory system without x-ray contrast
dyes and ionizing radiation. The ready availability of fMRI scanners has
resulted in a blossoming of studies that use fMRI to map brain function
during various mental activities.

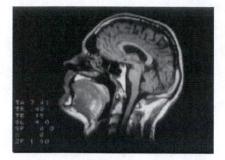

(a)

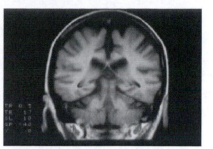

(b)

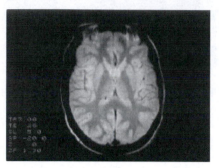

(c)

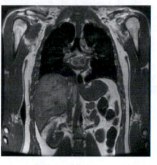

(d)

Figure 8.2 MRI scans can be taken at any orientation, including (a) sagittal, (b) coronal, and (c) axial cross-sectional images of the body (in this case, the head and brain). By contrast, CT is constrained geometrically to measuring axial images. (Reproduced with permission courtesy of Siemens Medical Systems.) (d) Scans of the abdomen and thorax reveal the excellent soft tissue contrast available with MRI, as shown in this coronal image. (Reproduced with permission courtesy of the National Library of Medicine's Visible Human Project, at http://www.nlm.nih.gov.)

MRI scanners work by using a subtle magnetic effect to detect the concentration and chemical environments of molecules, such as water and fat, in different regions of the body. We will see that it is possible to understand MRI's basic principles quite adequately with little mathematics, employing simple analogies to everyday magnets. For the moment, imagine that water, fat, and other molecules in the body act like numerous tiny radio stations when placed in an MRI scanner. Their broadcast signal strength indicates how much water or fat is present. Each location within the body broadcasts at a slightly different frequency, so by "tuning in" receivers to only one frequency, we can detect how much water or fat, for example, is at that location. While the body does not broadcast naturally by itself, it can be made to do so by placing it within a strong magnet while beaming in radio waves at just the right frequency. This simplified analogy will serve as a good starting point for the detailed descriptions to come.

How safe is MRI? Because MRI uses nonionizing radio waves, not ionizing radiation, it poses a very different set of potential problems than either x-ray or radioisotope imaging. Thus far, no evidence exists that the magnetic fields or radiation used in present clinical MRI scanners offer any risks to persons being examined. No human studies indicate any ill effects, and the type of animal and cell experiments that first signaled problems with x-rays bear out the safety of the radio power levels used in clinical scanners. Later, we will consider the complex issue of how the safety of MRI is evaluated, and the precautions necessary for its use.

To understand MRI's unique capabilities—and limitations—we must first take a temporary diversion to learn about the basics of magnetism and the magnetic properties of the atomic nucleus. We will then learn about the peculiar properties of the body that allow MRI to sensitively distinguish subtle differences in body tissue, and how a spatial map of the body is assembled. Finally, we will return to applications of MRI, including its use in sports medicine, the detection of breast cancer, and brain imaging.

> **Simple experiments to try:** To illustrate the exotic magnetic phenomena of magnetic resonance, we will describe some very simple experiments. You may either imagine these experiments or actually try them out for yourself. They require two bar magnets, a compass, and a toy top.

8.2 THE SCIENCE OF MAGNETISM

Since the same basic phenomenon underlies MRI and everyday applications of magnets in compasses, electric motors, and even the ubiquitous refrigerator magnet, we will begin by considering the properties of the simplest type, the **dipole** bar magnet shown in Figure 8.3. Each bar magnet has two ends with different magnetic properties; we call one end a **north pole** and the other a **south pole** to denote this difference. (We will see that this nomenclature comes about because the Earth itself acts like an enormous dipole magnet.) A quantity called the **dipole moment** is used to describe the magnitude and direction of a dipole's magnetism; its direction is defined to point from the south toward the north pole. Certain materials, called **permanent magnets**, can possess an inherent magnetic dipole moment when properly prepared. Many alloys of iron, including many steels, can form permanent magnets, as do samarium and cobalt alloys used to make extremely strong magnets for commercial uses.

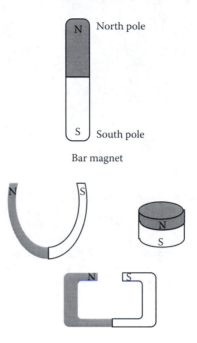

Figure 8.3 Each dipole magnet has a north and a south pole. Many shapes are possible, but each dipole magnet still has this basic structure.

If you have two dipole magnets at your disposal, try moving them near each other and noting the forces between the two for different orientations. The most noticeable feature of two dipole magnets' interaction with each other is that opposite poles attract (north attracts south), while like poles repel. Another easily observed effect is that two dipole magnets have a preferred orientation that they will assume when brought close together. If allowed to move freely, they experience forces that rotate them into place with the north pole near the other magnet's south pole (Figure 8.4a). This principle determines the operation of a compass. The needle of the compass is a tiny dipole magnet, mounted so that it can rotate freely in response to these attractive and repulsive forces until its north pole points "north." (That is, the needle points toward the Earth's magnetic south pole, which is close enough to the geographic north pole for most navigational purposes.)

We can express this by saying that two dipole magnets are in their state of lowest energy when oriented in opposite directions (Figure 8.4a). You must add energy to this system by exerting on the magnets **torques**, the rotational analog of force, defined by both a force and its orientation with respect to the axis of rotation, to make them assume other, higher energy configurations. To see this, hold the two dipoles in their preferred orientation, then carefully twist one 180° (Figure 8.4b). Notice that you had to

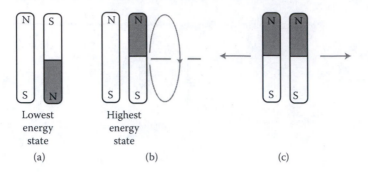

Figure 8.4 (a) For dipole magnets, like poles repel and unlike poles attract. The most favorable, lowest energy configuration for two dipole magnets is shown. (b) A torque (rotational force) must be applied to rotate the two dipoles into their highest energy configuration. (c) If unable to rotate, two dipoles in a high energy configuration (north poles and south poles in close proximity) will experience forces that accelerate them away from each other. This converts energy stored in their magnetic configuration into energy of motion.

exert a torque—and hence do work—on the magnets to make them assume the higher energy final orientation; your action of twisting the magnets into this orientation stores up energy. If the magnets cannot rotate when you place them on a smooth surface and release them, they will instead move away from each other, converting the stored magnetic energy into kinetic energy (Figure 8.4c). This process of adding energy to a magnetic system by reorienting it to a higher energy state, then allowing that energy to be released when it relaxes to its lowest energy state, lies at the core of MRI.

Remarkably, the forces magnets exert on each other extend to great distances, as you can see by moving your compass to different positions at varying distances around a dipole bar magnet. To describe the interaction between one magnet and another, we can define a new quantity called a **magnetic field**. The magnetic field at a particular location is defined as always pointing along the direction of the compass at that point, while its magnitude is a measure of the torque required to reorient the compass needle from this preferred orientation. We represent this graphically by drawing **magnetic field lines** with arrowheads pointing north everywhere (Figure 8.5a); the magnitude of the field is denoted by how closely the lines cluster. For example, in Figure 8.5(a) the field is strongest near the ends of the dipole, and relatively weak farther away.

The units for measuring magnetic field magnitude are the small **gauss** and much larger **tesla** (**T**): one tesla is equal to 10,000 gauss. At its surface, the Earth's magnetic field is roughly one gauss (10^{-4} T). A very strong refrigerator magnet can have fields as high as 250 gauss (0.025 T). Modern MRI magnets capable of advanced imaging typically use fields of 1.5 T (15,000 gauss). Lower fields can give good images and are employed in some

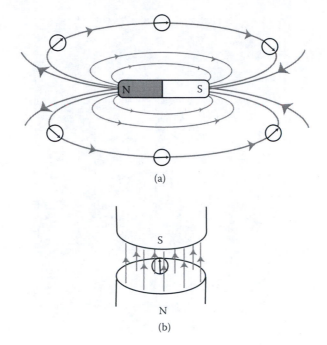

Figure 8.5 (a) The magnetic fields surrounding a dipole magnet have the orientation shown, with the field lines at a particular location lying parallel to the direction of a compass at that point. The magnetic field strength is greatest where the field lines are bunched most closely together, at the ends of the dipole in this case. Only a few of all possible field lines are drawn. All of the lines that originate from either pole loop back to the opposite pole. (b) The magnetic fields used for MRI must be very uniform in magnitude and orientation. One configuration for achieving this is to use a dipole magnet with its poles brought close together. (Fields outside the region of interest are not shown.) (c) "Open" MRI scanner using the magnetic field geometry shown in (b). (Reproduced with permission courtesy of Siemens Medical Systems.)

systems, while high fields of over 4 T are used in fMRI scanners. These values all refer to the **static** field, the magnetic field that is constant in time and present in the MRI scanner at all times. Imposed on this static field are **fluctuating** fields (those that change with time) of much lower field strength. The magnetic field in an MRI magnet is especially easy to understand. If you bring a north and south pole very close together, what results is a region in which the magnetic field's magnitude and direction both are very uniform (Figure 8.5b). If you were to hold a dipole magnet within such a field, you would feel no forces or torques as long as your magnet was in the orientation of the compass shown. Just as for the two dipole magnets, this would constitute the lowest energy configuration, and the configuration with the compass needle rotated 180° would be the highest energy state.

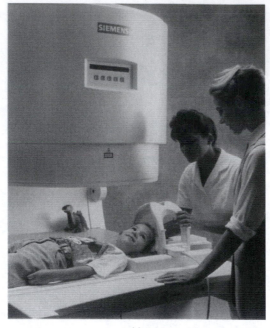

(c)

Figure 8.5 (continued).

MRI scanners can indeed be made using giant permanent magnets like the one shown in Figure 8.5(b), but because these are limited to fields on the lower end of that achievable for MRI magnets, they cannot perform some modern imaging techniques. However, this magnetic field geometry is used in "open" MRI scanners, which offer an environment less confining than standard scanners (Figure 8.5c). Instead, most MRI scanners employ **electro-magnets** (magnets formed using wires carrying electrical currents) to create magnetic fields. Electromagnets are also used in numerous common applications, including motors and loudspeakers. The electrical configuration needed to generate a dipole electromagnet is surprisingly simple: it simply involves passing an electrical current (a flow of electrical charge) through a loop of wire (Figure 8.6a). If a current circulates around the wire loop with the orientation shown in Figure 8.6(a), then its magnetic properties will be identical to those of a permanent dipole magnet (Figure 8.5a). To create the uniform magnetic field required for MRI, many current-carrying loops of wire are wound into a spiral to form a **solenoid** magnet (Figure 8.6b). This configuration is used because the resulting magnetic field within the **bore** (central opening of the cylindrical magnet) is highly uniform in both direction and magnitude. The characteristic cylindrical shape of most MRI scanners is determined by such a solenoid magnet (Figure 8.6c). For scans of the entire body, giant magnets roughly 2 meters long are used.

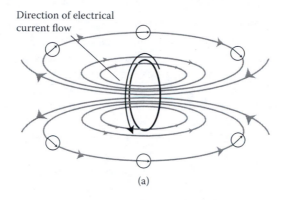

Direction of electrical current flow

(a)

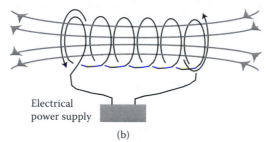

Electrical power supply

(b)

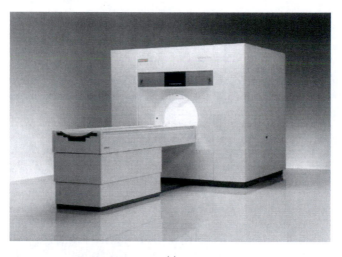

(c)

Figure 8.6 (a) A wire loop around which an electrical current (flow of electrical charge) flows has a magnetic field resembling that of a dipole bar magnet. (Compare to Figure 8.5a.) (b) If a long spiral of wire is used instead, the magnetic field strength within this solenoid magnet is very uniform in magnitude and direction. (c) Standard MRI scanner employing a solenoidal magnet for achieving the main magnetic field. (Reproduced with permission courtesy of Siemens Medical Systems.)

Superconducting magnets for MRI: If you plug too many appliances into an extension cord, the large flow of electrical current will cause noticeable heating of the cord. Similarly, the large flow of electrical current used to generate the enormous magnetic fields for MRI can cause appreciable heating if ordinary metal wires are used. Considerable electrical power is required to replace the energy lost to heat, as well as to cool the wires. However, MRI magnets can avoid this problem by taking advantage of a remarkable effect called **superconductivity**.

In an ordinary metal like copper, the electrons that flow to generate the current can be thought of as colliding with nuclei of metal atoms in constant thermal motion. These collisions transfer energy to the atoms, increasing their average energy of random thermal motion, and hence raising the metal's temperature in an effect called **Joule heating**. This effect has many practical applications, since it is the principle by which electric ovens, toasters, hairdryers, and other electrical heating devices work. By contrast, in superconductivity, interactions between the electrons and nuclei cause distortions in the nuclei's positions that ease the passage of the electrons. This cooperative motion of electrons and nuclei results in zero collisions and no heating. Because no energy is lost from the electrons' motion, the electrical current will circulate indefinitely with no need of additional electrical power. Wires made of alloys of the superconducting metals niobium and titanium can carry the currents in MRI magnets. To remain in the superconducting state, these wires must be kept below −250°C, using a cooling bath of liquid helium. Superconducting magnets give fields that are practically perfectly constant, with no fluctuations and with decreases of only a few gauss (10^{-4} T) every year.

8.3 NUCLEAR MAGNETISM

What would happen if we were to break a dipole bar magnet in two? You might reasonably expect that one north pole fragment and one south pole fragment would result. Surprisingly, two new *dipoles* are created, no matter how carefully we chop the original magnet (Figure 8.7a). If we further subdivide the new dipoles, the same thing happens: we just get smaller dipoles. In fact, this same phenomenon continues if we continue to divide until our magnets consist of individual atoms. By examining individual atoms, we would discover that even electrons, and the components of the nucleus—protons and neutrons—are inherently dipole magnets (Figure 8.7b).

In many experiments, electrons, protons, and neutrons also behave as though they were spinning about an axis. Consequently, they can be described as having a quantity called **spin**, which defines the magnitude and the direction of the axis about which they revolve. Since the spin is also

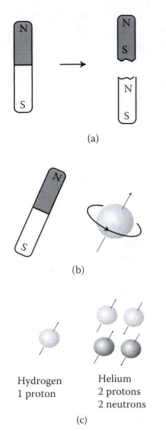

Figure 8.7 (a) If a bar magnet is broken in two, each fragment becomes a new dipole. Isolated north or south poles are never observed. (b) Tiny subatomic particles, such as protons, neutrons, and electrons, act like tiny dipole magnets. The orientation of their dipoles is given by the particle's spin orientation. (c) The nuclei of some elements, such as helium, have even numbers of protons and neutrons. The spins in these elements align to give zero net spin, so these nuclei do not act like magnetic dipoles. By contrast, the nucleus of hydrogen-1, with only 1 proton, does act like a nuclear dipole magnet.

(a)

(b)

Hydrogen
1 proton

Helium
2 protons
2 neutrons

(c)

related to the orientation of their magnetic dipole, the two terms are often used in describing the magnetism of atoms. A simple mechanical analogy can be used to justify this relationship: a spinning charged particle acts like a tiny electromagnet, because its rotation results in an electrical current with an associated magnetic dipole.

Even though most materials are not magnetic, their subatomic constituents are always magnetic. Much of the phenomena associated with magnetism results from the configurations of the dipoles of the *electrons* within materials. Within most atoms and molecules, the dipoles of electrons are paired north to south within each atomic orbital, so that their magnetic fields cancel out exactly. These materials are called **diamagnetic**. Magnetic fields have little or no effect on diamagnetic materials; water and almost all body chemicals fall within this nonmagnetic category. **Paramagnetism** results when one or more orbitals are filled with only one electron, so that a net atomic dipole results. When placed in another magnet's field, these atomic dipoles orient along the external field lines, thus increasing the total magnetic field. The pigment melanin, and some body chemicals containing iron, are paramagnetic. Permanent magnets also have unpaired electrons, and hence atomic dipoles. However, only in certain cases do interactions between the unpaired electrons promote the orientation of their dipoles in the same direction, creating a magnetic field even when no external magnet is present. This situation results in **ferromagnetism**; ferromagnetic materials are used to create permanent magnets.

However, MRI detects the magnetism of atomic *nuclei*, rather than that of electrons. If an atomic nucleus contains an even number of protons, their dipoles cancel exactly, and the same is true for neutrons (Figure 8.7c). Examples of nuclei with no net magnetic dipole include the most common isotopes of helium-4 (2 protons, 2 neutrons), carbon-12 (6 protons, 6 neutrons), oxygen-16 (8 of each), and calcium-40 (20 of each). However, if a nucleus has an odd number of either protons or neutrons, an overall net dipole remains from the unpaired nucleons. This **nuclear magnetism** gives dipoles 1000 times weaker than those due to electrons, so it is not a factor in the behavior of permanent magnets. Nuclei with net magnetic dipole moments include hydrogen-1 (with only 1 proton), phosphorus-31 (15 protons, 16 neutrons), and carbon-13 (6 protons, 7 neutrons).

In the absence of any magnetic field, a nucleus' magnetic dipole can point in any direction, and it has the same energy for any orientation. However, the quantum mechanical nature of the nucleus manifests itself when it is placed in a magnetic field like the one provided by an MRI scanner. While an ordinary bar magnet can point in any direction in a magnetic field and hence have any orientation energy, an atomic nucleus can assume only limited orientations. For most nuclei, the limited choices are either to point aligned with (spin up or parallel), or opposite to (spin down or antiparallel) the magnetic field, corresponding to a different energy for each orientation. Even more peculiarly, due to the effects of quantum mechanics, the nuclear dipole does not wholly align with the magnetic field, but lies at a fixed angle to it. Its direction perpendicular to the field is undetermined. To describe this situation, we can label an energy diagram for the nucleus' different orientation, just like the energy diagram for electron orbitals in Chapter 3, showing how the presence of the external magnetic field creates two energy levels (possible values of the nucleus' energy) (Figure 8.8a).

The nuclear magnetic dipole can flip its orientation by absorbing or emitting an energy exactly equal to the energy difference, ΔE, between states (Figure 8.8a). This energy difference depends on the magnetic field, as well as upon the exact makeup of the atomic nucleus. The exact value of this energy difference is given by:

$$\Delta E = 2 \times 2.79 \times \mu_n B \tag{8.1}$$

where B is the magnitude of the magnetic field in tesla, and μ_n is a number equal to 5.05×10^{-27} J/T, called the **nuclear magneton**. The factor of 2.79 is an experimentally determined value peculiar to the proton; for nuclei of other isotopes, a different number would be used in computing the energy difference.

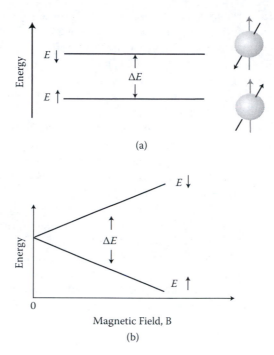

(a)

(b)

Figure 8.8 (a) Energy level diagram for a nucleus with spin placed in a uniform magnetic field of magnitude B. For a given value of B, nuclei oriented parallel to (spin up) and antiparallel to (spin down) have different energies, with the lower (more favorable) configuration corresponding to the spin up orientation. An energy difference, ΔE, is required to flip the nucleus between orientations. (b) The energy difference, ΔE, is proportional to B, so greater energy differences are achieved for higher magnetic fields.

Sample calculation: What is a typical energy spacing in eV between levels for proton in a magnetic field with strength 1.00 T, comparable to values used in MRI scanners? Using Equation 8.1, we get:

$$\Delta E = 2 \times 2.79 \times \mu_n B$$

$$= 2 \times 2.79 \times \left(5.05 \times 10^{-27} \text{ J/T}\right) \times 1.00\text{T} \times \left(1.0\text{eV}/1.60 \times 10^{-19}\text{J}\right)$$

$$= 1.7 \times 10^{-7} \text{eV}$$

The energy difference is only 0.176 millionths of an eV.

The energy difference is simply proportional to the magnetic field magnitude (Figure 8.8b); doubling the magnitude doubles the spacing, etc. For hydrogen nuclei, we saw above that this energy spacing is 0.176 *millionths* of an eV for a 1.00 T magnetic field, while the values for other isotopes within the body, such as phosphorus-31 and sodium-23, are even lower. To appreciate how extremely small these energies are, recall that x-ray photons have energies on the order of 1 keV or more, while chemical bond energies and photons of visible light both have energies on the order of eV. Consequently, nuclear magnetism does not play a role in the body's chemical processes, because it lacks the energy to influence chemical bond formation.

Photons with energies matching the differences between nuclear dipole orientations lie in the radio frequency (RF) regime of the electromagnetic spectrum, so nuclear dipoles can reorient by emitting or absorbing energy from RF photons. While we have very different associations with radio waves than with visible light and x-rays, they too are yet another form of electromagnetic radiation (Chapter 3). In addition to categorizing radiation by the energy carried by each photon, we can also consider the fluctuating electrical and magnetic forces induced when an RF wave sweeps by. Associated with the energy per photon is a characteristic frequency of these disturbances. The radio frequency gives the number of times per second the oscillating magnetic field associated with the radio wave fluctuates through an entire cycle (Figure 8.9).

The RF wave's frequency determines how it interacts with nuclear magnetic dipoles since nuclei have both a specific energy and frequency at which they absorb and emit RF waves. When a system responds preferentially to one characteristic frequency, we say it exhibits a **resonance**. Consequently, the selective absorption of only certain frequency waves by nuclear magnetic dipoles is called **nuclear magnetic resonance** (**NMR**). You can observe a simple example of magnetic resonance with a compass.

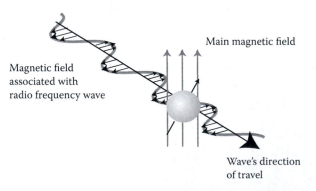

Figure 8.9 The magnetic field associated with a radio frequency (RF) wave oscillates both in space and as a function of time. The orientation between the exciting RF wave's magnetic field and the main magnetic field of an MRI scanner is shown.

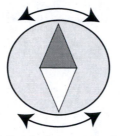

A disturbed compass needle
swings about its preferred orientation

(a)

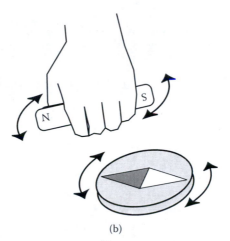

(b)

Figure 8.10 (a) Illustration of magnetic resonance with a compass. When undisturbed, the compass needle points steadily north. If deflected momen-
tarily, the needle oscillates (swings back and forth) around that
direction. The time between swings defines the compass' resonant
frequency. (b) Bringing a bar magnet nearby changes this resonant frequency. If the bar magnet is oscillated nearby, the compass needle
responses strongly only at its resonant frequency.

When undisturbed, the compass needle points steadily north. What if the
needle is deflected using a bar magnet and then allowed to recover? Rather
than immediately pointing north, the needle oscillates (swings back and
forth) around that direction (Figure 8.10). The time between swings defines
a **resonant frequency**, which is about one oscillation per second (1 Hz) for
most compasses. This frequency depends on the magnetic field experienced
by the compass, as you can see by bringing a bar magnet close and observing the higher frequency swings that result. The resonant frequency also
describes the optimal frequency for disturbing the needle. To see this, twist
your bar magnet back and forth regularly. For very slow or very rapid
twisting motions, the needle will not respond appreciably. However, if you

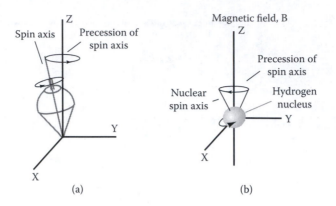

Figure 8.11 (a) Gravitational force will cause a top to fall over if it is not spinning. However, a spinning top precesses when it feels the pull of gravity. During precession, the axis about which the top spins itself rotates, tracing out a cone. (b) Nuclear spins also precess about the direction of an external magnetic field at their resonant (Larmor) frequency.

rotate the bar magnet at exactly the resonant frequency, the needle will swing wildly in response.

Nuclear dipoles also have a resonant frequency (called the **Larmor frequency**) at which they naturally oscillate. To visualize their more complex behavior, first imagine the analogous motion of a toy top. If you place a top on its end without setting it spinning first, it will fall over because of the downward pull of gravity. However, if you first set the top spinning, it will behave very differently when set on its end and released. Rather than making it fall over, the force of gravity unexpectedly causes the spinning top to **precess**—that is, the axis about which it spins slowly sweeps around in a cone (Figure 8.11a).

Similarly, a nuclear dipole does not *entirely* orient along an external magnetic field, but rather, lies at an angle with respect to the field direction. The upward force exerted on the spinning nucleus by the magnetic field causes the dipole to precess, sweeping around at a characteristic resonant frequency (Figure 8.11b), just as the downward force of gravity made the top precess. A single precessing dipole itself generates a time-changing magnetic field, which spreads outward from the nucleus as an RF wave. The nuclei in the body do not spontaneously broadcast radio waves when placed in a magnetic field, however. This is because the magnetic dipoles within a region are randomly oriented, so that their fluctuating magnetic fields cancel on average (Figure 8.12).

If we denote by f the Larmor frequency of the photon that can cause these spin-flipping transitions, then:

$$f = \Delta E/h = 2 \times 2.79 \times \mu_n B/h \tag{8.2}$$

where h is Planck's constant, 6.63×10^{-34} J-s. The latter expression holds true for protons; for another nuclear species, the factor of 2.79 would be replaced by an appropriate value. This equation relates the energy absorbed in the transition between different energy levels and the frequency of absorbed photons. The simplest case is for a hydrogen-1 nucleus containing a single proton. (We will often simply refer to hydrogen-1 nuclei as protons.) For hydrogen, the frequency is 42.5 MHz for B = 1.00 T. (Recall that the frequency and energy both depend directly on magnetic field strength.)

Sample calculation: We get this value by using a magnetic field of B = 1.00 T in Equation 8.2:

$$f = 2 \times 2.79 \times \mu_n B / h$$

$$= 2 \times 2.79 \times \left(5.05 \times 10^{-27}\,\text{J/T}\right) \times 1.00\text{T} \Big/ \left(6.63 \times 10^{-34}\,\text{J} \cdot \text{s}\right)$$

$$= 4.25 \times 10^7\,\text{s}^{-1} = 42.5 \times 10^6\,\text{Hz} = 42.5\,\text{MHz}$$

Thus, photons with a Larmor frequency of 42.5 MHz will have the correct energy to cause transitions between the up and down spin states of a proton.

The nucleus's resonant frequency is proportional to the energy difference between spin up and spin down orientations, so it depends on the nucleus under consideration and it is proportional to the magnetic field magnitude. For protons, the resonant frequency is 64 MHz for a 1.5 T magnetic field. Lower frequencies of 26 MHz are found for the nuclei phosphorus-31, and 17 MHz for sodium-23. (For comparison, your radio dial has an FM range of about 88 to 108 MHz and an AM frequency range of 0.54 to 1.60 MHz.)

During MRI scans, radio transmitters are used to broadcast RF electromagnetic radiation into the body. RF waves penetrate deep inside because water and other body chemicals absorb relatively little energy at those frequencies, so signals can easily be transmitted into and out of the body. Once inside, a small fraction of the RF photons with the appropriate resonant frequency are absorbed by nuclei. This process, called **excitation**, results in both absorption of energy from the RF wave and reorientation of the nuclear spins.

What happens to the nucleus when it experiences both the main magnetic field and an oscillating field due to the RF wave? To visualize its response, consider Figure 8.12. The RF waves used for MRI excitation have their magnetic field oriented perpendicularly to that of the main scanner magnet; such a situation can be produced by using an appropriately oriented radio transmitter built into the MRI scanner. The oscillation in time of

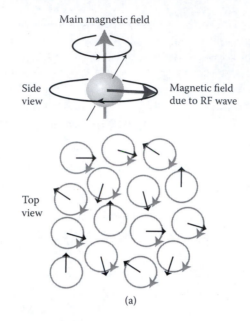

Main magnetic field

Side view

Magnetic field due to RF wave

Top view

(a)

Figure 8.12 (a) Before an RF pulse, nuclei in the body precess in such a way that, on average, their dipoles lie parallel to the main magnetic field. Since each nucleus ordinarily precesses with a random orientation *perpendicular* to the main field, there is no average time-changing magnetic field for an entire region. This means that no RF waves are emitted from the body before the RF pulse. (b) An RF wave can be generated so that its magnetic field at a fixed point rotates at the wave's radio frequency. When the RF wave's frequency coincides with the nucleus' resonant frequency, magnetic forces due to the wave will cause the dipole to tip over during the RF wave's duration. If the wave is turned off after the dipole has been tipped perpendicular to the main field, it is referred to as a 90° RF pulse. For spin flips of 180°, twice the RF pulse duration is required.

the RF waves results in a continual rotation of the magnetic field direction (Figure 8.12). This second, fluctuating field adds to the main magnetic field, but its value is too tiny to significantly alter the resonant frequency. It does, however, produce an additional force on the dipole, which tends to tip it over to greater angles. If the RF wave does not oscillate at the resonant frequency, this force averages to zero, just as the wrong frequency fails to disturb the compass significantly. For waves at the resonant frequency, the tipping forces constantly reinforce, causing the nucleus' spin to gradually tip over as it precesses (Figure 8.12). The angle by which the spin is tipped (called the **spin flip angle**) depends on how long the RF wave acts on it; MRI scanners often use pulses that flip the dipole by exactly 90° or 180°. We call the exciting RF signal a **pulse** because it is typically switched on for only a short period of time. Any spin flip angle can be achieved by applying a sufficiently long pulse of RF.

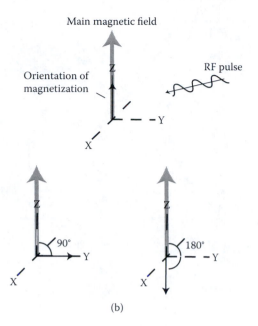

(b)

Figure 8.12 (continued).

After the RF pulse has been switched off, the nuclei continue to precess at the resonant frequency. If this process occurs inside an MRI scanner, the magnetic fields due to *all* of the nuclei in a region of the patient's body oscillate in synchrony. The nuclei act like radio transmitters, their oscillating magnetic field generating a new RF signal at exactly the resonant frequency. We call the emitted RF wave the **free induction signal** to distinguish it from the exciting RF wave that caused the precession in the first place.

The RF free induction signal (often referred to as just "the signal" here) is detected by the MRI scanner using a radio receiver. The receiving antenna consists simply of coils of wire placed near the body. The RF signal induces within the antenna time-changing voltages that can be measured to determine the frequency and magnitude of the free induction signal. Scanners have built-in receiving coils, but for some imaging applications, special receiving antennae are used. **Surface coils,** consisting of wires covered with plastic insulation and padding, are placed directly on the body over the parts of interest (Figure 8.13). These surface coils "listen in" only on broadcasting nuclei in a hemispherical region directly underneath. Their immediate proximity to the body allows them to more efficiently collect an RF signal to produce a better quality MR image from superficially located tissues. We will return to this subject later when considering imaging applications.

The strength of the free induction signal is proportional to the number of nuclei that respond to the exciting RF field. Since different nuclei have different resonant frequencies, a particular frequency of excitation singles

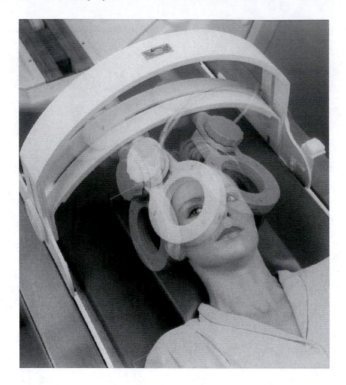

Figure 8.13 Special receiving antennae called surface coils are designed to collect RF signals from a small region of the body directly beneath the coil. Their use allows higher resolution scans of a specific part of the body such as the head or joints. (Used with permission courtesy of Siemens Medical Systems.)

out only one chemical species. Hydrogen nuclei are by far most commonly used for MRI, since most body tissues are roughly 75% water. Because each water molecule has two hydrogens, it follows that a perfect candidate for study is located naturally throughout the body. Molecules of fat also have many hydrogens, and provide another signal source. Since mineralized bone has only 10% water content, and the major isotopes of its calcium and oxygen have no net magnetic dipole, the skeleton is transparent to MRI. Because bones do not obscure other structures, even the bone marrow and spinal cord can easily be examined.

Because NMR can detect small changes in magnetic fields due to other atoms' magnetic dipoles, it is sensitive to the arrangements of atoms within molecules. One major application, **NMR spectroscopy** (called **MR spectroscopy** when performed in the body), analyzes chemical structure by detecting the different resonant frequencies characteristic of hydrogens in different chemical environments either in the laboratory or within the human body. The **chemical shift** is defined as the difference in resonant frequency between an isolated hydrogen and its value when bound to a specific site within a molecule. The chemical shift between fat and water hydrogens is only 220 Hz out of 63.9 *million* Hz for 1.5 T, typical of the parts per million frequency differences usually measured. Chemical NMR apparatuses can measure these subtle changes only by using an extremely uniform magnetic field whose strength varies by less than 1 part in 10 million over several centimeters.

In NMR spectroscopy, radio waves of various frequencies are beamed at a tiny sample of the chemical, and the absorption of energy at each frequency is noted. The frequencies of absorption indicate the chemical species with which the hydrogens are associated. While NMR spectroscopy is most frequently performed on hydrogen nuclei, other magnetic nuclei, such as phosphorus-31, are natural candidates for study, as we will consider later.

8.4 CONTRAST MECHANISMS FOR MRI

So far, NMR sounds like an ideal technique for probing the body: we need only measure the chemical shift everywhere within the body to detect the concentration of water, fat, proteins, etc., then use this information to map anatomy. Unfortunately, this simple concept cannot be used to generate detailed images. The extremely uniform fields used to distinguish the tiny chemical shifts are difficult to maintain over the entire body; equally important, MR spectroscopy by itself generates no spatial information about where the chemicals reside.

Instead, MRI scanners work by measuring signals from only one chemical species at once—almost always hydrogen nuclei—while using deliberately imposed changes in magnetic field strength to localize them. Thus, one would assume that the signals measured in MRI directly probe only regional **proton density** (hydrogen concentration). However, this brings us back to the problem that plagues x-ray imaging: virtually all soft tissues have very similar water (and hence proton) concentrations. While proton-density images indeed play a role in MRI, other magnetic properties of human tissue often prove more important. The other magnetic properties that MRI measures to overcome the limitations of proton-density images are so surprising, that we will consider a fanciful analogy before discussing them.

Imagine you are traveling in a foreign country whose language is wholly unknown to you. You are staying with friends who take care of all arrangements. One day, you accidentally become separated from them while in a distant part of the city. Your initial panic subsides when you remember that they have provided you with a map. However, on inspection, the map itself proves to be in their foreign tongue and none of the passersby knows your language. How will you find your way?

Fortunately, a map in a strange language can still be a good guide if you can gradually piece together which features in the landscape correspond to the labels on the map. For example, you could find nearby street signs and locate those streets on the map, then work outward from that starting point. As you progress, you would probably learn to associate words with types of places (for example, the word for post office or library).

In fact, this situation describes much of the history of biology. Cells are mostly transparent, so they do not reveal much of their structure under the microscope. Out of necessity, microscopists have traditionally employed stains—chemicals used to make structural distinctions visible. However, until recently, these stains were just found in practice to color one part of the cell and not another, and the reason why was not known. These stories all show how a map of some sort—*any* sort—can be helpful if you can piece together its meaning. This is relevant because much of MRI involves measuring peculiar magnetic quantities rather than those of immediate and obvious physiological importance. However, by associating these measurements with known anatomy, and by learning how they correspond to disease states, doctors have learned to interpret these seemingly arbitrary maps.

We now return to our discussion of what is actually measured in MRI. Once again, imagine disturbing a compass needle from its preferred orientation using a bar magnet, then watching it recover. At first, the needle oscillates at the resonant frequency. Then these oscillations decay gradually in time, leaving the magnet pointed along the local field (Figure 8.14). We call the time required for the magnet to reachieve a fixed percentage of its

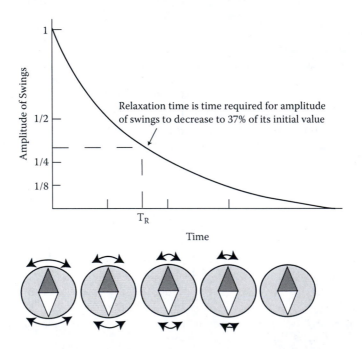

Figure 8.14 Simple example of relaxation times in magnetic systems. A compass needle disturbed from its preferred orientation will oscillate about that position, as described in Figure 8.10. The *amplitude* of the oscillations decays in time, with a characteristic behavior described by its relaxation time.

preferred orientation a **relaxation time**. MRI makes extensive use of these relaxation times, which are often a more sensitive probe of chemical environment than proton density by itself.

So far our discussion has considered how RF signals affect individual magnetic dipoles. However, an MRI scanner can only excite and detect RF signals from many nuclei at once. For this reason, we need to define a quantity called the **magnetization**, defined as the *net* magnetic dipole in a region containing many microscopic dipoles. A simple analogy would be to imagine that many magnets are nailed to a board in many different orientations. Then, a compass will respond to this array of magnets as if to an imaginary magnet with a dipole given by the board's magnetization (Figure 8.15). If the nuclei are oriented at random, their magnetic dipole contributions to the total magnetic field cancel so the magnetization is exactly zero at long distances. In the body, when no magnetic field is present, this cancellation always occurs, so all human tissues ordinarily have zero magnetization. An MRI scanner's main magnet induces a magnetization within the body, which points in the same direction as the main field. This is because the torques exerted on the individual magnetic dipoles tend to align them along the direction of the external field. This magnetization does not, however, result from a total alignment of all of the nuclear dipoles within the body. The nuclear magnetic dipoles in body tissue are always flipping over due to their random thermal motions, even in a very strong magnetic field—just as many compasses on a vibrating table would swing in all directions, with only a small bias toward pointing along the Earth's magnetic field. In fact, a field of 1 T is capable of aligning an excess of only

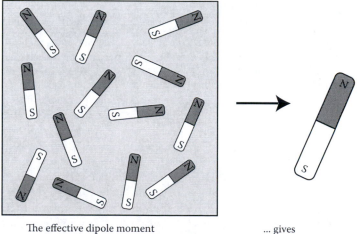

The effective dipole moment
of an assembly of dipoles...

... gives
the magnetization

Figure 8.15 The magnetization (right) gives the net effective dipole moment due to a collection of dipoles within a region of material, such as body tissue (left).

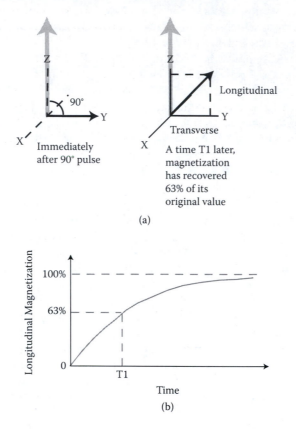

(a)

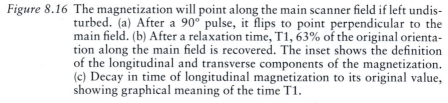

(b)

Figure 8.16 The magnetization will point along the main scanner field if left undisturbed. (a) After a 90° pulse, it flips to point perpendicular to the main field. (b) After a relaxation time, T1, 63% of the original orientation along the main field is recovered. The inset shows the definition of the longitudinal and transverse components of the magnetization. (c) Decay in time of longitudinal magnetization to its original value, showing graphical meaning of the time T1.

1 in every 290,000 nuclei! This tiny imbalance gives the magnetization that is detected in MRI.

The compass needle simply rotates in a plane, but the magnetization in a region of tissue precesses in a much more complex way. As a result, more than one relaxation time must be used to describe its decay to normal. To begin our discussion, consider the effect of an RF pulse that reorients the magnetization 90° from its initial value (Figure 8.16a). Nuclei excited by this RF signal gradually reorient themselves until all lie along the main field direction again in an exponential decay process (Chapter 6). The time it takes for this reorientation to be 63% complete is called **T1**, the **longitudinal relaxation time** (Figure 8.16). (Longitudinal means lying along, or parallel with, the main magnetic field.)

The processes that result in longitudinal relaxation are not driven by static magnetic fields (such as those due to small nonuniformities in the main magnet). However, the magnetic field around a nucleus contains fluctuating contributions from other atoms in ceaseless thermal motion, and these magnetic fields *can* shorten T1. In order to flip nuclei back to their preferred orientation, fluctuations in the local magnetic field at the resonant frequency are required. (Thus, the value of T1 *does* depend on the main magnetic field magnitude, since that value determines the Larmor frequency.) While the changing magnetic fields around the nucleus will take place at all frequencies, there will be a small contribution at exactly the resonant frequency. The nucleus can then absorb energy from this contribution, flipping back to its preferred orientation more quickly and thereby shortening T1. Thus, the value of T1 can depend significantly upon the local environment of a proton within the body.

Table 8.1 lists some characteristic relaxation times for various body tissues. For example, water molecules are small and mobile. Their rapid motion precludes the strong interactions at the Larmor frequency which would promote a rapid decay of the longitudinal magnetization. As a result, pure water has a long T1 in the range 2.5 to 3 seconds, and similar values are found for urine, for water fluids in cysts, and for cerebrospinal fluid in the brain and central nervous system. However, T1 values for most tissues are appreciably shorter, and vary considerably throughout the body. For example, the hydrogens in fat have a T1 of only 260 milliseconds at 1.5 T, because the long, chainlike fat molecules are slower moving and couple more effectively to their environment. Proteins, surfaces within cells, and meshlike protein gels can constrain the thermal agitation of nearby molecules, shifting more motions to lower frequencies, hence giving more motions at the resonant frequency. Effects like these allow extremely small concentrations of other body chemicals to cause T1 to vary significantly even between tissues with very similar water content, providing an excellent source of contrast between soft tissues.

Table 8.1 Typical MRI parameters for various body tissues

Type of tissue	Effective proton density	T1[a] (milliseconds)	T2 (milliseconds)
Fat	1.00	260	80
Gray matter	0.8	900	100
White matter	0.7	780	90
Cerebrospinal fluid	1.0	2400	160
Muscle	0.75	870	45
Liver	0.75	500	40

[a] T1 depends on magnetic field; values for 1.5 T only are shown.

Meanwhile, at the same time that the longitudinal component is growing, the **transverse component**—that component of the magnetization which is perpendicular to the main field—is shrinking (Figures 8.16 and 8.17). When the system is totally relaxed, the transverse component is equal to zero (Figure 8.16c). It may seem obvious that the time, **T2**, for **transverse relaxation** should merely be equal to T1, since the growth of T1 implies the decrease of T2. Indeed, the two times can have close to the same value; since the transverse magnetization also necessarily decays when the longitudinal part has returned to normal, T2 always must be equal to or less than T1. However, in the body, T2 can be much shorter than T1, so it provides another contrast mechanism for distinguishing body tissues.

To understand how T2 can be different from T1, consider Figure 8.17. Immediately after a 90° RF pulse, all of the nuclei in a region precess in synchrony, and they would continue to do so if the resonant frequency were the same for every spin (Figure 8.17a). However, what if local variations in the magnetic field cause the resonant frequency to vary throughout? The spins would then gradually get out of step, some rotating more quickly, some more slowly. After some time had passed, they would be oriented at random (become **decoherent**) (Figure 8.17b). The total RF signal detected by the receiving antenna contains contributions from each nucleus. At first, signals from every nucleus reinforce, giving a large starting RF signal. However, after they have fallen out of step, for every RF signal emitted by a nucleus with one orientation, another with exactly the opposite orientation emits an exactly opposite signal. On average, the signals cancel exactly, so even though the nuclei are still precessing, the region no longer emits a signal. The time for the signal to decrease by 63% of its original value defines T2 (Figure 8.17c). Thus, surprisingly, the signal can decay more rapidly than would be expected from T1 alone.

T2 also depends on chemical environment through variations in magnetic field induced by local atomic dipoles. Both the atoms and their organization matter. For example, liquid water has a very long T2 of 2.5 to 3.0 seconds, but the same water frozen into ice has such a short T2 that no signal can be detected. Because many of the hydrogens in the body will have such short T2 values that no signal is received from them, the proton density measured in MRI is really only a *partial* hydrogen concentration. Unlike the processes of energy absorption required to reorient spins for longitudinal decay, no energy is lost or gained in driving the spins out of synchrony. This also means that *any* frequency of fluctuation caused by thermal agitation can contribute to shortening T2, so in general, T2 is much shorter than T1.

The fluctuating magnetic fields created by the hydrogen's chemical environment also shorten T2 in a fashion characteristic of different types of tissues. Unfortunately, this interesting shortening of T2 is usually overwhelmed by variations due to imperfections in the main magnetic field. Because these variations have nothing to do with the body, a different name is given to the relaxation time that results from external magnetic field

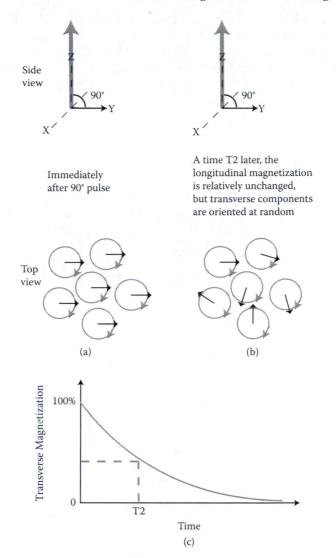

Figure 8.17 (a) Orientation of spins immediately after a 90° pulse, showing uniform direction of precession in-plane. (b) Even if the longitudinal magnetization is relatively unchanged, after a time T2 the transverse components lose coherence in their in-plane orientations. As a result, the free induction signal diminishes as the in-plane orientations become disordered and transverse magnetization decays in time. (c) Decay in time of the transverse magnetization from its original large value (just after the 90° pulse) to zero after several times the decay time T2.

variations: **T2***. Unlike T2, T2* is due only to field variations that do not change in time, a fact that MR scanners take advantage of to measure T2.

Different types of MRI scans yield images constructed by measuring either proton density (hydrogen concentration), or one of these relaxation times; images are said to be **weighted** by the measurement used. T1-weighted images show variations between tissues with different T1 values. If an organ has essentially the same value of T1 throughout, a T2-weighted image can be constructed instead. (In fact, the exact values of T1 and T2 detected depend upon the main field strength, further complicating matters.) To see how these abstract concepts are used to construct an actual MR image, we will now examine one major method for measuring MR contrast.

8.5 LISTENING TO SPIN ECHOES

The problem in trying to measure relaxation times is that the shortest relaxation time dominates the time behavior of the signal. Unfortunately, this is usually T2*, a quantity that has nothing to do with the body. To measure T1 or T2, a more sophisticated method must be used to separate out these more interesting time behaviors. To accomplish this, most imaging techniques use **pulse sequences**, many RF pulses emitted and detected in a series. The free induction signals emitted following several exciting RF pulses are measured in order to tease out information about T1 and T2. One commonly used pulse sequence technique is called **spin-echo imaging**. In understanding this method, you will gain an appreciation of the general ideas behind MR imaging. (Note that the "echoes" in question only share a name with those used in ultrasound imaging; the underlying physics is very different.)

The first step in spin-echo imaging involves using an exciting RF pulse that flips the spins by 90° (Figure 8.18a). After the pulse has ended the spins are left precessing in the orientation shown in Figure 8.18(a). The spins then rapidly fan out and become decoherent with a relaxation time, T2*, determined by static variations in the magnetic field (Figure 8.18b). Thus, while they initially emit a large RF signal, this signal decays rapidly to zero with a relaxation time, T2*.

The next step uses an RF pulse to flip the spins to the exact opposite direction (by 180°) (Figure 8.18c). However, this flip also exactly reverses the direction of the precession of the spins. The same constant variations in static magnetic field that caused the spins to get out of step in the first place now cause them to reconverge into a neat packet. (The spins behave in a fashion similar to race cars, which may leave the starting line at the same time, but which spread out as they travel at different speeds. If the cars were to *exactly* reverse their speeds and travel back to the start, they would once again line up.) When the spins reconverge to a single packet, their individual RF signals once again reinforce and give a large net RF signal, called the **spin echo** (Figure 8.18d and e). The elapsed time between the original pulse and the echo, called **TE**, is determined by the timing of the 180° pulse.

Of course, in the case of the nuclei, processes that relate to T2 relaxation also have been randomly speeding up and slowing down the spins. These

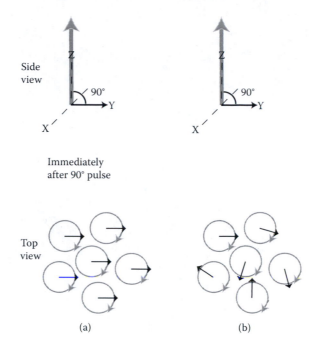

Side view

Immediately after 90° pulse

Top view

(a)

(b)

Figure 8.18 Steps in spin-echo imaging. The time sequences of pulses used and signals collected are illustrated schematically in (e), while (a)–(d) show the accompanying spin orientations. (a) Immediately after a 90° pulse, the spins are oriented perpendicular to the main magnetic field and they precess in the same direction. (b) After some time has elapsed, the effect of the decay of the transverse magnetization results in a progressive loss of the spins' in-plane orientation. (c) A 180° pulse is next used to flip the spins to the exactly opposite direction. This also results in the spins precessing with the opposite orientation. (d) As a result, the faster spins and slower spins precess so as to reconverge along their original direction in a time TE. The resulting enhanced signal is referred to as a spin echo. (f) Illustration of the pulse sequences used in spin echo imaging. The repetition time, TR, and time to echo, TE, are illustrated in relation to the various RF pulses applied and the signals generated.

random effects are *not* reversed by the 180° pulse, so, in fact, the spins do *not* reconverge to a single direction, but rather to a small spread of directions determined by T2. (This situation corresponds more closely to a motorboat race in which waves and changing currents buffet the motorboats at random. Even if the motorboats reversed their engines, these random effects would result in a spread of positions upon their return to the starting line.) Because the spins do not fully recover their original orientations, the RF signal emitted by the echoes is lower in intensity than the original by an amount that depends on both TE and T2 (Figure 8.18f). If the spins have largely lost synchrony by the time the echo is generated (that

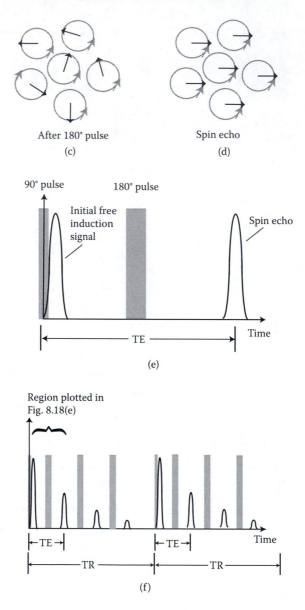

Figure 8.18 (continued).

is, T2 is less than TE), a weak echo results, while if T2 is much longer than TE, the echo will be fairly intense.

After the spin echo has been generated, the spins once again fan out. Another 180° pulse can be used to group them back into a second echo, and the same process can be repeated several times. The successively weaker RF signals emitted by the echoes primarily give a measurement of T2. TE must be chosen to be shorter than T2 for multiple echoes to be observed.

The intensity of the *initial* RF signal emitted by the nuclei is a measure of how many hydrogens respond, so it could be used to map proton density. For example, the MR image can be displayed using a gray scale that assigned brighter intensities to regions of the body corresponding to greater initial signals, hence higher proton densities; darker regions would correspond to those emitting smaller signals and having lower proton densities. On the other hand, the *change* in signal strength between the initial emitted signal and the echo gives a measurement of T2. In a T2-weighted image, this can be displayed using gray scale, so the MR image displays the variation of T2 within a region of the body. For example, regions of short T2 appear dark on a T2-weighted image, because the rapid decay of signals gives a weak echo; conversely, longer T2 gives brighter signals, and hence corresponds to bright regions on a T2-weighted image.

This method can be extended to allow the generation of T1-weighted images as well. So far, the pulse sequences have exhibited little dependence on T1, because T2 is typically so much shorter. In order to measure only T1 relaxation effects, a second string of pulses is generated a **repetition time, TR,** after the first echo sequence (Figure 8.18f). The resulting signals can best be understood by considering two extreme cases. If T1 is *short* compared to TR, then the situation at the beginning of the next pulse sequence is essentially identical to the original state of the spins, because the nuclei have had plenty of time to return to their normal state. Thus, a similar sequence of echoes, with similar intensities, results the second time. By contrast, for long T1, the spins are still precessing at large angles, but with a random spread of transverse magnetizations, at the start of the next sequence. Thus, they cannot absorb and emit RF radiation significantly, and so produce weaker echoes; this situation is also described by saying the spins have been **saturated** by the earlier pulse. T1-weighted images represent this information by using the relative echo intensity between sequences to determine the displayed brightness of regions on the image. Short T1 values correspond to bright regions, and those with long T1 appear dark, using this construction.

To summarize these results, we consider how to choose TR and TE values to produce images weighted by proton density, T1 or T2. The use of long TR and short TE results in proton density-weighted images if the TR used is longer than all the T1 relaxation processes. This ensures that the T1 relaxation processes can go to completion, and there is no T1 contrast. The selection of TE shorter than all relevant T2 values means that there is little effect from T2 relaxation processes. Hence, the signal strengths depend strongly only on proton density.

The choice of short TR and short TE gives T1-weighted images. As in the previous example, the short value of TE reduces the contrast due to T2. TR is chosen, for example, to lie between two T1 times of interest in order to distinguish the two tissues while giving optimal signal intensity. This works because the shorter T1 tissue recovers before the next pulse sequence, while the longer T1 time tissue is still saturated.

Finally, T2-weighting is accomplished by using long TR and long TE values (but with TE less than TR). The choice of long enough TR ensures that no T1 contrast is measured, while TE is selected, for example, to lie between T2 times of interest. Tissues with T2 values much shorter than TE will generate little signal compared to those with T2 longer than TE. (The remaining possibility, with TE longer than TR, is not used.)

MRI Contrast mechanisms—example: To understand how contrast mechanisms work in a typical MR image, consider Figure 8.19. In Figure 8.19, (a) and (b) are plotted, respectively, considering the decay with time of the longitudinal and transverse magnetization for different tissues in the brain. It can easily be seen that the magnetization (and hence the free induction signals) varies between the tissues at different times. This results in excellent contrast between various soft tissues in a typical MR image of the brain. This is illustrated in Figure 8.19(c), which shows the same axial view of the head (orientation shown in the inset) weighted by proton density, T1 and T2. These images differ in appearance even though they represent exactly the same tissues. For example, the ventricles of the brain contain cerebrospinal fluid (with relatively long T1 = 2400 millisecond and T2 = 160 millisecond). Since their value of T2 is longer than other T2 values in the brain (Table 8.1, Figure 8.19b), these regions show up bright (high in signal intensity) in the T2-weighted image. Their value of T1 is also longer than the other tissues (Table 8.1 and Figure 8.19b), so they are relatively dark (low in signal intensity) in the T1-weighted images in the same figure. Their relatively lower density results in a dark (low intensity) appearance in the proton density-weighted image as well. Since diseased tissues often have abnormally high levels of fluid, this identifying feature of fluids is an important clue to pathology.

The exact values for TE and TR are adjusted to create images with various types of weighting. For example, for T1-weighting, TE is chosen to be very short to minimize the effects of different T2 values, and several values of TR can be used to better determine T1. The time to take a complete scan also must allow for the system's inherent need to restore its dipoles to equilibrium. In practice, for complete relaxation to occur, TR must be equal to several seconds in order to be several times the longest value of T1. This has traditionally placed a constraint on how quickly MRI scans can take place. Several newer MRI techniques work by exciting only a fraction of the available magnetization, sometimes in combination with flip angles of less than 90°; both maneuvers result in a faster spin recovery, permitting faster scans. Turbo MRI techniques fall into this category. However,

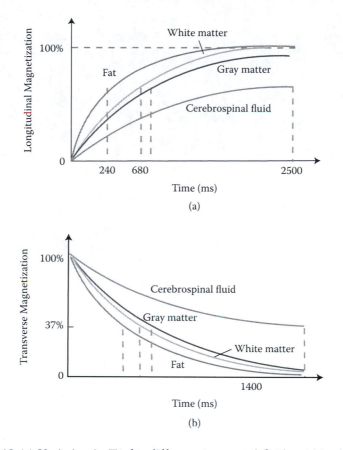

Figure 8.19 (a) Variation in T1 for different tissues and fluids within the brain, illustrated using the decay of the longitudinal magnetization with time. (b) Variation in T2 for different tissues and fluids within the brain, illustrated using the decay of the transverse magnetization with time. Note that different contrast levels will be achieved depending upon whether T1 or T2 is used to generate the MR image contrast. (c) Images taken in an axial plane through the head in the plane shown. Different contrast mechanisms were used to create MR images weighted by proton density (left), T1 (center), and T2 (right). Different soft tissue contrast results from the choice of imaging method.

by reducing scan times, these methods also lower the signals collected per slice, resulting in noisier, lower-quality images. At the end of this chapter we will discuss a method, echo-planar imaging, that allows reduced scanning times without sacrificing image quality.

Numerous other methods are used in modern MRI, but most build on ideas very similar to those explained in this section. We will now see how this idea can be extended to construct spatial maps of the weighting parameters throughout the body.

Proton density   T1   T2

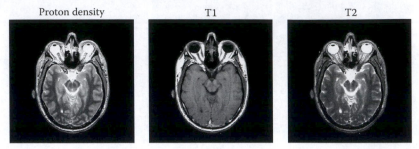

(c)

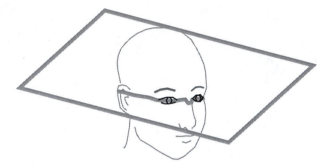

Figure 8.19 (continued).

8.6 HOW MRI MAPS THE BODY

As in CT, MRI images are inherently cross-sectional images of the body constructed from pixels, which represent volume elements of actual human tissue called voxels (Figure 5.30). The image matrices used for MRI can have varying numbers of voxels for the same field of view, with low values (64 × 64, 128 × 128) giving coarse spatial resolution, and much larger numbers (256 × 256, 512 × 512, or 1024 × 1024) giving very fine spatial resolution. As with CT, a trade-off exists between spatial resolution and the image's noisiness. However, increasing spatial resolution in MRI scans does not come at the cost of an increasing dose of ionizing radiation. Present-day MRI scanners boast spatial resolutions that depend upon the exact scanner and matrix size, ranging from several mm (for coarse scans for spectroscopy or functional imaging) to mm to below 0.25 mm (for microMRI of small body parts or small animals.)

So far we have considered how contrast is determined in MRI, but now we will see how spatial information is determined. Since MRI scanners use physics very different from CT, how does a proton signal its location within the body, and how does this information get converted into an image? In other types of imaging, the actual paths taken by the sound waves, x-rays, or gamma rays can be determined, then used to compute spatial information for reconstructing the image. However, MRI detects an RF signal emitted by the hydrogens themselves, and this signal is generated by an entire region of the body. The exciting radio waves cannot be produced as collimated beams to allow images to be formed as projections, as in radiography. (In fact, the large value of the RF wavelength would preclude their being used to make images in this fashion.) How, then, can it be possible to determine where in the body the RF signals come from?

To understand the answer, first consider what would happen if the *magnetic field itself* is varied throughout the body. The resonant frequency also changes because it depends upon the magnetic field. As a result, protons absorb and emit RF waves at different resonant frequencies that depend on the value of the field magnitude in each region of the body. MRI makes use of this effect by smoothly varying the strength of magnetic field throughout the body, as illustrated in Figure 8.20(a). In a **field gradient**, the magnetic field *direction* is the same everywhere, but its *magnitude* varies. By using only a very small range of RF frequencies for excitation, the scanner can stimulate only protons in a thin slice where their resonant frequencies coincide with the exciting frequency (Figure 8.20a); regions directly adjacent to the slice have resonant frequencies too high or too low to absorb energy from the RF exciting waves. In practice, these gradients are quite tiny, with typical values giving only a 0.01% change every cm for a 1.5 T magnet, but they enable a high degree of spatial localization on one dimension. Thus, the limiting dimensions of the slice imaged relate to the range of exciting RF frequencies used and the magnetic field gradient, *not* the wavelength of the RF radiation.

Gradients can be generated in MRI in three directions to map out locations within the body: head to toe (the Z-direction), right to left (the X-direction), and front to back (the Y-direction). We will now step carefully through how gradients can be used to further localize MRI signals in the body, by considering one possible imaging scheme in detail. (1) In imaging, a gradient field along the Z-direction (the **slice-selection gradient**) is first used to isolate only one slice of the body by selective absorption by the exciting RF (Figure 8.20a). (2) When both the Z-gradient and the exciting RF are switched off, only dipoles within this slice precess and emit signals at a resonant frequency determined only by the main magnet. (3) Next, a gradient along (for example) the X-direction is briefly applied. Since this will cause spins at different positions along X to rotate at different frequencies, the spin angles will gradually rotate to different positions within the slice (Figure 8.20b).

These different angles are referred to as **phase shifts**, so the gradient is termed the **phase-encoding gradient**. The gradient is quickly turned off, and the spins resume precessing at the same frequency everywhere, but with different phases. (4) Now a **frequency-selection gradient** is applied along, for example, the Y-direction (Figure 8.20c), again shifting the resonant frequencies within the slice very slightly, like a vibrating guitar string

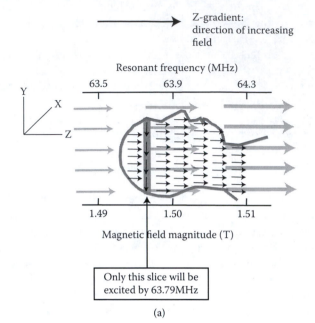

Z-gradient:
direction of increasing
field

Resonant frequency (MHz)

63.5   63.9   64.3

1.49   1.50   1.51

Magnetic field magnitude (T)

Only this slice will be
excited by 63.79MHz

(a)

Figure 8.20 Illustration of the steps involved in one scheme for mapping the body in MRI. (a) A magnetic field gradient along the Z-direction results in an increasing field magnitude in the same direction as the main magnetic field. The resonant frequency consequently also increases along this direction. This effect allows localization of RF excitation to a single slice within the body. For example, if an exciting RF signal of exactly 63.79 MHz is used, then only protons in a single slice with that resonant frequency will be excited and consequently emit RF signals. (The magnitude of the gradient is exaggerated compared to actual values used in imaging.) After excitation, the exciting RF and Z-gradient are switched off. (b) A second gradient along the X-direction shifts frequencies so that the protons at different positions within the slice precess at different frequencies. This phase-encoding gradient results in a variation in the phase of the protons along the X-direction. (c) A frequency-selection gradient along the Y-direction results in different values for the frequencies of the RF signals detected from each line within the slice. The location of each voxel within the plane of the slice is encoded in the phase and frequency of the emitted RF signals.

changing its pitch upon tightening. This gradient remains turned on for the rest of the measurement. Now each *line* within the slice of precessing tissue has a different characteristic frequency of RF emission. If a method existed for separating out each frequency in the confusing buzz emitted by the many precessing dipoles, the signal for only that line could be determined.

Indeed, just as a musician can distinguish different musical notes by ear, computers can be programmed to separate out the different frequencies emitted by each line within the slice, and can analyze the magnitude of the signal emitted at each frequency. (A very simple example of this is

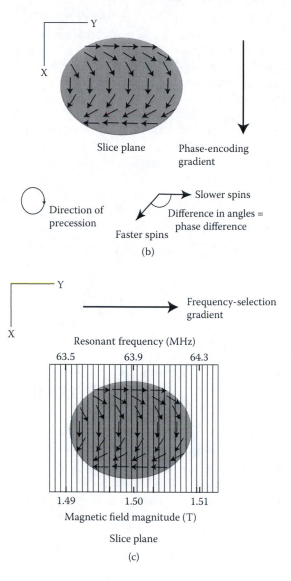

Figure 8.20 (continued).

the capability of radio tuners to tune in only one radio station's broadcast frequency at a time.) However, rather than listening to each line's frequency separately, MRI scanners monitor *all* of the emitted frequencies simultaneously. Thus, the signals of interest for imaging can be collected all at once, separated by position along the Y-direction.

RF signals from each line are measured only as the total contribution from that part of the slice, and the different phases cannot be directly separated to isolate each section of a line along the X-direction. However, the different phases of spins within each line do influence the total signal strength in a complex fashion. To get information along this remaining direction, the entire cycle can be repeated: (1) the Z-gradient is turned on and the same slice excited; (2) the Z-gradient and excitation signal are shut off; and (3) the phase-encoding gradient is applied within the slice briefly, *but so as to rotate the spins by a different amount*; then (4) the same frequency-encoding gradient again applied. Once again, the signals at different frequencies are separately measured, giving information about each line within the sample. Using the signal emitted by each line for many different phase-encoding gradient values, the spatial information along the remaining X-direction can be computed.

So far, the procedures described above result in the creation of only one slice. A cross-sectional image of a different region of the body can be compiled by using step (1) (the slice-selection step) to isolate a different plane within the body to scan, then repeating steps (2) through (4) to map the new slice.

The total scan time for this imaging scheme thus encompasses multiple measurements, with one complete set of multiple measurements required for each slice. Each measurement must allow the nuclear dipoles to recover fully, which takes seconds per separate spin-echo measurement. A large number of measurements are required to reconstruct a single cross section, with the exact number determined by the number of voxels. In addition to allowing spin relaxation to fully occur, collecting signals for longer times gives less noisy images. Thus, spin-echo imaging can take several minutes to gather enough information to reconstruct a detailed, good quality cross-sectional image.

The gradient magnetic fields require special electromagnets to generate them, one set for each direction. The gradient coils used to create Z-gradients can simply consist of circular coils of wire concentric with those of the main magnet (Figure 8.21a). The current in one coil circulates with the same orientation as that in the main solenoid magnet, so its magnetic field adds to the main magnetic field, while the second coil's current circulates in the opposite direction, diminishing the field strength at that end. A more complicated arrangement must be used to impose gradients in other directions. Semicircular **saddle coils** generate the X- and Y-gradients (Figure 8.21b). In these magnets, the straight sections play no role in generating the field gradient. The circular coils are powered so that the currents flow as indicated, giving an enhanced field due to one saddle magnet and a diminished field due to the other. The two contributions result in a gradient in a direction perpendicular to the main magnetic field direction.

The loud noises characteristic of MRI scanners have their origin in forces created by the constantly switching field gradients. Interactions between moving charges within a current-carrying wire and the magnetic field generate a force on the wire with the orientation shown in Figure 8.22(a). (The same effect is used to generate motions in electric motors and loudspeakers.)

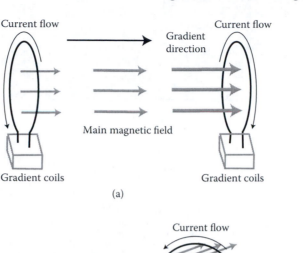

Figure 8.21 Illustration of the orientation of the field gradient coils required to create gradients along the (a) Z-direction (along the main magnetic field direction) and (b) directions perpendicular to the main magnetic field.

A gradient coil with current flowing in the direction shown in Figure 8.22(b) experiences forces pointing radially outward, and these forces abruptly change as the gradients are quickly switched on and off many times a second. Sound is generated as the coils flex in response to the changing forces. Ear protection, such as headphones or earplugs, and piped-in music can help patients screen out the associated noise.

The thickness of the slices used in imaging is set by the range of frequencies used in the exciting signal compared to the change of resonant frequency due to the slice selection gradient. The other dimensions of the voxels are determined in a more complex way by details of how the imaging information is extracted. By exchanging the order in which the gradients are imposed, the slices can be oriented in any plane desired, including the standard axial, coronal, and sagittal views used in describing anatomy (Figure 8.2). This flexibility in choosing viewing angles constitutes a major advantage of MRI over CT, since the only x-ray paths possible dictate

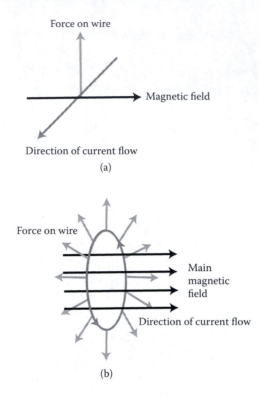

Figure 8.22 (a) Any current experiences a force in a magnetic field, with the direction indicated and a magnitude proportional to both the current and the magnetic field magnitude. (b) Gradient coils experience forces due to interactions between their currents and the main magnetic field. The time-changing deformations caused by these forces cause the loud banging noises heard during MRI scans.

taking axial CT images. Three-dimensional images can also be assembled from MRI scans, allowing further flexibility in the display of anatomical and functional images (Figure 8.23).

8.7 HOW SAFE IS MRI?

MRI has been in widespread clinical use since the early 1980s with no evidence of harmful effects. In contrast to the early history of x-rays in medicine, MRI was introduced at a time of much greater understanding of biology, medicine, and physics. Thus, the ongoing evaluation of MRI's safety can build on an existing body of knowledge about the interactions between different forms of radiation and the body.

No evidence exists that a single person has sustained injury or died from the biological effects of the static, gradient, or RF magnetic fields from the

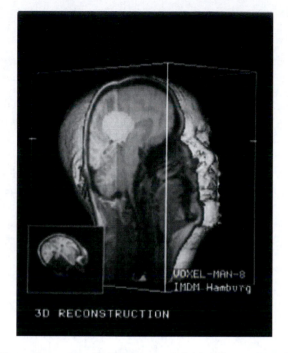

Figure 8.23 Three-dimensional MRI image of the head constructed from a series of scans. (Reproduced with permission courtesy of Siemens Medical Systems.)

hundreds of thousands of MRI exams administered so far. In addition, the picture that emerges from laboratory experiments on the effects of the magnetic fields and RF exposures used in MRI is very different from that for x-rays and other ionizing radiation. Experiments performed as early as the 1920s consistently showed that ionizing radiation could cause the genetic mutations that underlie its potential dangers. By contrast, for the magnetic fields and RF powers used in MRI, numerous experiments have found no sign of induced mutations over a much longer and more thorough period of experimentation. Thus, if any genetic risks from exposure to magnetic fields or RF exist, they are much smaller than those from ionizing radiation.

No one has performed large-scale population studies for MRI comparable to those available for ionizing radiation. However, studies of small numbers of people exposed to MRI have shown no signs of harmful effects on heart activity, brain functioning, pregnancy outcomes, or other physiological processes. It is not possible to rule out extremely small risks using population studies of such limited size. On the other hand, with MRI there is no reason to anticipate these risks from other evidence. By their very nature, the potential harmful effects of RF waves are expected to exhibit genuine thresholds—levels of intensity and exposure time below which no damage occurs. The main reason for these very different behaviors is the very different energies carried by RF and x-ray photons. The body absorbs energy from RF waves in imaging, but not in energy packets sufficient to break chemical bonds, and hence cause genetic mutations.

Nevertheless, other mechanisms exist by which magnetic field gradients and RF waves can interact with the body. Some of these definitely generate physiological effects, and some could conceivably cause bodily harm. While the RF energy absorbed by nuclei is much too small to present a danger, the body also absorbs radio waves by other means. All bodily fluids contain significant concentrations of ionized (electrically charged) chemical species, such as sodium, potassium, and chlorine, that can conduct a flow of electrical current through the body. Indeed, the conduction of nerve signals throughout the body is partly accomplished by this mechanism. The electrical and magnetic forces created when an RF wave travels through the body cause these ions to flow in oscillating currents that reverse their directions many times a second. Just as with the flow of electrons in a metal wire, these electrical currents in the body cause heating due to collisions between the ions and their environment.

Thus, the RF waves used in MRI can lead to heating of body tissues, with the exact temperature rise dependent upon details of the imaging scan and how well the body is able to dissipate the heat. Since the typical transmitter power during a pulse is appreciable, this is not a trivial concern. For example, lethal doses can be delivered to animals if they receive long enough exposures of very high RF intensities to cause their body temperature to rise more than 5°C. Indeed, heating causes most of the harmful effects that have been observed to result from exposure to radio waves. For example, elevated body temperatures during pregnancy are known to induce birth defects in laboratory animals, with the magnitude of the effect depending on the exact temperature increase. For this reason, FDA regulations for MRI scanners specify that temperature rises must not exceed 1°C (1.8°F), well below the threshold at which damage occurs. Measurements made on humans before and after they have undergone MRI scans have shown minimal increases of internal body temperature. A small number of thermal injuries due to more localized heating have been documented.

Both the exciting RF signals and gradient fields have the potential for interacting with the body's own electrical systems. Their changing magnetic fields inherently have the capability to generate electrical currents in body fluids. However, the currents caused by this effect are estimated to lie below those required to excite seizures or alter the heart rate. Studies performed to determine whether MRI scans alter brain function or damage the cardiovascular system have consistently shown no effects. However, these interactions definitely can cause short-term symptoms. While present clinical scanners do not generate such effects, they can occur in newer functional MRI modes that utilize faster gradient switching. For example, some persons have reported hallucinations—tapping sensations, flashing lights, and odd tastes—while being scanned in scanners with fields of 4 T or greater. Another neurological effect is RF hearing (faint noises sensed during exposure to RF), which are usually masked in MRI by much louder noises from the field gradients. While bizarre, these hallucinations are not observed to have lasting consequences.

The *known* risks associated with MRI actually do not involve biological effects of RF or magnetic fields. An MRI scanner's enormous static magnetic field can be hazardous for practical reasons: magnetic metal objects experience a force that draws them toward higher magnetic fields, just as nearby bar magnets are accelerated toward each other when released. This **missile effect** means that surgical tools, keys, or other metal objects could become lethal projectiles hurtling toward the opening if brought near the scanner. In addition, the MRI magnet is always producing a static magnetic field, so caution must be exerted in its presence at all times, not just during scanning. For this reason, all MRI facilities must be secured areas, where persons entering are screened carefully for metal. The combined necessity to isolate the MRI scanner from outside influences, and to ensure low magnetic fields in neighboring areas, places substantial restrictions on the siting and construction of scanner rooms. Fortunately, the magnetic fields outside a scanner drop rapidly to a value comparable to the Earth's magnetic field, so healthcare workers in the same room are chronically exposed only to weak fields of several gauss (10^{-4}T).

Equally serious is the concern that metal implants *within* the body would move or reorient themselves in the strong static magnetic field. Fortunately, the metals used in most surgical implants are now either nonmagnetic or very weakly ferromagnetic. However, the presence of metal pins, plates, clips on blood vessels, implants in the eye, prostheses, etc. can present serious problems. (Metallic dental alloys used in filling teeth are not magnetic, so they present no danger.) Physicians also avoid performing MRI on individuals who have cardiac pacemakers, implanted neurostimulators, cochlear implants to aid hearing, or other implantable electrical devices. In these cases, not only are metal parts used in their manufacture, the devices themselves are electrical circuits potentially sensitive to the changing gradient fields and RF signals used; in the case of some types of cardiac pacemakers, this interference could prove fatal.

Many MRI scanners use superconducting magnets that must be kept extremely cold in order to sustain their superconductivity. If such a magnet **quenches**—heats up enough to lose its superconductivity—the abrupt change in magnetic field strength can be very large. While such accidents are very unlikely to happen during imaging, in the early days of MRI some scientists raised concerns about possible physiological effects due to electrical currents induced within the body by extremely rapid field changes. Modern magnet designs allow for quenches with a gradual reduction in magnetic field over several seconds, thus reducing these risks. To date, no problems have been reported for unintended quenches in clinical settings. Another concern is that the cryogenic coolants used to keep the magnet cold are "boiled off" during a quench. MRI-scanning facilities are designed to properly vent the resultant gases outside the facility, in order to prevent the nontoxic fumes from displacing oxygen and thereby presenting a threat of suffocation.

Solenoid-type scanners present another practical problem—the discomfort experienced by many from the tunnel-like environment and noise. As mentioned earlier, MRI scanner manufacturers now market "open MRI" scanners designed with more sensitivity to the user's situation. Modern scanners incorporate a clearer field of view (which can be accomplished with a mirror positioned before the patient's face), relaxing music, and less confining geometries. The open MRI scanners present an alternative for imaging small children, the critically ill, or other persons who cannot tolerate confinement. They also permit interventional procedures to be performed simultaneously with the actual imaging.

8.8 CREATING BETTER CONTRAST

Now that we have a basic understanding of how MRI scanners operate, we can investigate its special diagnostic capabilities. Many of the advantages MRI offers have been mentioned earlier in the chapter: MRI can flexibly image in any plane, the different methods of weighting images can yield better soft-tissue contrast than can CT, it does not use ionizing radiation, contrast agents for MRI are safer than those used in x-ray imaging, bone and air-filled spaces do not obscure other tissues, and MRI promises to offer superior capabilities for imaging the major blood vessels, even in three dimensions.

One of the chief beauties of MRI is that it often does *not* require introducing foreign contrast media into the body, because many body tissues can be distinguished by their proton densities or T1 or T2 relaxation times. In a sense, naturally occurring body chemicals containing nuclei with a net spin play the role of radioactive tracers in radionuclide imaging. However, even with MRI, contrast agents are desirable in a large range of applications, principally to provide additional information when imaging body function.

Remarkably, blood itself can serve as an effective contrast agent. Blood in the circulatory system picks up fresh oxygen as it passes through the lungs. The heart then pumps the blood through the arteries to supply body tissues with the oxygen needed to convert food into energy. Finally, the oxygen-depleted blood returns to the heart via the veins. The blood protein hemoglobin, responsible for ferrying oxygen throughout the body, contains an iron atom that binds oxygen. The magnetic properties of this iron atom depend substantially upon whether the hemoglobin is bound to oxygen (oxyhemoglobin, which is *not* paramagnetic), or is not bound to oxygen (deoxyhemoglobin, which *is* paramagnetic). Arterial blood fresh from the lungs is 95% oxygenated, while blood returning in the veins has only 70% oxyhemoglobin. Similarly, stagnant blood largely contains deoxyhemoglobin.

Recall that paramagnets align with an external magnetic field so as to increase the total field. Because their magnetism results from unpaired electrons, it creates effects almost 1000 times stronger than those due to nuclear magnetism. Thus, the additional magnetic fields due to deoxyhemoglobin can strongly reduce relaxation times in blood. Because these interactions only affect nuclei quite close by, the main effect is to shorten local T2 values, decreasing the MRI signal from regions with high concentrations of deoxygenated blood. These effects can be used to detect blood flow, and hence to map out brain activity, a topic discussed further in the section on echo-planar imaging.

Another method, **flow-related enhancement**, provides contrast due to the passage of blood flowing from outside to inside the image slice. For example, during gradient echo pulse RF excitation, spins within the image plane become saturated. However, blood flow brings unsaturated (completely relaxed) spins into the image plane between RF excitations while it moves the region of blood containing saturated spins out of the slice (Figure 8.24a). The unsaturated spins transported into the slice by blood flow produce a greater signal than neighboring tissues; thus, the highest signal intensity regions correspond to the interior of blood vessels. Images acquired in this fashion can be compiled into a single three-dimensional

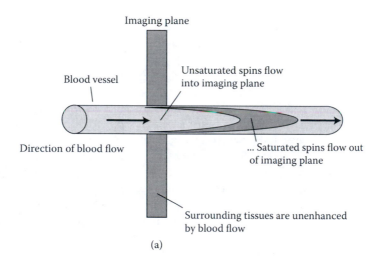

(a)

Figure 8.24 (a) In flow-related enhancement, spins within the image plane become saturated during gradient echo pulse RF excitation. Blood flow brings unsaturated (completely relaxed) spins into the image plane between RF excitations while it moves the region of blood containing saturated spins out of the slice. The unsaturated spins transported into the slice by blood flow produce a greater signal than neighboring tissues, so that the highest signal intensity regions correspond to the interior of blood vessels. (b) Images of the circulatory system can be compiled using such flow contrast imaging processes. Three-dimensional maps of the regions of maximum signal intensity can then be compiled into images in Magnetic Resonance Angiography (MRA).

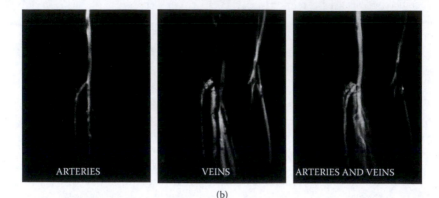

ARTERIES   VEINS   ARTERIES AND VEINS

(b)

Figure 8.24 (continued).

image of the blood vessels, permitting the study of blood vessels in
Magnetic Resonance Angiography (Figure 8.24b). MRI images of the circulatory system can be obtained relatively noninvasively, and assembled
into truly three-dimensional images of major blood vessels and the heart.
It can simultaneously provide the quantitative measures of heart function
yielded by radioisotope imaging, discussed in Chapter 5, as well as detailed
anatomical information.

In addition to the noninvasive techniques described above, MRI can also
make use of foreign tracer compounds similar to the radiopharmaceuticals
described in Chapter 5. Instead of radioactive labels, however, MRI contrast media incorporate magnetic atoms. For example, one commonly used
element, gadolinium (Gd), is strongly paramagnetic because of its seven
unpaired electrons, so it generates local magnetic fields almost 100,000
times those of deoxyhemoglobin. A gadolinium atom can accept multiple
chemical partners, which surround it in a cage of chemical bonds called a
chelate compound. Gadolinium is usually presented into the body tightly
bound in a chelate so as to render it nontoxic. The extremely strong local
magnetic field fluctuations caused by even minute concentrations of such
atomic paramagnets shorten T1 in their immediate neighborhood.

MRI contrast dyes can be used in cancer imaging, to study the circulatory system (including circulation in the brain), to examine kidney function, and in numerous other applications. For example, contrast agents can
enhance the ability of MRI to detect strokes and brain tumors because the
contrast dye will distribute itself anywhere the blood-brain barrier has been
breached (Figure 8.25). Just as in x-ray imaging, this technique can be used
to map out the function of an organ, such as the kidney, by detecting the
concentration and spatial distribution of the contrast medium and determining how it changes with time.

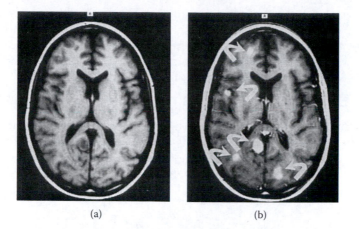

(a)   (b)

Figure 8.25 The effects of contrast enhancement with a magnetic tracer compound, called a paramagnetic gadolinium chelate, are shown in these T1-weighted images of the brain, shown in an axial cross section. On the left (a) is a scan taken without contrast medium. On the right image (b), taken on the same person with gadolinium chelate contrast, bright spots (arrows) indicate the presence of brain tumors that have spread from an existing cancer. (Reproduced with permission courtesy of Dr. Robert R. Edelman.)

8.9 SPORTS MEDICINE AND MRI

Another important area in which MRI excels is applications in orthopedics, where it provides a highly important tool for imaging injuries and disease of the musculoskeletal system. In sports medicine, MRI provides noninvasive diagnostic capabilities for examining injured joints, bones, and muscles. While it serves mainly as an adjunct to radiography for imaging broken bones, MRI has become an essential player in soft-tissue imaging. In orthopedics, MRI's high spatial resolution is augmented by special purpose surface coils, which permit the imaging of the knee, shoulder, spin and muscles, as well as small parts like the wrist, ankle, and elbow. Specialized micro-MRI scanners for small parts of the body can achieve very fine resolution by limiting the field of view to small regions, also allowing applications in such areas as osteoporosis screening (Chapter 5). The resulting images with large matrices, small fields of view, and correspondingly high spatial resolution can be formed in multiple planes for better imaging the complex anatomy of structures such as the knee (Figure 8.1).

MRI also provides uniquely high contrast for imaging the soft tissues of interest. A combination of T1- and T2-weighted images offer contrast between muscle, tendon, cartilage, fat, ligaments, and fluid (Figure 8.1). Gadolinium contrast compounds can also be injected into joints for further enhancement. Sports injuries to the soft tissues, such as bone bruises and stress fractures, can be imaged, as can traumatic injuries to muscles. Common athletic injuries, such as rotator cuff tears in the shoulder or tears in the cruciate ligaments in the knee, can be diagnosed in this fashion (Figure 8.1b). In addition to aiding in the diagnosis of injuries, MRI can help orthopedic surgeons evaluate the need for surgery and its likely effectiveness, then map out surgical procedures. For example, knee arthroscopy (Chapter 2) is the most common orthopedic procedure in the U.S., at 1.5 million operations per year, and surgeons routinely use MRI to determine whether patients require this surgery and to plan the details of each procedure. They can finally evaluate the process of healing and recovery after surgery, all without the need for invasive testing.

8.10 MAGNETIC RESONANCE BREAST IMAGING

In Chapter 5, we saw how mammograms (breast x-rays) can be used to help detect breast cancer. However, mammograms can give false negatives either because no sign of a tumor is visible on the mammogram, or its indications are slight or ambiguous on the x-ray image. Mammography also often yields false positives, incorrectly indicating that a tumor may be present. What is needed is a technique that is more sensitive to the presence of tumors, so that fewer are missed, and yet so specific that it does not confuse benign growths with cancer. In addition, mammograms only can detect tumors from small variations in x-ray absorption. Because ordinary breast glandular tissue and implants obscure the subtle variations in density resulting from a tumor, it is difficult to interpret mammograms obtained from women with very dense breasts (which includes most premenopausal women), women with scars from previous surgery, nursing mothers, and women with silicone breast implants.

Breast MR, the MRI version of mammography, overcomes many of these disadvantages, offering a valuable additional technique for breast imaging. Because MR imaging does not involve forming projections, true cross-sectional MR images of the breasts are not obscured by implants, surgical scars, or dense breast tissue. They also do not exhibit the overlap between different tissues that inevitably occurs in diagnostic x-rays. However, breast MR has lower spatial resolution than mammography, so it cannot resolve fine details, such as microcalcifications or the detailed shape of tumor boundaries. Breast MR can be performed with special, high-resolution RF surface coils positioned near the breasts. This allows the entire breast to be imaged in three dimensions. With surface coils, the confining geometry associated with full-body MRI scans is not necessary and the scan time can be kept to minutes. Breast tumors do not present a unique signature in terms of proton density, T1, or T2 when compared with normal tissues. However, physicians can use gadolinium contrast enhancement

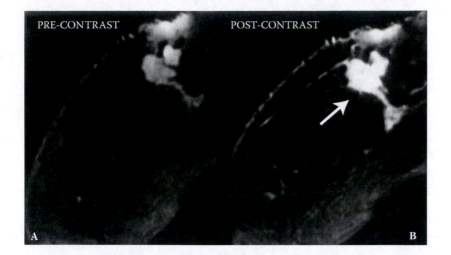

Figure 8.26 MR breast scan, showing a cross-sectional image of the breast. Special pulse techniques and gadolinium contrast compounds were employed to show the extent to which lesions (arrow) enhance (shows greater signal intensity) in images taken without contrast (A) vs. with contrast (B); the extent and rate of MRI contrast enhancement is an indication of the likelihood that a lesion is malignant. (Reproduced with permission courtesy of Dr. Steven Harms.)

to highlight regions of abnormal blood flow indicative of the presence of a tumor. This occurs in part because the neovascularization (abnormal growth of new blood vessels) promoted by the presence of a tumor concentrates these contrast agents, creating a signal that can be detected by MRI. Researchers are working to determine special RF pulse sequences and contrast enhancement techniques that will allow both highly specific and sensitive detection of breast tumors (Figure 8.26).

At present, breast MR has been show to be an extremely high sensitivity method for detecting breast cancer (here the term sensitivity is used in the technical sense of yielding very small numbers of false negatives.) Studies have shown that breast MR is 94 to 100% likely to detect all tumors in the breast. However, it has the failing of low specificity, ranging from 37 to 97%; that is, it also yields a high percentage of false positives. The higher cost of breast MR makes it unlikely to replace screening mammography any time soon. However, this imaging modality already is recommended in certain cases: for supplementary screening of women already at high risk for breast cancer, to make sure all tumors have been located when breast cancer has been found by other means, to guide some biopsies, and to plan surgery and follow therapy for breast cancer. These exams also allow the imaging of women for whom mammography is not a good option for the reasons mentioned above. MR spectroscopy, discussed in the next section, is one option presently being explored for harnessing our expanding knowledge of cancer biology to improve the specificity of breast MR.

8.11 MAPPING BODY CHEMISTRY
WITH MR SPECTROSCOPY

Just as chemists can use NMR spectroscopy to analyze a sample for its chemical constituents, MR spectroscopy can allow physicians to map the distribution of certain chemicals throughout the body. Ordinary MRI measures as a single quantity all RF signals emitted by different chemicals within the body. By contrast, the basic idea behind MR spectroscopy is to collect data from a voxel of body tissue while distinguishing between the frequencies emitted by different chemical species. The field gradients used for localizing signals shift the resonant frequency by about one part in 100,000 across a voxel with 1 mm edges, much more than typical chemical shifts of parts per million. This means that the very act of spatial mapping using gradients masks the important chemical information, so the MR signal of interest must be collected with a technique that involves switching off all magnetic field gradients. In addition, the concentrations of interesting body chemicals are 1000 to 20,000 times lower than those of the water and fat molecules that make up most of the proton MRI signal. Suppression techniques can allow these dominant fat and water signals to be reduced, but the signals due to interesting body chemicals are still small. If tiny voxels are used, too few nuclei emit signals to permit the collection of adequately low-noise images. Consequently, larger voxels, cm to an edge, must be used for spectroscopic imaging, leading to much blurrier images than obtained in standard MRI. The addition of MR spectroscopy to an MR imaging scan typically adds only 10 minutes to the procedure, but provides complementary information.

While spectroscopic imaging of protons (hydrogen) can be performed with high magnetic field clinical scanners, the different resonant frequencies of the other nuclei also require the use of special coils and electronics, making the technique generally more complex than standard scanning. The low signals present from molecules of interest in general necessitate using high magnetic field scanners because, as we saw in earlier sections of this chapter, the higher the static main magnetic field, the greater the separation between frequencies emitted by different chemical species. On the other hand, several chemical elements either important to body chemistry, or useful as chemical labels, can be detected in this way, including phosphorus-31, carbon-13, sodium-23, and fluorine-19, as well as hydrogen-1 itself, providing a wealth of potential chemicals to image by this means.

The exact resonant frequency at which protons precess depends upon chemical environment, so it is different for protons in several chemicals important to brain chemistry, such as choline (a chemical important to the construction of cell membranes, which typically increases in malignant tumors), NAA (n-acetylaspartate, a chemical found in healthy nerve cells), and many other useful chemical species. The strength of the radio frequency signal emitted from nuclei within a voxel of tissue hence measures quantitatively the local concentration of choline or NAA once it is broken down into the relevant frequency components. Many other chemical by-products of body metabolism can be detected in a similar fashion, allowing the mapping of body chemistry at the level of cm. Patterns of metabolic chemistry can be used to define the degree of malignancy in cancer imaging of the brain, breast, and prostate, to diagnose metabolic diseases and inflammation, and in various neurological applications.

8.12 BRAIN MAPPING AND FUNCTIONAL MRI

Spin-echo images constructed in the fashion described above are highly informative, but they are also inherently limited to fairly long scan times, placing significant constraints on MRI's speed and overall usefulness. However, the static anatomical information they provide can provide important information for a variety of neurological diseases. For example, MRI studies of multiple sclerosis have redefined the underlying assumptions about the disease by revealing lesions in the brain and central nervous system even in patients who are not experiencing the disease's characteristic symptoms. This information has played a major role in creating new, effective drug therapies that significantly reduce relapses and disability among a large population of sufferers from this condition.

However, anatomical studies of the brains of person suffering from various neurological conditions are informative, but do not offer functional information. In fact, the vast majority of early MRI applications involved imaging of the central nervous system and the musculoskeletal system because motions associated with the heartbeat, bowel, and respiration significantly blurred scans of the rest of the body. However, fast techniques such as **echo-planar imaging** (**EPI**) vastly reduce scan times to as low as a twentieth of a second for a complete cross-sectional image. This important innovation makes MRI a much more versatile and comprehensive technique without sacrificing its other advantages.

EPI utilizes the same gradient scheme for slice selection described earlier, but it deduces spatial information within the slice differently. Using spin-echo techniques similar to those described earlier, EPI crams the measurement of a complete cross-sectional image into the brief window of opportunity after an exciting RF pulse. Since the free induction signal only lasts a fraction of a second, this means the entire measurement is proportionately fast. A detailed description of EPI's scheme for applying gradients lies beyond the mathematical level of this book, but the basic idea involves using oscillating gradient fields within the slice to simultaneously map out both in-plane directions.

EPI and other fast MRI scanning techniques provide the important ability to prevent blurring due to motion, which opens up the possibility of MRI of any part of the body, including the heart and lungs, and time-resolved imaging of many body processes. Using fast scans, doctors can now visualize important organs like the liver, which were blurred in longer scan times due to respiration, or gather more information about body functions, such as the passage of a tracer through the urinary tract.

To image the heart with conventional MRI, physicians have used an idea called "**gating**." The electrical signal associated with each heartbeat (the electrocardiogram or EKG) is monitored, and used to take an MRI scan repeatedly only during a certain stage of the heartbeat. The total scan accumulates from many separate snapshots to reduce blurring, while gathering an image of adequate quality. However, this idea cannot be used with an irregular heartbeat and it does not totally eliminate blurring due to motion. EPI can freeze a very fast image of the heart, taking either scans of many different planes or rapidly compiling a film loop of the heart as it beats. These movie-loop images of the heart are taken at roughly the best speeds achievable with ultrafast CT (20 frames per second) and ultrasound (30 frames per second), though about four times slower than cardiac angiography with x-rays. (For comparison, ordinary video signals are 30 frames per second.) This ability to resolve fast motions also allows cardiologists to measure blood flow, to visualize regions of the heart's muscle with inadequate blood supply (a possible sign of impending heart attack), or to see abnormalities in blood flow associated with a defective valve.

Perhaps EPI's most impressive ability is mapping brain activity. Contrast agents introduced into the bloodstream can be used to map out blood volume increases associated with regions of brain activity. Alternatively, as discussed above, fresh, oxygenated blood gives a stronger MRI signal than depleted deoxygenated blood. This means that regions of brain activity present a characteristic MRI signal because of the enhanced blood flow required to meet their enhanced energy demands. Using either contrast mechanism, EPI presents opportunities for studying brain function during mental activities, at speeds faster than PET and with much better resolution and lower noise than that technique. MRI scanners capable of making these measurements also are widely available, and they yield images without the need for radioactive tracers.

What specifically is being measured in fMRI of the brain is the pattern and degree of brain activity measured during simple mental tasks. Such information can be combined with high spatial resolution scans to establish the relationship between function and anatomy. For example, the pattern of brain activation during specified motor tasks or sensory stimulation can be observed to determine which parts of the brain are involved (Figure 8.27). The spatial resolution of this technique is fairly large compared to the nerve cells involved in detailed mental processes, so only a coarse map of acti-vated regions of the brain can be produced. However, it suffices to locate entire structures involved in, for example, language production or vision. Experiments have concentrated on questions similar to those discussed in Chapter 5, involving mapping out which areas of the brain are involved with simple mental tasks such as recalling words or listening to music. Statistical comparisons of diseased and healthy patients' brains performing similar tasks can be used to identify subtle differences in brain function that would not be manifested in overall anatomical changes. Mental processes stud-ied using fMRI have included language (including the conversion of heard speech into meaning), memory, and vision (such as the recognition of faces). For example, fMRI has allowed the noninvasive study of visual process-ing in living human subjects, rather than animal models. Using techniques such as fMRI and PET, it has been possible to show that visual perception (in which a person sees an object) and visual imagery (in which the person *imagines* seeing the same object) activate many of the same brain processes. The capability for mapping the functionality of the brain also allows fMRI to permit detailed determination of diseased and healthy regions for use in preoperative planning of brain surgery. This capability and the continual development of increasingly specific MRI contrast agents promises to extend the explosive growth of MRI yet further.

Figure 8.27 gives an excellent illustration of how fMRI can be used to perform noninvasive basic research in neuroscience. These images were drawn from research performed to investigate a form of congenital blind-ness caused by a mutation that interferes with the functioning of the retina in humans and animals. The study examined blind dogs born with this muta-tion, using fMRI to determine whether their visual cortex responded after retinal gene therapy to restore light sensitivity; this research aimed at deter-mining whether the lack of retinal stimulation during development resulted in compromises to the optical nerve and brain that would prevent such therapy from being effective. The coronal MRI scans shown here were per-formed on a dog with normal vision ("WT canine" top row) and the same congenitally blind dog under three different conditions ("RPE65-mutant canine," three lower rows), using fMRI to measure blood oxygenation lev-els indicative of brain activity. For the blind dog, the top row shows MRI scans before gene therapy, while the bottom-most two rows show results 1 and 2 months post-gene therapy, respectively. The color-mapped signals superimposed on structural MRI scans (in gray scale) indicate increasing levels of brain activity in the visual cortex after gene therapy; the dog with normal vision and congenitally blind dog 2 months post-therapy have simi-lar fMRI levels. Human subjects also were studied using structural MRI to show that they had normal optical nerve and visual cortex anatomy. Taken

WT Canine [E946]

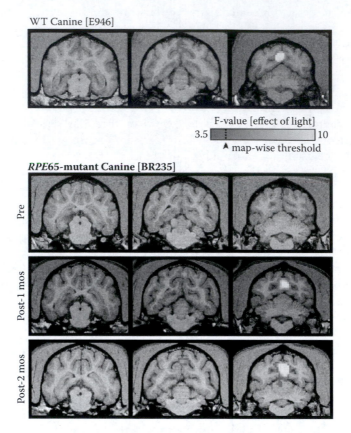

F-value [effect of light]
3.5 ⬛⬛⬛⬛⬛⬛⬛⬛⬛⬛ 10
▲ map-wise threshold

*RPE*65-mutant Canine [BR235]

Pre

Post-1 mos

Post-2 mos

Figure 8.27 (*See color figure following page 78.*) Functional MRI scans (fMRI) scans have been used to study whether gene therapy can restore vision to humans and dogs born with a mutation causing blindness. The coronal MRI scans shown here were performed on a dog with normal vision ("WT canine" top row) and the same congenitally blind dog under three different conditions ("RPE65-mutant canine," three lower rows), using fMRI to measure blood oxygenation levels indicative of brain activity. For the blind dog, the top row shows MRI scans before gene therapy, while the bottom-most two rows show results 1 and 2 months post-gene therapy, respectively. The color-mapped signals superimposed on structural MRI scans (in gray scale) indicate increasing levels of brain activity in the visual cortex after gene therapy; the dog with normal vision and congenitally blind dog 2 months post-therapy have similar fMRI levels. These results indicate that gene therapy indeed holds hope of restoring vision in these cases of congenital blindness. (Reproduced with permission from Canine and Human Visual Cortex Intact and Responsive Despite Early Retinal Blindness from RPE65 Mutation, Aguirre GK, Komáromy AM, Cideciyan AV, Brainard DH, Aleman TS, et al. *PLoS Medicine* Vol. 4, No. 6, e230 doi:10.1371/journal.pmed.0040230.)

together, these results suggest that gene therapy may someday restore vision to sufferers from this form of congenital blindness, an elegant example of how studies in animals and humans can elucidate basic questions in brain function while also investigating the effectiveness of new therapies.

SUGGESTED READING

MRI texts

(See also the texts listed in Chapter 1.)

Robert J. Gillies, ed., *NMR in Physiology and Biomedicine*. Academic Press, San Diego, 1994.

Donald W. McRobbie, Elizabeth A. Moore, Martin J. Graves and Martin R. Prince, *MRI from Picture to Proton*. Cambridge University Press. Cambridge, U.K., 2003.

References on issues pertaining to the safety of MRI

Frank G. Shellock, *Reference Manual for Magnetic Resonance Safety, Implants, and Devices*. Biomedical Research Publishing Group, Los Angeles, 2008.

The website of the Institute for Magnetic Resonance Safety, Education and Research: http://www.imrser.org/Default.asp.

QUESTIONS

Q8.1. Which of the following isotopes could be used for radioisotope imaging with a gamma camera? For PET? For MRI? For cancer therapy? The answer may be none, one, two, three, or all of the possible choices. Explain your reasoning in each case.

Isotope	Decay product	PET	MRI	Cancer therapy	Radioisotope imaging
Carbon-11	Positrons				
Carbon-12	Stable (doesn't decay)				
Carbon-13	Stable (doesn't decay)				
Gold-198	Gamma rays and electrons				
Fluorine-19	Stable (doesn't decay)				
Fuorine-18	Positrons				
Cobalt-60	Gamma rays				

Q8.2. What are the best spatial resolutions presently achievable in clinical settings for MRI? For PET? For ultrasound imaging? For radiography and CT?

Q8.3. Why does MRI utilize the relaxation times T1 and T2 for contrast rather than exclusively relying on proton density weighted images?

Q8.4. Explain the differences between the relaxation mechanisms that result in the decay of the transverse and longitudinal magnetizations after a 90° pulse. Use sketches to illustrate your reasoning.

Q8.5. What advantages over CT does MRI hold in imaging the brain?

Q8.6. Make a drawing explaining how the slice-selection magnetic field gradient should be oriented to image (a) coronal and (b) sagittal cross sections.

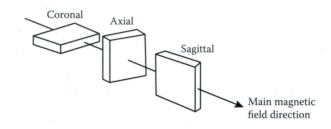

Q8.7. The wavelength of the radiation used presents a limitation on spatial resolution for imaging with visible light (Chapters 2 and 3), and with sound waves in Chapter 4, but not for MRI. Explain what wavelengths of radiation are used in this technique, and explain why the actual spatial resolution can be much greater than the wavelength.

Q8.8. Explain how MRI contrast agents based on gadolinium compounds work.

PROBLEMS

P8.1. (a) For a 4.0 T research MRI scanner, what would the proton resonant frequency be? The resonant frequency for phosphorus-31? (b) What photon energies (in eV) do these frequencies correspond to? How do they compare to typical chemical bond energies in the body, and typical x-ray photon energies? Comment on the medical importance of this last calculation.

P8.2. (a) The main magnetic field in a 1.00 T MRI scanner varies by 0.01% per cm along the slice-selection gradient direction. The range of frequencies used to excite the protons in the body of a person being scanned is 42.5711 MHz to 42.5689 MHz. What is the thickness of the slice excited? (b) If the static magnetic field of a MRI scanner varies by 15 to 40 parts per million over the standard MRI field of view, by how much does the proton Larmor frequency vary?

P8.3. If the difference in resonant frequencies due to the chemical shift between water and fat protons is roughly 210 Hz, and the gradient in a 1.5 T MRI scanner's main magnet is $1.5 \times 10{-4}$ T/cm, the fat protons will appear to be in a different position than water protons. (a) Explain why this is true using a sketch. (b) By how much do their apparent locations differ? (c) By how much would their frequencies differ in a lower field, 0.5 T scanner? Use this result to explain why high fields are used in MR spectroscopy.

P8.4. Explain how you might choose TR to distinguish on a spin-echo image two different tissues with the values of T1 shown in Figure P8.4. Use the plot in Figure P8.4 to explain your answer.

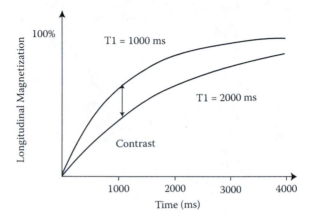

Figure P8.4

P8.5. Explain how you might choose TE to distinguish on a spin-echo image two different tissues with the values of T2 shown in Figure P8.5. Use the plot in Figure P8.5 to explain your answer.

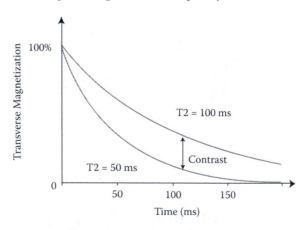

Figure P8.5

P8.6. Spin-echo imaging is used to generate MRI scans of the tissues listed in Table 8.1. Explain what relative signal intensity for each you would expect on (a) a T1-weighted image and (b) a

T2-weighted image. State any assumptions you make in order to explain your answers.

P8.7. It is desirable to reduce the large signal due to fat in some scans. Techniques to do this "fat suppression" can allow better contrast for the other soft tissues being imaged. Taking into account the information provided in Problem P8.3, explain how you could accomplish this task. Assume you can utilize an exciting RF source that can emit RF radiation at a very specific frequency to generate spin-flip angles of any desired value, and that you have the ability to perform spin-echo imaging. (Hint: Consider what happens in spin-echo imaging with TR much shorter than T1.)

Index